Dose Optimization in Drug Development

DRUGS AND THE PHARMACEUTICAL SCIENCES
A Series of Textbooks and Monographs

Executive Editor

James Swarbrick
PharmaceuTech, Inc.
Pinehurst, North Carolina

Dose Optimization in Drug Development

edited by

Rajesh Krishna
Merck & Co., Inc.
Rahway, New Jersey, U.S.A.

informa
healthcare

New York London

FIRST INDIAN REPRINT, 2014

Informa Healthcare USA, Inc.
52 Vanderbilt Avenue
New York, NY 10017

International Standard Book Number-10: 1-5744-4808-0 (Hardcover)
International Standard Book Number-13: 978-1-5744-4808-5 (Hardcover)

This book contains information obtained from authentic and highly regarded sources. Reprinted material is quoted with permission, and sources are indicated. A wide variety of references are listed. Reasonable efforts have been made to publish reliable data and information, but the author and the publisher cannot assume responsibility for the validity of all materials or for the consequences of their use.

Library of Congress Cataloging-in-Publication Data

Dose optimization in drug development / edited by Rajesh Krishna.
    p. ; cm. -- (Drugs and the pharmaceutical sciences ; no. 161)
    Includes bibliographical references and index.
    ISBN-13: 978-1-5744-4808-5 (alk. paper)
    ISBN-10: 1-5744-4808-0 (alk. paper)
    1. Drugs--Dose-response relationship. 2. Drugs--Dosage. 3. Drug Development.
    [DNLM: 1. Pharmaceutical Preparations--administration & dosage. 2. Pharmacokinetics.
    3. Dose-Response Relationship, Drug. QV 38 D7224 2006]

    RM301.8.D67 2006
    615'.19--dc22   2005046645

To Mom,
for always encouraging me to pursue my ambitions,
to Dad, for his strong belief that anything is achievable,
and to my wife,
for sharing and surmounting life's challenges together.

Foreword

Arguably the most difficult aspect of drug development, once proof-of-concept is achieved for a novel mechanism, is defining the "right" dose. Indeed, the question rapidly expands to right for whom? An individual? A population? A specific disease? A unique demographic? The answers can yield a dizzying array of alternatives. Yet pressures to rapidly realize the benefits of a new compound often limit time spent in early development (Phase I/II) when such questions have traditionally been explored. To more efficiently address the problem of defining the optimum dose, new approaches are being applied across the disciplines of drug development.

The present volume, *Dose Optimization in Drug Development*, in the series Drugs and the Pharmaceutical Sciences, provides a timely overview of emerging knowledge in this field. This knowledge encompasses techniques for exploring individual as well as population dose optimization including the definition of dose-concentration-response relationships, modeling based on these PK/PD relationships, clinical trial simulations, and application of pharmacogenomic principles. One aspect of this research which should not be lost is the requirement for more highly integrated interactions between the clinicians, kineticists, and statisticians addressing these problems.

Dr. Rajesh Krishna, the editor of the present volume, has assembled an extraordinary group of contributors. He has succeeded in identifying the critical newly emerging capabilities in drug development as applied to dose finding and generated a volume of enormous power. The authors, for their part, address the fundamental issues of the day with respect to dose optimization—translational research, methodology development, clinical trial modeling, PK/PD simulations, biomarker identification and validation, and application of novel clinical trial designs—in a manner that is of both sufficient depth and general applicability as

v

to be of practical utility to the reader. This volume will become an indispensable reference work for anyone interested in applying these state of the art principles for dose optimization to the science of drug development.

Barry J. Gertz, M.D., Ph.D.
Executive Vice President
Clinical and Quantitative Sciences
Merck Research Laboratories
Rahway, New Jersey, U.S.A.

Preface

Advancements in various aspects of clinical science have resulted in remarkable improvement in scientific drug development, specifically with respect to quality of new drug applications. Despite these small and perhaps case-dependent improvements, the promise of biomarkers, new clinical methodologies and technologies, the "omic" sciences and the pharmacostatistical approaches to advanced modeling of biodynamic systems and trial simulations have all yet to significantly modulate the quality of new candidate selection, clinical optimization, and characterization, and thus profoundly reduce late stage development attrition. Fundamentally, all of these powerful tools and methodologies individually retain enormous potential to result in a better understanding of the new drug candidate's behavior in various patient populations, in understanding exposure–response relationships, and in quantitatively delineating risk versus benefit. The latter developmental aspect is a singularly worrisome gap in many drug development programs, sometimes resulting in complicated and prolonged regulatory reviews and, in rare cases, drug product withdrawals.

In considering the aspect of risk versus benefit further, one relatively underutilized concept is surprisingly the scientific basis of dose selection, focus, and optimization. It is surprising because dose selection is still largely empirical and not rationally scientific, at least to the extent that could be possible. Dose selection is hardly trivial and is intimately linked to risk versus benefit as it quantifies the therapeutic window for a given new chemical entity within the context of the disease it is being developed for.

The realities of new product development took a turn for the better when the U.S. Food and Drug Administration recently released a report entitled "Innovation/Stagnation: Challenge and Opportunity on the Critical Path to New Medical Products" on March 16, 2004, aimed at modernizing drug development. This is the first major step in recent years that a federal authority has taken to further identify the deficiencies in new drug development from a regulatory standpoint. Fortunately, this key regulatory initiative, or rather a formal recognition of a persistent problem, has fueled considerable interest in integrating knowledge that would contribute productively to new drug development, gain a better understanding of the drug candidate's behavior in patient populations, while increasing the probability of success for new chemical entities. The emphasis on dose optimization has also encouraged research and discussion on performing more innovative Phase I/II trials to seek evidence of target engagement earlier rather than later, thereby reducing failure rates attributable to poor efficacy. These considerations have played a central role in the conceptualization and development of this book.

The theme of this volume is dose selection and optimization, specifically as they relate to new drug development. When conceptualizing this volume, the editor identified those specific areas that contribute to the rational scientific basis for dose selection. Those areas leverage the first principles of pharmacokinetics and pharmacodynamics, which in the editor's opinion are fundamental to drug development. The concepts presented here are intentionally somewhat advanced and may appeal favorably to those who are familiar with basic pharmacokinetics and clinical pharmacology. The book is not designed as a formal study course textbook, but more along the lines of presenting perspectives from expert scientists drawn from the pharmaceutical industry, academia, and regulatory agencies. The perspectives are intended to be thought-provoking and designed to elicit sustained interest and discussions on dose selection and its broader impact on various elements of risk-versus-benefit and model-based drug development.

The editor recognizes that there are two key interfaces in new drug development: first, the transition from preclinical to Phase I clinical development (so-called early or translational development), and second, the transition from establishing pharmacological proof-of-concept in Phase IB/IIA development to pivotal efficacy Phase IIB/III trials (so-called late development). The interplay of biomarkers, novel clinical trial designs, pharmacogenomics, and new technologies overlapping these two transition events will be emphasized. Aspects of dose adjustment necessitated by both intrinsic and extrinsic considerations will also be discussed, although this is not the focus of this volume. The volume is intentionally not all-encompassing, focusing only on those opportunities which in the editor's perspective, if leveraged successfully, will positively influence drug development dose decisions.

It is hoped that the book will appeal to drug development scientists, particularly those who are clinical pharmacologists, pharmacokineticists, clinicians, and regulators. Advanced students of medicine, pharmacy, and allied health sciences may also benefit if their primary interests lie in new drug development. The book will appeal to anyone who would like to appreciate how integration of sciences facilitates meaningful changes in delineating risk versus benefit and ultimately in the selection of safe and effective doses.

Rajesh Krishna

Contents

Contributors

James Bolognese   Departments of Clinical Pharmacology and Biostatistics and Research Decision Sciences, Merck Research Laboratories, Merck & Co., Inc., Rahway, New Jersey, U.S.A.

Stephan Chalon   Lilly Research Laboratories, Eli Lilly & Company, Indianapolis, Indiana, U.S.A.

Lois M. Freed   Division of Neurology Products, Center for Drug Evaluation and Research, United States Food and Drug Administration, Silver Spring, Maryland, U.S.A.

Jogarao V. S. Gobburu   Pharmacometrics, Office of Clinical Pharmacology and Biopharmaceutics, United States Food and Drug Administration, Silver Spring, Maryland, U.S.A.

Mathangi Gopalakrishnan   Department of Mathematics and Statistics, University of Maryland, Baltimore, Maryland, U.S.A.

Peter H. Hinderling   Office of Clinical Pharmacology and Biopharmaceutics, Center for Drug Evaluation and Research, United States Food and Drug Administration, Silver Spring, Maryland, U.S.A.

Rajesh Krishna   Department of Clinical Pharmacology, Merck Research Laboratories, Merck & Co., Inc., Rahway, New Jersey, U.S.A.

Patrick J. Marroum   Office of Clinical Pharmacology and Biopharmaceutics, Center for Drug Evaluation and Research, United States Food and Drug Administration, Silver Spring, Maryland, U.S.A.

Markus Müller   Department of Clinical Pharmacology, Medical University of Vienna, Vienna, Austria

Vladimir Piotrovsky Clinical Pharmacology and Experimental Medicine, Johnson & Johnson Pharmaceutical Research & Development, Beerse, Belgium

Diether Rueppel Global Metabolism/Pharmacokinetics, Sanofi-Aventis Deutschland GmbH, Frankfurt, Germany

John-Michael Sauer Elan Pharmaceuticals, Inc., South San Francisco, California, U.S.A.

Wolfgang M. Schmidt Department of Clinical Pharmacology, Medical University of Vienna, Vienna, Austria

Jun Shi Clinical Pharmacology and Drug Dynamics, Forest Laboratories, Inc., Jersey City, New Jersey, U.S.A.

Paolo Vicini Department of Bioengineering, University of Washington, Seattle, Washington, U.S.A.

John A. Wagner Department of Clinical Pharmacology, Merck & Co., Inc., Rahway, New Jersey, U.S.A.

Willi Weber Global Metabolism/Pharmacokinetics, Sanofi-Aventis Deutschland GmbH, Frankfurt, Germany

Jennifer W. Witcher Lilly Research Laboratories, Eli Lilly & Company, Indianapolis, Indiana, U.S.A.

1

Introduction to Dose Optimization in Drug Development

Rajesh Krishna

*Department of Clinical Pharmacology, Merck Research Laboratories,
Merck & Co., Inc., Rahway, New Jersey, U.S.A.*

INTRODUCTION

On average, it now takes approximately at least 10 years of pharmaceutical research and development time and approximately $1.7 billion to bring a new molecule to bridge the gap of growing demands of unmet medical needs (1–8). It is also interesting to note that there is a failure rate of approximately 50% in Phase III late stage development in the industry (1,5,7). A schema on the drug development value chain is presented in Figure 1. Drug development proceeds in stages, as a molecule moves from preclinical to clinical development, eventually through registration and, in the process, valuable knowledge on the preclinical and clinical properties is gained that is consistent with the learning and confirming paradigm. It takes even more to keep the drug as a viable option for therapy post-approval as new information becomes available on the safety and efficacy of the drug in a wider patient population (8). As an example of post-marketing events, Table 1 lists the drugs withdrawn from the market due to safety-related reasons. The promise of new technologies that have spanned the entire breadth and width of drug development from combinatorial chemistry approaches to high throughput screens and the advances in genomic sciences appear not to have made a significant impact on the drug development statistics yet (6). This is reflected in the declining number of new molecular (or chemical) entities received by the United States Food and Drug Administration (FDA) as compared to the early 1990s (1). The scope of

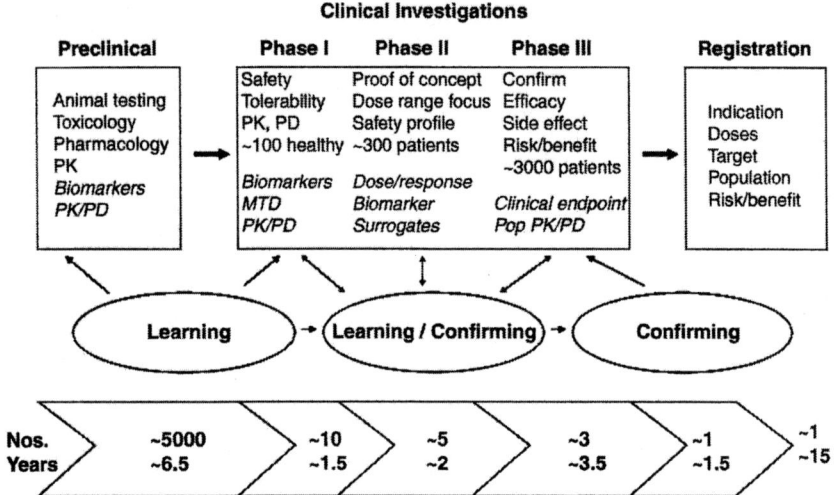

Figure 1 Drug development value chain from preclinical development through registration. The schema also illustrates compound attrition rate and development time.

knowledge-based drug development is illustrated in Figure 2, one recurring aspect of which, namely dose optimization, is the theme of this book.

CHANGING FACE OF REGULATORY ENVIRONMENT

The regulatory environment has also been rapidly changing as new information on the safety of an approved molecule arises from the wider patient population and additionally as long-term outcome trials on risk factors for disease dictate drug development and approval. This has had particular impact on drug withdrawals from the market in the past decade or two. Brewing in the midst of this cycle of innovation and stagnation, two schools of thought have emerged. One aims to critique the drug development as being too slow in bringing promising medical breakthroughs to the care of patients who deserve them faster than currently is the case, while the other aims to critique that the current drug development trials are insufficient to generate adequate safety and efficacy data to support a new molecule's broader use in a patient population.

The declining rate in approval of new molecular entities has been a subject of debate for a number of both scientific and business forums in the understanding of why pharmaceutical innovation is on the decline. The FDA Modernization Act of 1997, implying that a single adequate and well-controlled investigation with confirmatory evidence was sufficient for drug approval, triggered additional thought and public debate (9–16). A hypothesis on this issue was presented by Carl Peck, Donald Rubin, and Lewis Sheiner, which appeared

Table 1 Partial List of Drugs Withdrawn from the Market (1971–2005) Due to Safety Reasons

Drug	Reason for withdrawal
Azaribine	Thromboembolism
Ticrynafen	Liver and kidney toxicity
Benoxaprofen	Liver toxicity
Encainide	Mortality
Nomifensine	Hemotological effects
Suprofen	Kidney toxicity
Temafloxacin	Haemolytic-uraemic syndrome
Triazolam	Psychiatric effects
Zomepirac	Anaphylactic reactions
Apa	Anaphylactic reactions
Dilevalol	Liver damage
Fenclofenac	GI and skin toxicity and carcinogenicity
Feprazone	GI toxicity
Indoprofen	GI toxicity
Indomethacin-in-OROS	GI toxicity
Metipranolol	Granulomatous anterior uveitis
Perhexiline	Peripheral neuropathy and liver damage
Terodiline	Torsades de pointes
Zimeldine	Peripheral neuropathy
Flosequinan	Increased deaths
Fenfluramine	Heart valve disease
Terfenadine	Fatal arrhythmia
Bromfenac	Liver toxicity
Mibefradil	Fatal arrhythmia
Grepafloxacin	Fatal arrhythmia
Astemizole	Fatal arrhythmia
Troglitazone	Liver toxicity
Alosetron	Ischemic colitis
Cerivastatin	Muscle damage leading to kidney failure
Rapacuronium	Severe breathing difficulty
Etretinate	Birth defects
Levomethadyl	Fatal arrhythmia
Rofecoxib	Heart attack, stroke
Valdecoxib	Skin disease

Source: Adapted from Refs. 8, 45.

in *Clinical Pharmacology and Therapeutics* in June 2003 (17). The authors argued against the perception of lowered standards for drug effectiveness and stated that drug development will be more efficient in the end with a single clinical trial with confirmatory evidence of effectiveness.

Recognizing the apparent deficiencies in drug development and regulatory approval, the U.S. Food and Drug Administration put forth a white paper on

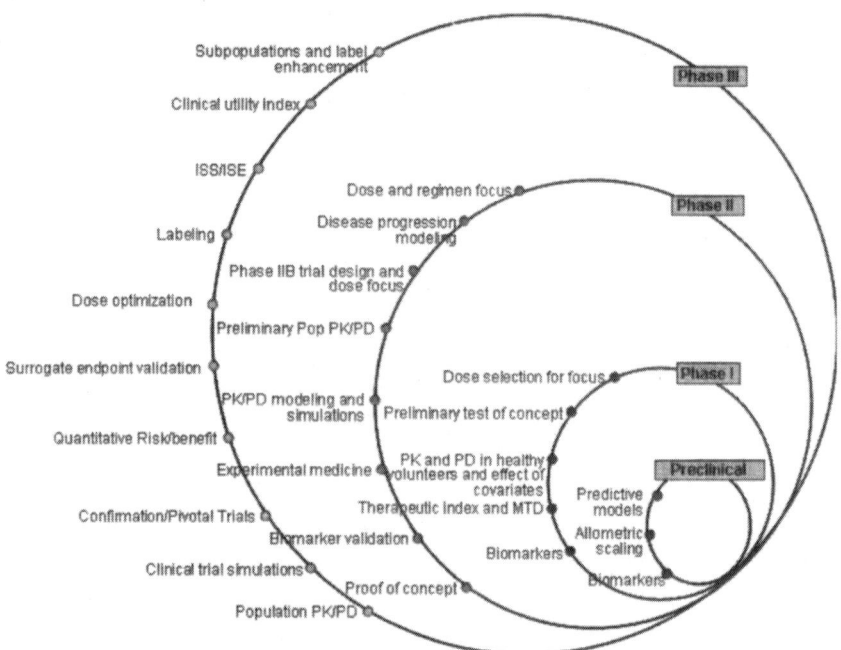

Figure 2 Scope of knowledge-based drug development (modified from the original, courtesy Dr. Jeff Barrett, University of Pennsylvania).

challenge and opportunity on the critical path to new medical products, in March 2004 (1). The white paper calls for an increased emphasis on methodologies that can reliably predict the safety and effectiveness of a drug and also novel clinical evaluation approaches to increase the efficiency of the so-called bottleneck of drug development, the clinical development (18). According to the white paper, the critical issue impeding successful development is the inability to predict safety and efficacy failures early in the process, such that the clinical development path (Phases I through III) is optimized for molecules with high probability of success to regulatory acceptance and approval. The FDA hopes to create new publicly accessible methodologies on modeling, simulation, biomarkers, and clinical endpoints to streamline the path to regulatory approval and has initiated a number of initiatives within and external to the agency to help make this vision a reality. A regulatory perspective is presented in Chapter 9.

NEW TECHNOLOGIES FOR DRUG DEVELOPMENT

Biomarkers

The integration of biomarkers in a drug discovery and development program provides valuable insights into a mechanism of action for a desired therapeutic intervention (19–40). These biological or biochemical markers of efficacy and/or safety will aid in the development of appropriate exposure/response relationships and can be implemented as early as preclinical pharmacology studies are performed in the drug discovery stage. Together with allometric scaling of pharmacokinetics (PK), exposure margins from toxicological data, and prediction of drug behavior in humans, they present the first opportunity to elucidate the projected clinically relevant dose range in translational development for assessment in the first human trial.

Typically, early biomarker identification and applications involve those biomarkers that are implicated in the normal course of disease progression, such that measurement of the marker provides some understanding of the pharmacological responses to a desired effect.

It is not uncommon to use the early phase of clinical development to investigate the viability of multiple markers of disease progression and/or safety. Biomarkers are particularly useful in the transition from preclinical to clinical development and also at the interface of early clinical and late stage clinical development. Their application in translational and early clinical (Phase I) development is in the selection of doses and/or regimens to be initially assessed.

Disease progression is discussed in Chapter 2 while biomarker validation and qualification are discussed in Chapter 3. Surrogate endpoints (discussed in Chap. 6) are generally those biomarkers that are intended to substitute for a particular clinical endpoint; clinical endpoints are those that represent functional or survival attributes (21–40). Specific definitions for the terminology used have been proposed by the biomarkers definitions working group listed in Table 2 (20).

Informative biomarkers and surrogate endpoints add value to drug development not only for deciding on comparative efficacy among lead candidates and a basis for termination or continuance of a program, but they are amenable to elucidating PK/pharmacodynamic (PD) assessments, thus aiding in target validation, providing early scope for risk/benefit, dose selection, focus and optimization, and in identifying a subset of the target population who may respond to a specific treatment option more favorably. In addition, they can aid

Table 2 Terminology for Biomarkers and Endpoints

Term	Definition
Biomarker	A characteristic that is objectively measured and evaluated as an indicator of normal biological processes, pathogenic processes, or pharmacologic responses to a therapeutic intervention.
Clinical endpoint	A characteristic or variable that reflects how a patient feels, functions, or survives.
Surrogate endpoint	A biomarker that is intended to substitute for a clinical endpoint. A surrogate endpoint is expected to predict clinical benefit (or harm or lack of benefit or harm) based on epidemiologic, therapeutic, pathophysiologic, or other scientific evidence.

Source: Adapted from Ref. 20 (Biomarkers Definition Working Group).

Table 3 Partial List of Biomarkers and Clinical Endpoints

Disease	Biomarker	Clinical endpoint
Alzheimer's disease	Entorhinal cortex volume by MRI	Cognitive testing
Asthma	Lung function tests	Respiratory distress
Cancer	Tumor size	Survival, progression
Diabetes	Fasting plasma glucose, HbA1c	Nephropathy, retinopathy
Glaucoma	Intraocular pressure	Visual acuity
Hyperlipidemia	Serum cholesterol	Myocardial infarction
Hypertension	Blood pressure	Stroke, myocardial infraction
Multiple sclerosis	Lesion incidence, volume	Neurologic manifestations
Osteoporosis	Bone mineral density	Fractures
Rheumatoid arthritis	c-reactive protein, joint space, erosion	Pain, mobility
HIV	CD4 levels, viral load	Survival
Congestive heart failure	Cardiac output, ejection fraction	Survival

Source: Adapted from Refs. 19–40.

in the design of efficient clinical trials and in the approval of new molecules, using an accelerated approval program. A good example of an accelerated approval based on a surrogate endpoint is from the infectious diseases therapeutic area (26,30,34–36). CD4 lymphocyte count is widely acknowledged and applied as a surrogate endpoint for AIDS progression. Zidovidine was first approved in 1987 based on survival data at 17 weeks. DDI, on the other hand, was approved in 1991 based on the CD4 as a surrogate endpoint for use in cases where AZT therapy failed, and ddC became the first molecule approved under the accelerated approval paradigm in 1992. Many drugs against HIV have since been approved. Based on a review of the recent accelerated approvals for drugs against HIV, the endpoint has been either the change of CD4, time-averaged change of CD4, HIV change from baseline, or HIV RNA <400 and/or <50 copies/mL. Table 3 lists the biomarkers, and surrogate and clinical endpoints for a few other disease segments. The role of pharmacogenomics in dose optimization is presented in Chapter 8.

Modeling and Simulation

PK characterization of a new molecule involves the quantitative description of the time course of a new molecule in the biological system, enabling elucidation of key PK parameters, such as half-life, volume of distribution, clearance, and so on. Similarly, PD characterization of a drug quantitatively describes the biological effects of drugs and mechanism of action. When PK is integrated with PD, valuable information on concentration versus effect relationships can be obtained, which has important implications in drug development. Simple and empirical exposure/response relationships can guide many aspects of drug discovery and development decisions such as dose selection, effect of exposure alteration on desired pharmacological response, defining target effect concentration margins, and prediction of response for a given concentration/exposure. Notably, PK/PD models can aid in elucidating the biological plausibility of various biomarkers early in drug development while providing an opportunity to accelerate drug development when integrated with biomarkers, surrogate, or clinical endpoints (12,17,41,42).

Over the last two decades, a new dimension of PK/PD modeling has emerged, in part borrowed from advanced engineering and business decision analysis fields (42). While probably still in infancy, the emerging science of pharmacometrics offers a quantitative basis for the principles of clinical pharmacology and therapeutics to an extent perhaps greater than that which has been accomplished in the past. This involves the application of complex computational and statistical principles in development of more mechanistic exposure/response relationships, integration of population PK/PD modeling, and stochastic simulation analysis incorporating Monte Carlo simulation paradigm, which have opened doors to a more quantitative outlook on clinical pharmacology. With the available programming and simulations software, these complex modeling and simulations approaches have already begun to have a positive impact on drug development. More importantly, their core application has been in forecasting the uncertainty in attaining a desired probability of success for a given therapeutic endpoint for large Phase II–III trials, thereby adding value to the design of clinical trials and dose and regimen optimization. This is possible by modeling the time course of disease progression based on available data on the progression of disease, outcome trials, and epidemiologic database, thus providing an opportunity to assess drug effects on disease progression. Virtual trials can be performed essentially in-silico and can assess the factors that influence the PK or PD of a given molecule against the backdrop of typical events that occur in an actual trial setting. Many of these concepts are applied and presented in Chapters 10–12.

Clinical Trial Design

In recent years, clinical trial designs have been a subject of numerous discussions and scientific debates. Given the increasing number of ineffective new molecular entities, failed clinical trial outcomes, and escalating trial costs, it has become increasingly apparent that novel clinical study designs would benefit from a redesign with an aim to improve upon the efficiency of clinical trials in selecting the winners, while minimizing exposing trial subjects to ineffective treatments. In general, for the purposes of discussion, there are two types of clinical designs based on flexibility. One is a frequentist design that is a *P*-value-based fixed allocation design, while the other is an evidence-based Bayesian approach evaluating subject-specific dose/response relationships. The latter design leverages prior information to decide on trial continuance or termination or reallocation, such that knowledge is updated as trial progresses. In statistical terms, this encompasses updating the prior estimate of the probability of an event to a posterior probability as new information becomes available. Adaptive clinical trial designs maximize the understanding of dose/response and contribute to selection of appropriate doses. Novel study designs are discussed more extensively in Chapter 5.

RISK VERSUS BENEFIT ASSESSMENT

A quantitative assessment of risk and benefit relates the desired therapeutic endpoint with the undesired effects for a given new molecule. Delineation of risk versus benefit enables a greater appreciation of the therapeutic index and safety margins, thus enabling dose selection to be optimized. A risk versus benefit profile can be leveraged by an understanding of the PK properties of a given drug and exposure/response relationships for safety and efficacy. A conceptual framework for risk/benefit leveraging of a biomarker approach for safety and efficacy is presented in Figure 3.

It is quite common to encounter undesired safety issues for a new molecule in Phase I development where super-pharmacological doses are used to aid in the

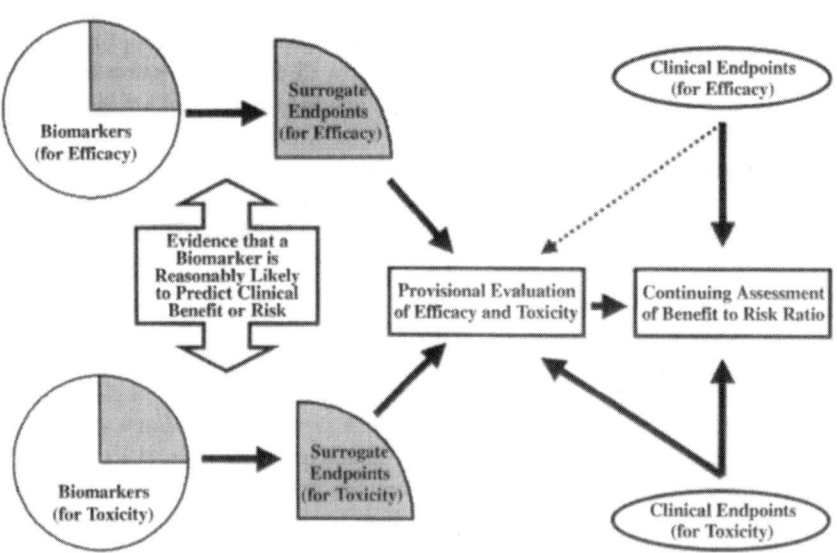

Figure 3 Assessment of risk/benefit. *Source*: Adapted from Ref. 20. Courtesy of the American Society for Clinical Pharmacology and Therapeutics.

assessment of dose-limiting tolerability/safety findings. With the integration of biomarkers for safety and efficacy, one could leverage the information quantitatively with the aid of PK/PD modeling approaches, and as new data become available, the model can be further updated. These analyses can guide the development of the therapeutic index for a given molecule and provide dose focus for later Phase II/III trials, allowing for a more precise evaluation of toxicity and efficacy using an iterative process.

An example of a biomarker for safety is the QTc interval prolongation as a predictor for torsades de pointes. A PK/PD modeling approach can predict the extent of prolongation for a given molecule in the target population if sufficient information is available on the factors influencing the PK and/or PD variability for a drug response. A therapeutically meaningful dose or range of doses can then be identified by maximizing the efficacy while minimizing the risk for an observed incidence of QTc prolongation. An example for PK variability would be the increased exposure to a drug metabolized by CYP3A in a subject with hepatic insufficiency or in a subject with concomitant administration of ketoconazole, a CYP3A inhibitor. Chapter 7 illustrates the role of PK and PD variability in dose optimization.

Advances in mechanism-based modeling have allowed the flexibility of incorporating underlying pathophysiological processes for an observed PD response. In addition to providing a characterization of the concentration/effect relationship, these approaches enable an effective delineation of risk/benefit by providing a measure of potency/activity and undesired effects.

A good example of an application of mechanistic modeling in quantitative risk/benefit assessments comes from the literature on inhaled corticosteroids (43,44). While inhaled corticosteroids present a viable therapeutic option for asthma, there have been questions on their long-term safety. Specifically, these concerns stem from their potential to suppress development of the adrenal function. Consequently, a clear delineation of the benefit (for asthma) and risk (clinical adrenal suppression) is necessary for development of newer inhaled corticosteroids. Here the benefit is a conglomeration of all favorable attributes of a molecule, including optimal PK properties, drug delivery properties, and increased residence in the lung, which may likely contribute to a more favorable systemic side-effect profile. An assessment of a quantitative risk/benefit value would entail the use of cortisol levels in plasma as a biomarker of the suppression in adrenal function. PK/PD modeling can then be performed integrating the biomarker, incorporating circadian rhythm, and any influence of down regulation. A model-based approach here would provide information on the degree of cortisol suppression for a range of efficacious doses and, thus, a therapeutic dose at which there is negligible cortisol suppression can then be identified.

Early identification of delineation of factors influencing risk and benefit is very useful as a clinical utility index is developed for a new molecule. This information may aid in the design of additional trials to further elucidate risk or benefit or add value in compound progression decisions.

IMPLICATIONS ON DOSE OPTIMIZATION

There are two crucial transition points in the drug development value chain. One is in the transition from preclinical pharmacology/toxicology to initial introduction to humans and the other is in the transition from Phase IIa to IIb/III. These crucial transition points emphasize the learning and confirming aspects of modern drug development. The selection of doses presents an important challenge during both transition points—specifically, the doses to be evaluated in the introduction to human study (Chap. 4), proof-of-concept study, and pivotal efficacy studies. Suboptimal dose selection can adversely influence program timelines, increase uncertainty in drug development probability of success, and elicit a poor understanding of exposure/response and, ultimately, risk/benefit. The goal of the early development program is to gain a robust understanding of PK, PD, safety and preliminary pharmacological activity, and hence key information on the maximum tolerated doses, minimum effective dose, and therapeutically relevant dose range is discerned. The influence of covariates (age, gender, special populations, concomitant drugs, renal status, and so on) on the PK or PD of a drug has important implications for dose adjustment recommendations. The availability of new methodologies and technologies, including biomarkers, surrogate endpoints, and genomic sciences, as well as the computational advances in modeling and simulations, have all made elucidating exposure/response relationships more informative in clinical drug development. Importantly, these technologies have improved our ability to understand disease progression and in delineation of risk and benefit by improving the predictive power of a desired effect or an undesired effect. It is hoped that these advantages translate into a productive and informed basis for dose selection in preclinical pharmacology studies and in transition to initial clinical trial in humans, while providing dose focus and refinement for later clinical trials and, ultimately, a range of doses for registration. Positive changes in the regulatory climate as evidenced by newer regulatory initiatives offer better dialogue between the regulatory agency and the sponsor on issues central to dose optimization by leveraging exposure/response relationships at key points in the value chain, consistent with the scope illustrated in Figure 2. The availability of drug disease model libraries will further streamline drug development and further refine the key transition points in drug development, such that late stage attrition can be reduced.

REFERENCES

1. Challenge and opportunity on the critical path to new medical products. United States Food and Drug Administration, 2004.
2. Tufts Center for the Study of Drug Development, Backgrounder: How New Drugs Move Through the Development and Approval Process. Boston, November 2001.
3. Niblack JF. Why are drug development programs growing in size and cost? A view from industry. Food Drug Law J 1997; 52(2):151–154.

4. Gilbert J, Henske P, Singh A. Rebuilding Big Pharma's Business Model, In Vivo, the Business & Medicine Report, Windhover Information, Vol. 21, No. 10, Nov 2003.

5. Lloyd I. New Technologies, Products in Development, and Attrition Rates: R&D Revolution Still Around the Corner. In: PARAXEL'S Pharmaceutical R&D Statistical Sourcebook, 2002/2003.

6. Boston Consulting Group. A Revolution in R&D: How Genomics and Genetics Will Affect Drug Development Costs and Times. In: PAREXEL's Pharmaceutical R&D Statistical Sourcebook, 2002/2003.

7. Duyk J. Attrition and translation. Science, Vol. 302, October 24, 2003.

8. Abraham J, Davis C. A comparative analysis of drug safety withdrawals in the UK and the US (1971–1992): implications for current regulatory thinking and policy. Soc Sci Med 2005; 61(5):881–892.

9. Peck CC. Drug development: improving the process. Food Drug Law J 1997; 59(2):163–168.

10. Woodcock J. An FDA perspective on the drug development process. Food Drug Law J 1997; 52(2):145–161.

11. Food and Drug Administration Modernization Act of 1997, Pub. L. No. 105–115, 111 Stat. 2295, 1997.

12. Peck CC, Wechsler J. Report of a workshop on confirmatory evidence to support a single clinical trial as a basis for new drug approval. Drug Inf J 2002; 36:517–534.

13. Peck CC. Streamlining and modernizing drug development: hearings before the Subcommittee on Health and Environment of the House Committee on Commerce, 104th Cong., 2nd Sess., May 2, 1996.

14. Peck CC. Modernizing effectiveness testing in drug development. Hearings before the Senate Labor and Human Resources Committee. Feb 21, 1996.

15. Peck CC. Clinical drug development may soon be accomplished in less than 3 years: will FDA and the pharmaceutical industry be ready? Hearings before the Subcommittee on Health and Environment of the House Committee on Commerce, 105th Cong., 2nd Sess., April 23, 1997.

16. Temple R. Experiences with single trials leading to section 115 of FDAMA and May 1998 evidence document: the use of the single, adequate and well-controlled efficacy trial (SCT) to support approval. Presented at Drug Information Association, The Use of the Single, Adequate and Well-Controlled Efficacy Study to Support Approval. Washington DC, Jan 22–23, 2001.

17. Peck CC, Rubin DB, Sheiner LB. Hypothesis: a single clinical trial plus causal evidence of effectiveness is sufficient for drug approval. Clin Pharmacol Ther 2003; 73(6):481–490.

18. Sheiner LB. Learning versus confirming in clinical drug development. Clin Pharmacol Ther 1997; 61:275–291.

19. Colburn WA. Selecting and validating biologic markers for drug development. J Clin Pharmacol 1997; 37(5):355–362.

20. Biomarkers Definitions Working Group. Biomarkers and surrogate endpoints: preferred definitions and conceptual framework. Clin Pharmacol Ther 2001; 69: 89–95.

21. Blue JW, Colburn WA. Efficacy measures: surrogates or clinical outcomes? [editorial]. J Clin Pharmacol 1996; 36(9):767–770.

22. Boissel JP, Collet JP, Moleur P, Haugh M. Surrogate endpoints: a basis for a rational approach. Eur J Clin Pharmacol 1992; 43(3):235–244.
23. Cannon CP. Clinical perspectives on the use of composite endpoints. Control Clin Trials 1997; 18(6):517–529; discussion 546–549.
24. Daniels MJ, Hughes MD. Meta-analysis for the evaluation of potential surrogate markers. Stat Med 1997; 16(17):1965–1982.
25. De Gruttola V, Fleming T, Lin DY, Coombs R. Perspective: validating surrogate markers—are we being naive? J Infect Dis 1997; 175(2):237–246.
26. Deyton L. Importance of surrogate markers in evaluation of antiviral therapy for HIV infection. J Am Med Assoc 1996; 276(2):159–160.
27. Ellenberg SS. Surrogate end points in clinical trials [editorial; comment]. Br Med J 1991; 302(6768):63–64.
28. Ellenberg SS. Surrogate endpoints [editorial]. Br J Cancer 1993; 68(3):457–459.
29. Fleming TR, DeMets DL. Surrogate end points in clinical trials: are we being misled? Ann Intern Med 1996; 125(7):605–613; comment 126(8):667.
30. Hughes MD, DeGruttola V, Welles SL. Evaluating surrogate markers. J Acquir Immune Defic Syndr Hum Retrovirol 1995; 10(suppl 2):S1–S8.
31. Lagakos SW, Hoth DF. Surrogate markers in AIDS: where are we? Where are we going? [editorial]. Ann Intern Med 1992; 116(7):599–601; comment 117(7):619.
32. Lee JW, Hulse JD, Colburn WA. Surrogate biochemical markers: precise measurement for strategic drug and biologics development. J Clin Pharmacol 1995; 35(5):464–470.
33. MacGregor JT, Farr S, Tucker JD, Heddle JA, Tice RR, Turteltaub KW. New molecular endpoints and methods for routine toxicity testing. Fundam Appl Toxicol 1995; 26(2):156–173.
34. Machado SG, Gail MH, Ellenberg SS. On the use of laboratory markers as surrogates for clinical endpoints in the evaluation of treatment for HIV infection. J Acquir Immun Defic Syndr 1990; 3(11):1065–1073.
35. Mildvan D, Landay A, De Gruttola V, Machado SG, Kagan J. An approach to the validation of markers for use in AIDS clinical trials. Clin Infect Dis 1997; 24(5):764–774.
36. Pozniak A. Surrogacy in HIV-1 clinical trials. Lancet 1998; 351(9102):536–537; comment 543–549.
37. Prentice RL. Surrogate endpoints in clinical trials: definition and operational criteria. Stat Med 1989; 8(4):431–440.
38. Rolan P. The contribution of clinical pharmacology surrogates and models to drug development—a critical appraisal. Br J Clin Pharmacol 1997; 44(3):219–225.
39. Wittes J, Lakatos E, Probstfield J. Surrogate endpoints in clinical trials: cardiovascular diseases. Stat Med 1989; 8(4):415–425.
40. Buyse M, Molenberghs G. Criteria for the validation of surrogate endpoints in randomized experiments [published erratum appears in Biometrics 2000; 56:324]. Biometrics 1998; 54:1014–1029.
41. Sheiner LB, Steimer JL. Pharmacokinetic/pharmacodynamic modelling in drug development. Annu Rev Pharmacol Toxicol 2000; 40:67–96.
42. Holford NH, Kimko HC, Monteleone JP, Peck CC. Simulation of clinical trials. Annu Rev Pharmacol Toxicol 2000; 40:209–234.

43. Kelly HW. Establishing a therapeutic index for the inhaled corticosteroids: Part I. Pharmacokinetic/pharmacodynamic comparison of the inhaled corticosteroids. J Allergy Clin Immunol 1998; 102(4, Pt 2):S36–S51.
44. Derendorf H. Pharmacokinetic and pharmacodynamic properties of inhaled corticosteroids in relation to efficacy and safety. Respir Med 1997; 91(suppl A):22–28.
45. CDER Report to the nation 2004. Improving public health through human drugs. US Department of Health and Human Services. Food and Drug Administration, 2004.

2

Bridging Preclinical and Clinical Development: Disease Progression Modeling in Translational Research

Paolo Vicini

*Department of Bioengineering, University of Washington,
Seattle, Washington, U.S.A.*

INTRODUCTION

The rate of growth of available information about biomedical and biological systems is exponential. In fact, available information has already gone far beyond human ability to synthesize, analyze, and predict. The biomedical information torrent is now a continuously growing set of exceedingly intricate knowledge about complex, large dynamic systems. Against this background, one of the most urgent challenges to the biomedical research community, with direct impact on drug development, seems to be to develop approaches to analyze this extremely large amount of data to discover *patterns* (1) or useful information that may be available in the data but not apparent through simple inspection. This integration aspect has always been a challenge in drug development, where data are continuously gathered at a variety of scales and sizes through the preclinical and clinical development programs. Recently, academic and health sciences research has also become aware of the importance of this very challenge. The National Institutes of Health (NIH) Roadmap for medical research in the 21st century states that:

> Today's biomedical researcher routinely generates an amount of data
> that would fill multiple compact discs, each containing billions of

bytes of data. [A byte is approximately the amount of information contained in an individual letter of type on this page.] There is no way to manage these data by hand. What researchers need are computer programs and other tools to evaluate, combine, and visualize these data. In some cases, these tools will greatly benefit from the awesome strength of supercomputers or the combined power of many smaller machines in a coordinated way but, in other cases, these tools will be used on modern personal computers and workstations (2).

Clearly, the storage and retrieval alone of these data sets poses formidable challenges, along with synthesis and visualization tools. However, another aspect of the biomedical data deluge poses an even more daunting test: biological and biomedical data are, almost without exception, only noisy and corrupted ghostly images of underlying phenomena which cannot be gauged directly. These underlying phenomena are the features of interest. As a very straightforward example, pharmacokinetics (PK) is usually gauged from measurements of drug levels in blood plasma and/or in urine. However, the concentration time course so obtained is not of primary interest. Much more relevant, easy-to-use, and simpler-to-grasp are the (kinetic) parameters that can be distilled from it, such as clearances and apparent volumes of distribution. Any distillation of information from data, such as pharmacokinetic data, requires a model, that is, a construct, hopefully with a mechanistic underpinning, which requires data as input and returns relevant, useful parameters as output. This is the *model as probe* concept (3), a potentially very useful paradigm for biomedical data analysis and synthesis. Within this framework, compartmental and non-compartmental approaches to data analysis, for example, deal with the same issue of information extraction.

Without a doubt, the main question is how do we measure *usefulness* in this context? Are all measured variables, parameters, or model outputs useful per se? Clearly, this is not the case. There have to be some basic requirements, having to do with physiological plausibility and predictive power, that these variables and parameters have to obey. In other words, estimated parameters should be as close as possible to the hidden, unknown feature they aim at measuring. When this is true, features of the model, such as, for example, predicted time courses, parameter values, or mechanistic structure, become *model-based biomarkers*, or (indirect) measures of biological processes conditional on both a mathematical and statistical (sometimes called *pharmacostatistical* in drug development) model assumption. Which particular features these parameters gauge depends on the application: volumes of distribution, clearance rates, production or secretion fluxes, sensitivity to intervention, response times, and time-to-event estimates, are all possible features amenable to this approach. Given the context, it should be apparent that model-based approaches are not just one way, they are *only* way to extract useful information from much of today's biomedical data. The reasons are multiple, but let us summarize only three.

First of all, a model-based analysis allows mitigation of the consequences of poor signal-to-noise ratio (the model can be seen as a data smoother, or filter), which all biological data suffer in various degrees. Secondly, as we have already mentioned, the sheer size of biological databases, both in the private and public sectors, nowadays by far outstrips human capacity. It is probably fair to say that no human will ever be able to wholly appreciate modern datasets like those coming out of proteomics research, which are starting to intrude in the petabyte range (a petabyte is comprised of 2 to the 50th power bytes, already much larger than the "monstrous" 2 to the 40th power bytes that comprise a terabyte). A model is thus not only a useful tool for prediction (at least potentially), but also for synthesis of available knowledge. A third reason is that more often than not, models have a mechanistic underpinning: their structure resembles the structure of the biological system they purport to represent. When this happens, then the model may allow for relevant inference on the short- and long-term behavior of the system under analysis, since the likely future behavior can be inferred from the combination of model structure and informative data.

Accepted biomarker classification (4) nowadays distinguishes between biomarkers and surrogate endpoints: the former is a larger class, while the latter classification requires independent validation and testing. Surrogate endpoints are harder to come by, but when they are available, they have an incredible potential to guide therapy design and the selection of optimal tests. Most valuable is the situation when:

- The biomarker/surrogate endpoint is amenable to mechanistic modeling, and
- It has been gathered over time, so as to give insight on temporal disease progression.

It would be most desirable for the biomarker to have a clear causal connection with the disease mechanism (5); regrettably, this is not always the case. However, while this is a shortcoming for mechanistic disease models, from a pragmatic standpoint the causal connection does not have to be there; in a sense, the marker needs only to be a monitor, or a probe of the disease process, without necessarily having to be in the causal chain.

BIOMARKERS AND DISEASE PROGRESSION MODELING

Since its introduction in clinical pharmacology and pharmacostatistical modeling (6), the idea of representing disease progression as a fundamental component of the quantitative representation of the PK and pharmacodynamics (PD) of a drug has made considerable strides. This paradigm shift has also made academic and industrial research and development entities closer than ever. The main reason is as follows. In this era of evidence-based medicine (7), where scientific findings are routinely used to make policy decisions, it is only natural that drug development makes aggressive use of the same body of scientific knowledge utilized by regulators and policymakers worldwide to make decisions that potentially affect the health and well-being of millions. It has now become quite clear that a computer model of disease progress, tightly integrated with a quantitative representation of the drug distribution and PD, has a previously untapped potential to streamline drug development at many levels. The cost of drug development has risen severalfold over the past decade, and the process is staggeringly expensive and far from efficient: only five out of 5000 candidate compounds reach the human experimentation stage, and only one out of these five will be approved by the FDA (8). There is a role for quantitative, testable, and queryable models of the drug-disease system that incorporate current knowledge, together with population variation and outcome mapping. The interest in these topics is starting to cross disciplines, from traditional mathematical biology to drug development, for example, as a recent mechanistic study about the effect of imatinib (Gleevec™) (9) testifies.

There seems to be a strong preference these days for biomarkers that are easy to measure, preferably univariate, and that have at least the potential to diagnose and predict therapy outcome for diseases that are at the worst multifactorial (10). In practice, this is going to be a lot trickier than it seems. We will neglect for now the role of environmental factors, but we will come back to them later. Straightforward diagnosis and obvious needs, even when coupled with a knowledge of the disease mechanism, such as for some monogenic diseases, do not necessarily translate into successful therapies. On the other hand, a lot of promise may lie in revisiting existing treatments or compounds, with the increased awareness that comes from a better understanding of the drug-disease system and its working mechanisms. An example is acute lymphoblastic leukemia, where significant increases in cure rates have been achieved largely through "the optimization of the use of existing drugs, rather than by the discovery of new agents" (11). Needs are multiple: while it is important to clearly discriminate the genetic basis of a disease, it is also important not to overlook disease aspects, which are more related to gross phenotypes, such as demographics, dosing extent, delivery, and timing of administration. Optimization of therapeutic conditions is also required, together with the development of novel genetic or molecular paradigms. The challenge with these systemic events is that they are best addressed from a holistic, or system-wide, point of view. The questions need to be posed in a specific language, and the grammar of the language is made of seemingly abstruse concepts, such as differential equations and probability densities, while its vocabulary consists of parameter values and regression techniques. Its end results are readily understood, since they are phrased in terms of dosing recommendations and effectiveness predictions.

A ROLE FOR INFORMATICS AND COMPUTATIONAL BIOLOGY

Interestingly, the modeling and simulation technology to achieve these goals has been available for decades (12) and originated from within multiple disciplines almost simultaneously (13); its practitioners used to be few and far between, but this corpus of techniques is now achieving something of a renaissance (14). Some companies have made this an integral part of their approach to drug development and candidate selection (15). These seemingly disparate technologies are necessary if we are to solve the problems that are listed here related to disease diagnosis and therapy, as applied to drug development.

- Most diseases are multifactorial, caused by several simultaneous mutations that are not amenable to direct quantification or prediction: one example for all is the prevalence of diabetes type 2 and its links to obesity and the metabolic syndrome. However, it may be difficult to translate even "simpler" causative links to promising therapeutic strategies. Moreover, most diseases may be caused by a combination of genetic and environmental factors, with the former providing predisposition and the latter providing the triggering of the adverse condition. It may not be appropriate to rely on either one or the other for predictive purposes, and especially for individualized medicine; rather, both need to be taken into account.

- There is a perceived excessive reliance on animal models and on otherwise simplified disease components, as opposed to an increased understanding of the disease mechanisms in humans. While cancer research has been recently singled out (16), the case could be made for other diseases as well. Preclinical models are often oversimplified, difficult to scale to humans (17), ultimately irrelevant, or all of these. This issue deeply affects both academic and governmental research and private R&D labs.

- A related issue with modern biomedical research is attention to the functional aspects of collected biological information. There appears to be a disconnection between the databasing and cataloging effort ongoing in bioinformatics and related fields and the translation of these findings into action items relevant for human health. While it is true that the knowledge base about human pathophysiology has increased severalfold, it is less clear how much of this knowledge is actually relevant and can be turned into lifesaving treatments or blockbuster drugs or both. The accumulation of knowledge may not be regarded as sufficient for much longer, as both the public and investors clamor to see tangible results of time spent or venture capital supplied.

- The lack of a common language between biologists and quantitative scientists, such as engineers, mathematicians, and statisticians, may be the single most important obstacle to the progress of biomedical research. If available, this language could be used for predictive statements and integration of data and experiment, but its absence is a major flaw. It has been said that, in the biological sciences, "you're not licensed to theorize unless you put the time in and get the data" (18), which seems a hardly efficient approach to science, since individual researchers' strengths and weaknesses may prevent such approaches. In a recent commentary, the author argues this very point, and goes on to state that it is "common experience that once the number of components in a system reaches a certain threshold, understanding the system without formal analytical tools requires geniuses, who are so rare even outside biology. In engineering, the scarcity of geniuses is compensated, at least in part, by a formal language that successfully unites the efforts of many individuals, thus achieving a desired effect, be that design of a new aircraft or of a computer program. In biology, we use several arguments to convince ourselves that problems that require calculus can be solved with arithmetic if one tries hard enough and does another series of experiments" (19).

With regard to the last statement, a possibility is that the most powerful and important role for bioinformatics and computational biology is not at all where everyone thinks it is. While databasing and the collection of genetic information and sequence results may be important per se in the end, the real promise for drug development will lie in their integration with predictive, quantitative models of drug-disease systems. Such models have concentration and effect measurements as inputs, often linked with biomarkers, demographic variables, genetic information and the like, and as outputs they return dosage information and probabilistic statements of outcomes. These models are now arising in a variety of areas, and their results in the determination of what we have called *model-based biomarkers* earlier are worth sharing here. Instead of focusing on drug development per se, we review recent findings in a few areas, discussing also validation aspects, or tests that can be conducted on a biomarker to evaluate whether it is measuring something of value. The commonality here is the great potential for *translational research*, that is, the generation of testable hypotheses or therapies from basic science research.

FINDING AND VALIDATING MODEL-BASED BIOMARKERS

Validation of model-based biomarkers is a fundamental issue, particularly when the potential exists for them to become surrogate endpoints. Measurement quality, statistical significance, and predictive power are all relevant in this context, since model-based biomarkers are by their very nature indirect measurements, and thus proxies for the actual biological parameter that would be of interest. In the examples we describe here, taken from the medical, pharmaceutical, and physiological literature, validated models have been used to either increase our understanding of the pathophysiological mechanisms at play, or they have allowed the indirect monitoring of biomedically relevant events. The endocrinology literature is replete with examples of this, in particular when considering the glucose-insulin system, which we will cover in some detail. The attempt to describe one individual's metabolic identity, or the state of an individual's regulatory pathways, with a relatively small set of parameters was a major thrust for this area of research, and has generated intriguing and important results. The basic approach undertaken may be extensable to other areas with little modification.

Model-Based Biomarkers in Gene Expression Studies

Microarray technology has gone from being an expensive and poorly understood technique to one of the most popular tools for the analysis of the genetic basis of biological systems (20). In these experiments, at least in theory, several thousands of gene expression levels following a certain stimulus can be assayed simultaneously. Microarrays thus allow tremendous efficiency in experimental design and allow to broadly examine a vast spectrum of how a biological system responds to an external change or stimulus. The approach is mostly used to determine which genes among this very large number are *differentially expressed* when experimental boundary conditions change. The underlying hypothesis is that, if a subset of gene expression levels changes dramatically, there is a high chance that these genes are somehow responsible for the behavior of the biological system or pathway under analysis (21). While the technology is very promising, issues regarding its broad applicability remain, both experimental and analytical in nature. Experimental issues include a relatively poor understanding of all the sources of error in the experiment and of the reproducibility properties of microarray experiments. Analytical issues arise when trying to decide what constitutes a significant change in expression level, and whether this is biologically relevant. Reliable differences in expression of genes are currently extracted through a variety of methods, including, for example, qualitative observations and heuristic rules (22), model-based probabilistic determination (23), and generalized likelihood analysis (24).

The basic problem with most of these approaches is that they lack a mechanistic background, so that changes in expression levels are, most of the time, examined in terms of size-fold difference. There could be, however, other aspects of the dynamic changes in expression levels that ultimately prove to be of interest. For example, the speed (rate) at which a certain cluster of genes reacts to a stimulus may relate more closely to the disease mechanism than the amplitude of the change in expression levels. A mechanistic model of expression changes could thus potentially provide much valuable insight, in that it describes the underlying relationships between system components that give rise to the observed behavior. Against this background, the parameters of a mechanistic model informed by the kinetics of gene expression could be a veritable treasure trove of information on the system. Conceivably, this model-based analysis method could provide a deeper understanding of the multiple reasons

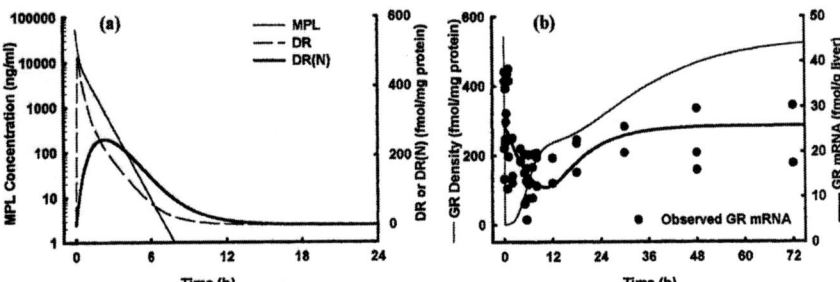

Figure 1 This figure shows the temporal evolution of components of a fifth-generation model of MPL pharmacokinetics and receptor dynamics developed in ADX rats. The *left panel* shows the time profiles of MPL concentration and the change of the cytosolic drug-receptor complex, DR, and the drug-receptor complex in nucleus, DR(N). A 50 mg/kg MPL i.v. injection was simulated. The GR density and mRNA are shown in the *right panel*, together with a plot of observed GR mRNA. *Abbreviations*: MPL, methylprednisolone; GR, glucocorticoid receptor. *Source*: From Ref. 26. Courtesy of The American Society for Pharmacology and Experimental Therapeutics.

behind gene expression changes and, ultimately, a mechanistic insight on the orchestration on the relationships between genes in a living system.

With application to PK-PD, Jusko et al. have demonstrated the integration of model-independent methods, such as cluster analysis (25) and model-guided inference (26), to study corticosteroid pharmacogenomics (Fig. 1 shows an example of their work). In this kind of work, traditional PK-PD comes together with more sophisticated pharmacogenomic quantitative constructs, in an integrated PK-PD-pharmacogenomic model for this class of drugs. The innovative aspect of this line of investigation is that biological inference is made on the basis of mechanistic conclusions about the likely working mode of the system, as opposed to inspection of the raw data and fold-change analysis of expression levels. Further work by the same group focused on related mechanistic aspects of this particular model system (27). Similar approaches bridging preclinical to clinical data and inference have been taken in other areas of research as well (28). Ideally, in vitro models should be followed by in vivo models (29) that generalize and amplify the findings possible in a controlled experiment.

Model-Based Biomarkers in Functional Imaging Studies

The quantitative aspects of imaging technology and its mechanistic underpinnings make it quite suitable as a tool for the extraction of model-based biomarkers. Positron emission tomography (PET) is one of the earliest functional imaging technologies. Through monitoring of a positron-emitting tracer, often a glucose analog, [^{18}F]FDG, unparalleled insight has been provided about the inner workings of organs like the brain or the heart. What is not necessarily appreciated is that the analysis of PET experiments has always required a mechanistic model of blood–tissue exchange to maximize the information extracted from this kind of study. The model was developed over many years (30) and has been subject to many modifications (31) and updates that extended the application of the technology to a variety of organs (32). Disease states have also been a focus, with studies demonstrating the interplay between transport and phosphorylation of glucose in diabetes through imaging (33), but also tracer studies (34). An intriguing study focusing on giant cell tumors (35) provides several hints as to how useful biomarkers can be extracted from these kinds of studies. The investigators focused on [^{18}F]FDG PET studies. They used standard compartmental analysis techniques to analyze [^{18}F]FDG kinetics in this kind of tumors. They also looked at determining the fractal dimension of the [^{18}F]FDG curve to measure its heterogeneity (the curve seems to have a fractal dimension of 1.3). Most interestingly, they correlated kinetic model parameters and the fractal dimension with gene expression levels. They were able to demonstrate that transport and uptake parameters, together with vessel density (all parameters of the standard [^{18}F]FDG model), correlated with the expression of genes known to be associated with angiogenic processes (Fig. 2). This is an interesting idea that relates the functional (model parameters) and genetic (expression levels) aspects of a dynamic imaging study.

Let us go back to parameters such as the fractal dimension (36) for a moment. The promise of such summary parameters is to summarize relevant aspects of a complex data set (such as an imaging data set) in a reduced array of values. This is of interest in image analysis (37) and time series (38), both of which exhibit difficulty in characterizing fluctuations. It has been put forth that fractal phenomena are ubiquitous in nature and especially in physiological systems (39). A summary parameter, such as the fractal dimension or approximate entropy (40), which characterize different functional aspects of the time series in a biologic recording or the spatial heterogeneity in a biomedical image, is very useful as a potential biomarker of disease progression, although care must be exercised to rigorously characterize the limitations of the analysis (41) and *what is being measured* (42).

Dynamic-contrast-enhanced magnetic resonance imaging (DCE-MRI), in conjunction with macromolecular contrast agents, is another recently proposed tool for monitoring microvasculature permeability, in particular, angiogenic processes. The time course of the DCE-MRI contrast agent will be measured as it leaves the vasculature (administration is usually intravenous) and permeates surrounding tissues. The rate of permeation, at least as stated currently, depends on the capillary fenestrations, which happen to be larger (either in number or size) in the presence of angiogenic events. Kinetic analysis of data gathered in animal models has provided promising results (43). In particular, the output of a blood–tissue exchange model applied to the dynamic imaging sequence was correlated with independent histological information (Scarff-Bloom-Richardson SBR histological scoring). Preliminary evidence showed increased capillary

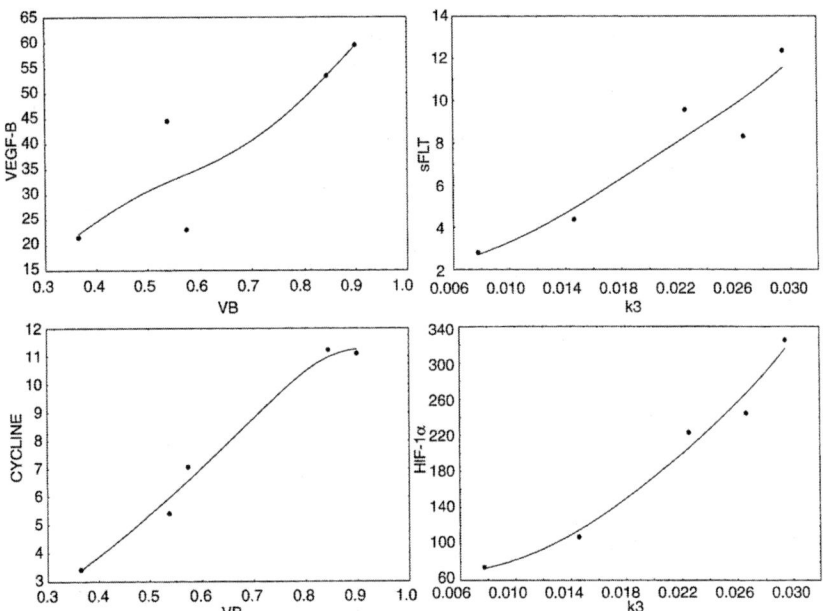

Figure 2   Correlations between compartmental model parameters and gene expression in giant cell tumors. (*left panel*): the compartmental model parameter VB, related to local tissue vascularization, is regressed against VEGF-B precursor (*top*) and cyclin E (*bottom*). (*right panel*): k3, a compartmental model parameter related to phosphorylation of [^{18}F]FDG, is regressed against sFLT kinase and HIF-1, the former related to the activity of VEGF-A and the latter related to tumor growth. Correlations were all significant with regression coefficient *r* greater than 0.87. *Abbreviations*: VEGB-B, vascular endothelial growth factor B; sFLT, soluble Fms-like tyrosine; HIF-1, hypoxia-inducible factor 1. *Source*: From Ref. 35. Courtesy of the Society of Nuclear Medicine.

permeability correlated with high SBR scores. It may be worthwhile to point out that the model, in this case, not only diagnoses the presence of a condition, but it provides a scaled measure of the degree of the condition—moreover, the measure is non-invasive.

Recently, these approaches have been applied to human trials as well (44). While sensitivity of the model-based biomarker remains to be evaluated, studies such as this provide an interesting avenue for exploration. Others have pointed out that, although these parameters are composites, they seem superior to the so-called "semi-quantitative" parameters that can be directly calculated from dynamic imaging data, but suffer from various limitations and are harder to generalize (45). The need is widespread and urgent; the Center for Biomarkers in Imaging (46) at the Department of Radiology of the Massachusetts General Hospital is cataloging imaging biomarkers in a variety of conditions and acts as a repository of knowledge about biomarkers, including a memorandum of understanding with the FDA (47). An interesting aspect is that imaging studies may help decrease our reliance on "soft" markers, such as cognitive or functional impairment. A recent review (48) suggests that biomarkers from MRI can be used to monitor brain lesions over time and thus can provide surrogate endpoints for clinical trials.

Model-Based Biomarkers in Intermediary Metabolism

What we have called "model-based biomarkers" have been investigated quite intensely in endocrinology over the past 25 years or so. Lessons for drug development that can be communicated through this body of work include:

- The need to gather data on the intact, in vivo system as soon as possible, as opposed to conducting in vitro studies;
- The necessity to explicitly represent biological fluxes that change with time, and their cross talk and interactions;
- The presence of non-linear control fluxes and signals, which have to be accommodated even in the most basic endocrinology model;
- Having to predict the kinetic behavior of remote compartments, such as peripheral or signaling compartments.

These aspects have increased in importance when studying biotechnology products: a majority of protein products are produced by the body under normal conditions, so one has to deal with the presence of endogenous fluxes and their regulation (49).

Many contributions have been made to the field of endocrinology by model-based analyses, also along the lines of time series investigations, such as those we have mentioned earlier (50). We will focus here on glucose kinetics and its control by insulin. A comprehensive review of the field is outside of our scope, but it has been carried out elsewhere (51). The appeal of glucose-insulin regulation, apart from its role in maintaining the crucial process of glucose homeostasis, is that it is a classical example of negative feedback control, with a few twists. Basically, high levels of glucose, such as those achieved after ingestion of a meal or a carbohydrate drink, cause an increase in secretion of the hormone insulin by the pancreatic beta-cells. Insulin then stimulates both the uptake and metabolism of glucose in muscle cells, thereby returning its concentration close to the original baseline. Metabolic diseases linked to pancreatic hormones result from one or more defects in all these processes, and sometimes just a subset. For some time now, it has been known how the responsiveness of tissues to insulin levels and pancreatic secretion of insulin lie on a hyperbola (52), that is, when one increases, the other decreases to compensate, and vice versa, and this maintains their product (often called the disposition index) approximately constant. One question, then, is how are these metabolic parameters *actually measured*, since they both cannot be assessed directly, but only indirectly, that is, through other means. The hyperbolic relationship seems to be largely independent of which particular approach is taken to measure beta-cell function and insulin sensitivity; it becomes particularly significant *across disease states*, as shown elsewhere (53). There are requirements that a measurement of these metabolic indices should satisfy across disease states. It should be:

- *Sensitive*: working equally well for patients with low- and high-sensitivity to insulin and insulin-secretory function;
- *Straightforward*: simple to implement in clinical practice, not too demanding or time-consuming;
- *Safe*: unlikely to generate side effects and suitable to application in large epidemiological studies.

The intravenous glucose tolerance test (IVGTT), as it is currently administered, is based on the administration of an intravenous bolus and glucose and the subsequent monitoring of glucose and insulin concentrations over time (54). Basically, the intravenous administration bypasses the absorption sites, and provides the *impulse response* (in engineering lingo) of the glucose system. The original protocol has been subject to many proposed modifications, motivated by the need to enhance the response of the system after a glucose challenge in highly insulin-resistant states; in these patients, secretory response may be blunted, and thus the effect of insulin on glucose disappearance is hard to discern. The most common modification is an exogenous administration of insulin (55). A third variable is often measured, the connecting peptide C-peptide. C-peptide is secreted equimolarly with insulin, but it is not extracted by the liver like insulin is; as such, its concentration in plasma is directly related to prehepatic insulin secretion. It turns out, as we will see later, that C-peptide availability is crucial for the determination of beta-cell secretory profiles.

The main difficulty in simultaneously modeling glucose and insulin time courses is related to the fact that changing levels of one influence the levels of the other by triggering signals that modulate production and secretion rates. The full feedback model that would be necessary to represent this complex signaling network should take into account glucose's effect on insulin secretion and insulin's effect on glucose production, in addition to insulin's effect on its own secretion and glucose's effect on its own production. The introduction of partition analysis (56) facilitated the scope of the work. Partition analysis artifactually opens the closed loop by analyzing the effects of insulin on glucose separately from the effects of glucose on insulin. What one loses is the development of a fully integrated feedback model, but the decreased generality that was brought forth in this case increased the robustness in the determination of individual metabolic indices.

The model concerned with one half of the feedback cycle, the effect of insulin on glucose disappearance, is simply called the glucose minimal model (57), and it has been highly successful in research and epidemiological settings. The minimal model uses two joint differential equations to model the time course of glucose concentration and of insulin action (the insulin signal acting on glucose disappearance) during an IVGTT. Based on the model equations, the action of insulin on glucose loss takes place from a signaling compartment [possibly related to interstitial fluid (58)], very similarly to the usual pharmacodynamic formulation of "effect site concentration" (59). Insulin concentration acts as a forcing function on the model, that is, it is assumed known without error. One of the parameters of the model (traditionally indicated as S_I) has the interpretation of tissue sensitivity to insulin, that is, it measures the effect of insulin on glucose disappearance. Low values of S_I and/or low time courses of insulin action indicate that the effect of insulin is blunted; this occurs in the diabetic syndrome, especially in diabetes type 2. This approach to determining the effect of insulin can also be applied to designer insulins (60), not only to human insulin. Early validation studies (61) have focused on the estimate of S_I across the spectrum of glucose tolerance states (62), between normal and various degrees of impairment (63). Insulin sensitivity ranges where the model appears not to be sensitive enough (64) have also given useful hints for patient classification. Despite its complexity, S_I also seems to predict cardiovascular disease risk better than other, simpler, and more straightforward measures of insulin resistance (65). Validation of time courses in glucose regulation has also been attempted (66). Ideally, this kind of validation should be attempted across populations and across degrees of disease, but, due to the related experimental challenges and the ambiguities related to the identification of suitable validation variables (especially in in vivo studies), such studies are few and far between.

Interestingly, the last five years have seen a surge of approaches that are related to the minimal model approach, but aim to alleviate some of its shortcomings. The minimal model was born as a research tool, and its sampling schedule, invasiveness of the intravenous protocol, and uncompromising simplifications of the underlying physiology are at the basis of current efforts. Improvements have focused on the design of tests that are even easier to administer and shorter, based on ingestion of either glucose (in the oral glucose tolerance test, OGTT) or a meal of known composition (as in the meal tolerance test, MTT). Just like in a pharmacokinetic study based on oral dosing, the main complication now is to account for absorption kinetics. Not much is known about glucose absorption in vivo, and the kinetics of absorption are likely quite variable across individuals. Also, without a concomitant IV administration, it is impossible to segregate the absorption profile alone. Extensions of the modeling paradigm were limited to healthy subjects (67), and used MTT data. Validation studies have also been conducted on a larger scale (68) in a variety of age groups. The agreement with the IVGTT estimates was quite good. More recently, the time course of absorption (69) (actually, the rate of appearance of glucose in plasma) was also subject to validation, and further contributed to the evaluation of metabolic indices at the same time.

Validation of time courses is most challenging. However, there are other studies where time courses have been validated by comparisons with independent measures of the same process. In general, in addition to matching the prediction of drug amounts in accessible compartments, multistate pharmacokinetic models also provide estimates of time-variant concentration in inaccessible compartments, or system locations. While these estimates are conceptually interesting, they present a substantial challenge for validation, since the actual levels in these spaces cannot be measured. In an interesting classic contribution (70), a mathematical model of tracer glucose kinetics was trained on measurements in serum. Given that the model had three compartments, or physiological spaces, that were needed to account for the data (serum, the accessible space, and a slow- and fast-exchanging compartment), a natural question is whether the levels predicted in these remote spaces, conditional on the model structure, are physiologically *valid*, that is, if they reflect actual measurements, or are just mathematical abstractions. In this particular case, thoracic duct lymph measurements were available in the animal model as a surrogate of the fast-exchanging compartment. Measurements agreed very well with the predicted time course, even if they were not trained on it specifically. Thus, the time course of tracer glucose could be accurately predicted in a peripheral, or remote, compartment, based only on data gathered in a different, accessible compartment.

We have not talked about the beta-cell secretion component of the system yet. This is even more important for the diagnosis and classification of, for example, diabetes type 1. The key aspect here is the availability of C-peptide, which, as we mentioned, has the same secretory profile as insulin but is not retained by the liver. C-peptide plasma measurements are thus an obvious choice to estimate prehepatic insulin secretion, provided a model for the kinetics of C-peptide can be established. Just like the minimal model, the model was first developed in animal studies (71), with promising results. A model for the secretory process is difficult to establish, and more polished representations are periodically proposed (72). Recent contributions seem to show that secretion parameters can be estimated from the simplified oral tests (73) we mentioned earlier (IVGTT and/or MTT tests), which may broaden the model's domain of applicability. These paradigms also brought forth novel candidate biomarkers, such as secretory response times (74) to glucose increases and decreases (75), which can be estimated by modeling the control of glucose rate of change (76) on the secretory process. In conclusion, these approaches to dissecting a complex intact system demonstrate that it is possible to estimate *both* insulin sensitivity (action) and secretion from just one glucose administration, thus opening up a potentially very wide spectrum of novel biomarkers and indirect measures.

CONCLUSION

Regrettably, independent validation of parameter estimates, but especially of time courses, is usually very burdensome, and independently designed experiments are required to carry it out (77). The gold standard for validation would be a paired evaluation of the model-based biomarker and a direct measure of the same quantity: this measure has to be obtained independently, and must have been already validated through other means. Difficulties include the design of the reference experiment, achieving a large enough sample size, recruiting subjects, safety considerations, and data analysis. Perhaps the most challenging aspect is to somehow demonstrate that the same physiological process, or metabolite level, or flux, is being measured by both the model and the reference experiment. As such, one can notice how this challenge is not terribly different from the one usually addressed in bioassay validation.

What sophisticated models of physiological systems actually accomplish is, in a sense, the removal of the existing division between PK and PD. All the models we have described represent distributional events, and so they are *kinetic* models, but we also have shown that their parameters shed light on *dynamic* effects (78). A validated model can be just as useful as a bioassay, in that it measures (albeit indirectly and through regression methods) parameters that have a direct physiological interpretation, whose changes over time can be monitored to provide insights into the progression of a disorder. An interesting aspect is that these models are all mechanistic. In conclusion, the case studies described here demonstrate that model-based biomarkers are difficult to validate and may generate controversy over their acceptance, but also that the drug development process may greatly benefit from the results they may bring.

ACKNOWLEDGMENT

This work was partially supported by NIH Grant P41 EB-001975.

REFERENCES

1. Stewart I. Nature's Numbers: the Unreal Reality of Mathematics. New York: BasicBooks, 1995.
2. The NIH Roadmap, Bioinformatics and Computational Biology, http://nihroadmap. nih.gov/bioinformatics/index.asp (accessed August 4, 2005).
3. Cobelli C, Caumo A. Using what is accessible to measure that which is not: necessity of model of system. Metabolism 1998; 47(8):1009–1035.
4. Lesko LJ, Atkinson AJ Jr. Use of biomarkers and surrogate endpoints in drug development and regulatory decision making: criteria, validation, strategies. Annu Rev Pharmacol Toxicol 2001; 41:347–366.
5. Schatzkin A. Problems with using biomarkers as surrogate end points for cancer: a cautionary tale. Recent Results Cancer Res 2005; 166:89–98.
6. Chan PL, Holford NH. Drug treatment effects on disease progression. Annu Rev Pharmacol Toxicol 2001; 41:625–659.
7. Dixon-Woods M, Agarwal S, Jones D, et al. Synthesising qualitative and quantitative evidence: a review of possible methods. J Health Serv Res Policy 2005; 10(1):45–53.

8. Davies K. Counting the cost of drug discovery. BioIt World, July 11, 2002, http://www.bio-itworld.com/archive/071102/firstbase.html (accessed August 4, 2005).
9. Charusanti P, Hu X, Chen L, et al. A mathematical model of BCR-ABL autophosphorylation, signaling through the CRKL pathway, and gleevec dynamics in chronic myeloid leukemia. Discrete and Continuous Dynamic Systems, Series B, 2004; 4:99–114.
10. Park JW, Kerbel RS, Kelloff GJ, et al. Rationale for biomarkers and surrogate end points in mechanism-driven oncology drug development. Clin Cancer Res 2004; 10(11):3885–3896.
11. Pui CH, Relling MV, Evans WE. Role of pharmacogenomics and pharmacodynamics in the treatment of acute lymphoblastic leukaemia. Best Pract Res Clin Haematol 2002; 15(4):741–756.
12. Sheiner LB, Rosenberg B, Melmon KL. Modelling of individual pharmacokinetics for computer-aided drug dosage. Comput Biomed Res 1972; 5(5):411–459.
13. Berman M. Kinetic analysis of turnover data. Prog Biochem Pharmacol 1979; 15:67–108.
14. Colburn WA. Biomarkers in drug discovery and development: from target identification through drug marketing. J Clin Pharmacol 2003; 43(4):329–341.
15. Parrott N, Jones H, Paquereau N, Lave T. Application of full physiological models for pharmaceutical drug candidate selection and extrapolation of pharmacokinetics to man. Basic Clin Pharmacol Toxicol 2005; 96(3):193–199.
16. Leaf C. Why we're losing the war on cancer. Fortune 2004; 76–97.
17. Bonate PL, Howard D. Prospective allometric scaling: does the emperor have clothes? J Clin Pharmacol 2000; 40(6):665–670; discussion 671–676.
18. Bray D. Reasoning for results. Nature 2001; 412(6850):863.
19. Lazebnik Y. Can a biologist fix a radio? Or, what I learned while studying apoptosis. Cancer Cell 2002; 2(3):179–182.
20. Hess K, Zhang W, Baggerly K, et al. Microarrays: handling the deluge of data and extracting reliable information. Trends Biotechnol 2001; 19:463–468.
21. Wang K, Gan L, Jeffery E, et al. Monitoring gene expression profile changes in ovarian carcinomas using cDNA microarray. Gene 1999; 229:101–108.
22. DeRisi J, van den Hazel B, Marc P, et al. Genome microarray analysis of transcriptional activation in multidrug resistance yeast mutants. FEBS Lett 2000; 470:156–160.
23. Long A, Mangalam H, Chan B, et al. Improved statistical inference from DNA microarray data using analysis of variance and a Bayesian statistical framework. Analysis of global gene expression in *Escherichia coli* K12. J Biol Chem 2001; 276:19937–19944.
24. Ideker T, Thorsson V, Siegel A, Hood L. Testing for differentially-expressed genes by maximum-likelihood analysis of microarray data. J Comput Biol 2000; 7:805–817.
25. Almon RR, DuBois DC, Pearson KE, et al. Gene arrays and temporal patterns of drug response: corticosteroid effects on rat liver. Funct Integr Genomics 2003; 3(4):171–179.
26. Jin JY, Almon RR, DuBois DC, Jusko WJ. Modeling of corticosteroid pharmacogenomics in rat liver using gene microarrays. J Pharmacol Exp Ther 2003; 307(1):93–109.

27. Jin JY, DuBois DC, Almon RR, Jusko WJ. Receptor/gene-mediated pharmacody-namic effects of methylprednisolone on phosphoenolpyruvate carboxykinase regu-lation in rat liver. J Pharmacol Exp Ther 2004; 309(1):328–339.

28. Panetta JC, Wall A, Pui CH, et al. Methotrexate intracellular disposition in acute lym-phoblastic leukemia: a mathematical model of gamma-glutamyl hydrolase activity. Clin Cancer Res 2002; 8(7):2423–2429.

29. Panetta JC, Yanishevski Y, Pui CH, et al. A mathematical model of in vivo methotrex-ate accumulation in acute lymphoblastic leukemia. Cancer Chemother Pharmacol 2002; 50(5):419–428.

30. Sokoloff L. [1-14C]-2-deoxy-d-glucose method for measuring local cerebral glucose utilization. Mathematical analysis and determination of the "lumped" constants. Neurosci Res Program Bull 1976; 14(4):466–468.

31. Phelps ME, Huang SC, Hoffman EJ, et al. Tomographic measurement of local cer-ebral glucose metabolic rate in humans with (F-18)2-fluoro-2-deoxy-D-glucose: vali-dation of method. Ann Neurol 1979; 6(5):371–388.

32. Williams KV, Bertoldo A, Mattioni B, et al. Glucose transport and phosphorylation in skeletal muscle in obesity: insight from a muscle-specific positron emission tomogra-phy model. J Clin Endocrinol Metab 2003; 88(3):1271–1279.

33. Williams KV, Price JC, Kelley DE. Interactions of impaired glucose transport and phosphorylation in skeletal muscle insulin resistance: a dose-response assessment using positron emission tomography. Diabetes 2001; 50(9):2069–2079.

34. Bonadonna RC, Del Prato S, Bonora E, et al. Roles of glucose transport and glucose phos-phorylation in muscle insulin resistance of NIDDM. Diabetes 1996; 45(7):915–925.

35. Strauss LG, Dimitrakopoulou-Strauss A, Koczan D, et al. 18F-FDG kinetics and gene expression in giant cell tumors. J Nucl Med 2004; 45(9):1528–1535.

36. Mandelbrot B. The Fractal Geometry of Nature. New York: W.H. Freeman and Co., 1977.

37. Nagao M, Murase K, Kikuchi T, et al. Fractal analysis of cerebral blood flow distri-bution in Alzheimer's disease. J Nucl Med 2001; 42(10):1446–1450.

38. Goldberger AL. Fractal variability versus pathologic periodicity: complexity loss and stereotypy in disease. Perspect Biol Med 1997; 40(4):543–561.

39. Bassingthwaighte JB, Liebovitch LS, West BJ. Fractal Physiology. New York, London: Oxford University Press, 1994.

40. Pincus SM. Assessing serial irregularity and its implications for health. Ann NY Acad Sci 2001; 954:245–267.

41. Jelinek HF, Fernandez E. Neurons and fractals: how reliable and useful are calculations of fractal dimensions? J Neurosci Methods 1998; 81(1–2):9–18.

42. Kuikka JT. Fractal analysis of cerebral blood flow distribution in Alzheimer's disease. J Nucl Med 2002; 43(12):1727–1728.

43. Daldrup H, Shames DM, Wendland M, et al. Correlation of dynamic contrast-enhanced MR imaging with histologic tumor grade: comparison of macromolecular and small-molecular contrast media. Am J Roentgenol 1998; 171(4):941–949.

44. Daldrup-Link HE, Rydland J, Helbich TH, et al. Quantification of breast tumor micro-vascular permeability with feruglose-enhanced MR imaging: initial phase II multicen-ter trial. Radiology 2003; 229(3):885–892. Epub Oct 23, 2003.

45. Miller JC, Pien HH, Sahani D, et al. Imaging angiogenesis: applications and potential for drug development. J Natl Cancer Inst 2005; 97(3):172–187.

46. http://www.biomarkers.org (accessed August 4, 2005).
47. http://www.biomarkers.org/NewFiles/news_archive/news_fda_hst.html (accessed August 4, 2005).
48. Schmidt R, Scheltens P, Erkinjuntti T, et al. White matter lesion progression: a surrogate endpoint for trials in cerebral small-vessel disease. Neurology 2004; 63(1):139–144.
49. Krudys KM, Dodds MG, Nissen SM, Vicini P. Integrated model of hepatic and peripheral glucose regulation for estimation of endogenous glucose production during the hot IVGTT. Am J Physiol Endocrinol Metab 2005; 288(5):E1038–E1046.
50. Veldhuis JD. Nature of altered pulsatile hormone release and neuroendocrine network signalling in human aging: clinical studies of the somatotropic, gonadotropic, corticotropic and insulin axes. Novartis Found Symp 2000; 227:163–185.
51. Bergman RN, Steil GM, Bradley DC, Watanabe RM. Modeling of insulin action in vivo. Annu Rev Physiol 1992; 54:861–883.
52. Kahn SE, Prigeon RL, McCulloch DK, et al. Quantification of the relationship between insulin sensitivity and beta-cell function in human subjects. Evidence for a hyperbolic function. Diabetes 1993; 42(11):1663–1672.
53. Ferrannini E, Mari A. Beta cell function and its relation to insulin action in humans: a critical appraisal. Diabetologia 2004; 47(5):943–596. Epub Apr 23, 2003.
54. Bergman RN. Pathogenesis and prediction of diabetes mellitus: lessons from integrative physiology. Mt Sinai J Med 2002; 69(5):280–290.
55. Finegood DT, Hramiak IM, Dupre J. A modified protocol for estimation of insulin sensitivity with the minimal model of glucose kinetics in patients with insulin-dependent diabetes. J Clin Endocrinol Metab 1990; 70(6):1538–1549.
56. Bergman RN, Cobelli C. Minimal modeling, partition analysis, and the estimation of insulin sensitivity. Fed Proc 1980; 39(1):110–115.
57. Bergman RN, Ider YZ, Bowden CR, Cobelli C. Quantitative estimation of insulin sensitivity. Am J Physiol 1979; 236(6):E667–E677.
58. Yang YJ, Hope I, Ader M, et al. Dose–response relationship between lymph insulin and glucose uptake reveals enhanced insulin sensitivity of peripheral tissues. Diabetes 1992; 41(2):241–253.
59. Holford NH, Sheiner LB. Pharmacokinetic and pharmacodynamic modeling in vivo. CRC Crit Rev Bioeng 1981; 5(4):273–322.
60. Osterberg O, Erichsen L, Ingwersen SH, et al. Pharmacokinetic and pharmacodynamic properties of insulin aspart and human insulin. J Pharmacokinet Pharmacodyn 2003; 30(3):221–235.
61. Beard JC, Bergman RN, Ward WK, Porte D Jr. The insulin sensitivity index in nondiabetic man. Correlation between clamp-derived and IVGTT-derived values. Diabetes 1986; 35(3):362–369.
62. Saad MF, Anderson RL, Laws A, et al. A comparison between the minimal model and the glucose clamp in the assessment of insulin sensitivity across the spectrum of glucose tolerance. Insulin Resistance Atherosclerosis Study. Diabetes 1994; 43(9):1114–1121.
63. Coates PA, Luzio SD, Brunel P, Owens DR. Comparison of estimates of insulin sensitivity from minimal model analysis of the insulin-modified frequently sampled intravenous glucose tolerance test and the isoglycemic hyperinsulinemic clamp in subjects with NIDDM. Diabetes 1995; 44(6):631–635.

64. Haffner SM, D'Agostino R Jr, Festa A, et al. Low insulin sensitivity (S(i) = 0) in diabetic and nondiabetic subjects in the insulin resistance atherosclerosis study: is it associated with components of the metabolic syndrome and nontraditional risk factors? Diabetes Care 2003; 26(10):2796–2803.

65. Howard G, Bergman R, Wagenknecht LE, et al. Ability of alternative indices of insulin sensitivity to predict cardiovascular risk: comparison with the "minimal model." Insulin Resistance Atherosclerosis Study (IRAS) Investigators. Ann Epidemiol 1998; 8(6):358–369.

66. Vicini P, Zachwieja JJ, Yarasheski KE, et al. Glucose production during an IVGTT by deconvolution: validation with the tracer-to-tracee clamp technique. Am J Physiol 1999; 276(2 Pt 1):E285–E294.

67. Caumo A, Bergman RN, Cobelli C. Insulin sensitivity from meal tolerance tests in normal subjects: a minimal model index. J Clin Endocrinol Metab 2000; 85(11):4396–4402.

68. Basu R, Breda E, Oberg AL, et al. Mechanisms of the age-associated deterioration in glucose tolerance: contribution of alterations in insulin secretion, action, and clearance. Diabetes 2003; 52(7):1738–1748.

69. Dalla Man C, Caumo A, Basu R, et al. Minimal model estimation of glucose absorption and insulin sensitivity from oral test: validation with a tracer method. Am J Physiol Endocrinol Metab 2004; 287(4):E637–E643. Epub May 11, 2004.

70. Gastaldelli A, Schwarz JM, Caveggion E, et al. Glucose kinetics in interstitial fluid can be predicted by compartmental modeling. Am J Physiol 1997; 272(3 Pt 1): E494–E505.

71. Toffolo G, Bergman RN, Finegood DT, et al. Quantitative estimation of beta cell sensitivity to glucose in the intact organism: a minimal model of insulin kinetics in the dog. Diabetes 1980; 29(12):979–990.

72. Toffolo G, De Grandi F, Cobelli C. Estimation of beta-cell sensitivity from intravenous glucose tolerance test C-peptide data. Knowledge of the kinetics avoids errors in modeling the secretion. Diabetes 1995; 44(7):845–854.

73. Breda E, Cavaghan MK, Toffolo G, et al. Oral glucose tolerance test minimal model indexes of beta-cell function and insulin sensitivity. Diabetes 2001; 50(1):150–158.

74. Breda E, Toffolo G, Polonsky KS, Cobelli C. Insulin release in impaired glucose tolerance: oral minimal model predicts normal sensitivity to glucose but defective response times. Diabetes 2002; 51(suppl 1):S227-S233.

75. Ehrmann DA, Breda E, Cavaghan MK, et al. Insulin secretory responses to rising and falling glucose concentrations are delayed in subjects with impaired glucose tolerance. Diabetologia 2002; 45(4):509–517.

76. Toffolo G, Breda E, Cavaghan MK, et al. Quantitative indexes of beta-cell function during graded up&down glucose infusion from C-peptide minimal models. Am J Physiol Endocrinol Metab 2001; 280(1):E2–E10.

77. Steil GM, Hwu CM, Janowski R, et al. Evaluation of insulin sensitivity and beta-cell function indexes obtained from minimal model analysis of a meal tolerance test. Diabetes 2004; 53(5):1201–1207.

78. Agerso H, Vicini P. Pharmacodynamics of NN2211, a novel long acting GLP-1 derivative. Eur J Pharm Sci 2003; 19(2–3):141–150.

3

Bridging Preclinical and Clinical Development: Biomarker Validation and Qualification

John A. Wagner

Department of Clinical Pharmacology, Merck & Co., Inc., Rahway, New Jersey, U.S.A.

INTRODUCTION

Dose optimization requires careful pharmacokinetic (PK) and pharmacodynamic (PD) analyses. Biomarkers are the basis of PD assessments and, more generally, are of increased interest to enhance decision-making in drug development. The focus of this chapter is on selected components of a suitable biomarker research plan, critical for the development and success of biomarkers, especially novel biomarkers. The elements that must be addressed by the research plan include both method validation and biomarker qualification. Method validation is the process of assessing the assay and its measurement performance characteristics, and determining the range of conditions under which the assay will provide reproducible data meeting the individual study objectives. Qualification is the evidentiary process of linking a biomarker with biological processes and clinical endpoints. For distal or disease-related biomarkers, there are four general categories of increasing levels for qualification: exploration, demonstration, characterization, and surrogacy. A biomarker research plan, like the validation and qualification activities it describes, is a graded, "fit for purpose" process dependent on the intended application. A biomarker research plan can describe activities leading to one or more purposes, or may be iterative in nature, evolving with the use of the biomarker.

Biomarkers have many current and potential roles in the setting of drug development. One critical use of biomarkers is to provide a rational basis for early decision-making in drug development (1,2). Importantly, the use of biomarkers is critical for dose optimization of new therapies (3,4). Early decision-making and dose optimization with the use of biomarkers are expected to provide significant cost and time saving in drug development. Traditional outcome-based drug development is a long, expensive, and uncertain process (5). Refined drug development decision-making can translate to large financial savings and substantial time savings in bringing new medicines to patients (6–10). Investigation of biomarkers in the setting of drug development may also aid in determining or refining the mechanism of action of new or existing therapeutics. Along similar lines, investigation of biomarkers may help determine or refine pathophysiology. Finally, if a particular biomarker qualifies for use as a surrogate endpoint, then such use can aid in interactions with regulatory agencies for review and approval of new therapeutics, and may ultimately benefit medical practice by allowing the use of new diagnostic tests.

There are many important issues relevant to a discussion of biomarkers. First, there are many different systems of biomarker nomenclature, based on different types of biomarkers. Second, there are different uses of biomarkers, which range from exploratory hypothesis generation to definitive go/no-go decision making in late-phase drug development. Third, there is a plethora of different technology platforms for biomarker assays, which range from immunologic assays to expression profiling to imaging. Fourth, there are different strategies for validation (assay or method validation) and qualification (clinical validation) of biomarkers in the context of a biomarker research plan. Finally, the regulatory needs for scientific consensus and a robust dataset highlight the potential for collaboration in biomarker development.

Biomarkers have been the subject of several important recent initiatives. One of the most important was the Biomarkers Definitions Working Group, with members from the Food and Drug Administration (FDA), the National Institute of Health (NIH), academia, and industry (3). The consensus definitions that arose from this working group are discussed next. A more recent on-going effort is the one that was originated by the American Association of Pharmaceutical Scientists (AAPS), and it focuses on gaining consensus around method validation for biomarker assays (11). In addition, the "Road Map," announced in 2003 by the NIH (12), highlights the critical need for the pharmaceutical industry to improve the productivity of its drug development process and the wide-ranging initiative by the FDA supports improvements in the efficiency of pharmaceutical development by augmenting the role of biomarkers in drug evaluations and decision-making (10). A major goal of all the recent initiatives is to foster a dialog on important biomarker issues.

DEFINITIONS

The definitions of the biomarkers and their related terms were refined by the Biomarkers Definitions Working Group with members from FDA, NIH, academia, and industry (3). Table 1 reviews the definitions of biomarker terms, including biomarkers, PD markers, surrogate endpoints, and clinical endpoints. The term biomarker is the most general case; it refers to any useful characteristic that can be measured and used as an indicator of a normal biologic process, a pathogenic process, or a pharmacologic response to a therapeutic agent (3). Of particular interest in dose optimization, a PD marker specifically refers to a biomarker of pharmacologic response. A clinical endpoint actually quantifies a characteristic related to how a patient feels, functions, or survives, and a surrogate endpoint is a biomarker that is meant to substitute for a clinical endpoint. There are relatively few biomarkers that qualify for the evidentiary status of surrogate endpoints. The primary examples of surrogate endpoints are

Table 1 Definitions

Biomarker	Characteristic that is objectively measured and evaluated as an indicator of normal biologic processes, pathogenic processes, or pharmacologic response(s) to a therapeutic intervention.
PD marker	Biomarker of pharmacologic response.
Surrogate endpoint	Biomarker that is intended to substitute for a clinical endpoint and is expected to predict clinical benefit (or harm or lack of benefit or harm) based on epidemiologic, therapeutic, pathophysiologic, or other scientific evidence.
Clinical endpoint	Characteristic or variable that reflects how a patient feels, functions, or survives.
Proximal biomarker	Biomarker that occurs early in a pathophysiologic cascade and informs on the physical or biological interactions with the molecular target of the drug. Also known as target engagement biomarker.
Distal biomarker	Biomarker that occurs late in the pathophysiologic cascade and is linked to clinical benefit.
Validation	Assessing the assay or measurement performance characteristics including sensitivity, specificity, and reproducibility.
Qualification	The evidentiary process of linking a biomarker with biological processes and clinical endpoints.

Abbreviation: PD, pharmacodynamic.

also PD markers, but it is important to note that this is not necessarily the case. Surrogate endpoints are also referred to as surrogate markers in the biomarker literature. The Biomarkers Definitions Working Group has pointed out that the term surrogate endpoint is preferred because the use of this term properly connotes that the biomarker is being used to substitute for a clinical endpoint (3).

Validation and qualification are other key terms used for discussion of biomarkers, and will be discussed in more detail below. Validation is the process of assessing the assay and its measurement performance characteristics, and determining the range of conditions under which the assay will provide reproducible data meeting the individual study objectives, including sensitivity, specificity, and reproducibility. Qualification, or evaluation, is the evidentiary process of linking a biomarker with biological processes and clinical endpoints, such that it can be used as a surrogate endpoint. The biomarker literature occasionally uses validation and qualification or evaluation synonymously; however, this should be avoided because the validation and qualification processes must be distinguished and the term validation does not adequately describe the qualification process (13).

Another useful distinction is shown in Figure 1. Pathophysiology is typically a multistep cascade. If a biomarker is directly involved in the pathophysiology of a disease, it may occur early or late in the cascade. Biomarkers that occur early in the pathophysiologic cascade are known as mechanism of action (MOA) or proximal biomarkers. Proximal biomarkers inform on physical or biological interactions with the molecular target of the drug. Biomarkers that occur late in the pathophysiologic cascade are known as disease-related or distal biomarkers. Qualified distal biomarkers are capable of prediction of clinical benefit. Thus, in Figure 1, putative biomarker A is identical to the one in the early pathophysiologic steps leading to the disease outcome, and is designated as a proximal biomarker. Putative biomarker B substitutes for one of the late pathophysiologic steps leading to the disease outcome, and is designated as a distal biomarker.

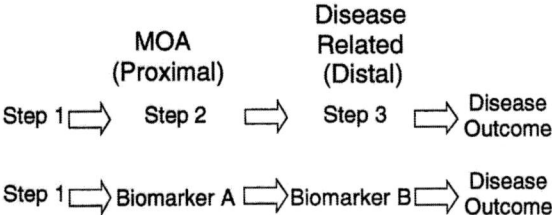

Figure 1 Pathophysiology is typically a multistep cascade. If a biomarker is directly involved in the pathophysiology of a disease, it may occur early or late in the cascade. Biomarkers that occur early in the pathophysiologic cascade are known as MOA, proximal, or target engagement biomarkers (*Biomarker A*). Biomarkers that occur late in the pathophysiologic cascade are known as disease-related or distal biomarkers (*Biomarker B*). *Abbreviation*: MOA, mechanism of action.

VALIDATION AND QUALIFICATION

A crucial distinction should be made between biomarker validation (assay or method validation) and qualification (or clinical validation or evaluation). Method validation is the process of assessing the assay or measurement performance characteristics and qualification is the evidentiary process linking a biomarker with biological processes and clinical endpoints. There are a series of issues relevant to this distinction, including differences between biomarker and PK assays, novel biomarker and diagnostic assays, the role for "fit for purpose" biomarker method validation and qualification, and the interaction between validation and qualification.

There are important differences between biomarker method validation and PK assay and also diagnostic assay validation. The goals and processes for biomarker assay validation are different from the PK validation. The FDA has issued detailed guidance for the industry on bioanalytical method validation. This guidance focuses on validation of assays for small molecule drugs and is not directly related to the biomarker assay validation. Another distinction should be made between diagnostic laboratory validation and novel biomarker validation. The laboratories that perform diagnostic assays are certified under the Clinical Laboratory Improvement Amendments of 1988 (CLIA), and there is an exemption under CLIA for research, such as novel biomarker assays. Thus, there is a lack of regulatory guidance on requirements for biomarker assay validation. Because of the diverse purposes of biomarker research, the FDA regulations, bioanalytical drug assays guidance, and the CLIA guidelines all fail to meet the needs of novel biomarker study purposes.

Biomarker method validation is the process of assessing the assay or measurement performance characteristics. Method validation should demonstrate that a particular method is "reliable for the intended application" and, thus, the rigor of method validation depends on the purpose. Generally, the rigor of method validation increases from the initial validation proposed mainly for exploratory purposes to more advanced validation dependent on the evidentiary status of the biomarker and/or the use of the results. There are two general categories of method validation in clinical drug development (11): (*i*) exploratory validation with crucial components including accuracy, recovery, precision, relative selectivity, initial target ranges, analyte integrity in matrix, and dilutional linearity, and (*ii*) advanced validation with graded addition of other necessary components, including additional specificity, sensitivity, parallelism, expanded reference range, extended stability, method robustness, and document control. For each biomarker project, the objectives and potential issues of the method should be identified in a specific validation plan to meet the objectives. Different applications of biomarkers require targeted method validation, that is, method validation should be considered as an iterative and an evolving process. For example, a biomarker for a purely exploratory objective in a Phase I study may be subject to exploratory method validation, whereas a well-qualified biomarker for a primary objective in a Phase I study may be subject to advanced method validation. Suitable biomarkers will typically require advanced method validation.

The primary distinction between biomarkers and surrogate endpoints is evidence. This is a point that has been highlighted by recent literature and also regulatory guidances. Many biomarker nomenclature systems categorize biomarkers according to their evidentiary status. For example, in AIDS research, one early nomenclature scheme includes: (*i*) Type 0 markers of natural history, (*ii*) Type 1 markers that assess biologic activity, and (*iii*) Type 2 markers that act as surrogate endpoints for clinical outcome of therapy (14). In addition, selected FDA guidances emphasize the evidentiary status in biomarker classifications. For example, in the exposure–response guidance, the FDA indicates that "biological marker (biomarker) refers to a variety of physiologic, pathologic, or anatomic measurements that are thought to relate to some aspect of normal or pathological biologic processes" and "these biomarkers include measurements that suggest the etiology of, the susceptibility to, or the progress of disease; measurements related to the mechanism of response to treatments; and actual clinical responses to therapeutic interventions" (15). Furthermore, in the exposure–response guidance, the FDA had classified biomarker types by their relationship to the intended therapeutic response or clinical benefit endpoints: (*i*) valid surrogates for clinical benefit (such as blood pressure, cholesterol, viral load), (*ii*) candidate surrogates reflecting the pathologic process (brain structure in Alzheimer's disease, brain infarct size in stroke, or radiographic and isotopic tests of function), (*iii*) measurement of drug action but of uncertain relation to clinical outcome (e.g., inhibition of ADP-dependent platelet aggregation or even angiotensin- converting enzyme inhibition in hypertension), and (*iv*) biomarkers that are remote from the clinical benefit endpoint (e.g., degree of binding to a receptor or inhibition of an agonist-provoked response). The FDA has also provided insight into its view of biomarkers through guidance on pharmacogenomic data submissions that shows it is likely to further distinguish into "probable valid biomarkers" and "known valid biomarkers," depending on the weight of the supporting evidence.

This evidentiary distinction between biomarkers and surrogate endpoints leads directly to the concept of qualification. Biomarker qualification is a graded evidentiary process linking a biomarker with biological processes and clinical endpoints, dependent on the intended application (13). When considering a distal or disease-related biomarker, it is instructive to conceptualize four general categories of qualification, as shown in Figure 2: (*i*) exploration biomarkers are research and development tools accompanied by in vitro and/ or preclinical evidence, but with no consistent information linking the clinical outcomes of the biomarker in humans, (*ii*) demonstration biomarkers are associated with adequate preclinical sensitivity and specificity and linked with clinical outcomes, but have not been reproducibly demonstrated in clinical studies, (*iii*) characterization biomarkers are associated with adequate preclinical

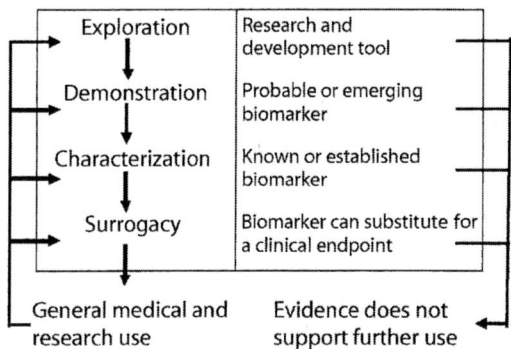

Figure 2 Life cycle of qualified biomarkers.

sensitivity and specificity and reproducibly linked clinical outcomes in more than one prospective clinical study in humans, and (*iv*) surrogacy reflects a holistic evaluation of the available data demonstrating that the biomarker can substitute for a clinical endpoint. The demonstration biomarker category corresponds to the "probable valid biomarker" in nomenclature suggested in the guidance from the FDA. The characterization biomarker category corresponds to the "known valid biomarkers" in nomenclature suggested in the guidance from the FDA. The surrogacy category and designation of a biomarker as surrogate endpoint requires agreement with regulatory authorities. Similar graded categories for biomarker qualification have previously been proposed for different purposes (16,17).

Figure 2 also illustrates the life cycle of qualified biomarkers. A novel biomarker may be progressively qualified from an exploratory biomarker to a surrogate endpoint for the purpose of drug development. Biomarkers may also enter the qualification pathway from general medical practice or research. Hemoglobin A1C is an important example of a biomarker that was in general medical use prior to its role in drug development. Importantly, biomarkers can also be "disqualified" if evidence no longer supports their use (i.e., runs of asymptomatic VT amidst normal sinus rhythm). Although the rationale exists for the suppression of intermittent ventricular tachyarrhythmias as a biomarker for suppression of ventricular arrhythmia and reduction of mortality following myocardial infarction, a well-controlled clinical study disqualified suppression of intermittent ventricular tachyarrhythmias as a biomarker for this purpose. In fact, the results of the Cardiac Arrhythmia Suppression Trial revealed that mortality was *increased* by anti-arrhythmic therapy following myocardial infarction (18).

The focus on evidentiary status for biomarkers also highlights an interesting observation about clinical endpoints relative to surrogate endpoints. Clinical endpoints are defined as a characteristic or variable that reflects how a patient feels, functions, or survives, and surrogate endpoints are defined by an evidentiary link between a biomarker measurement and a clinical endpoint. It is interesting to reflect that clinical endpoints also require an evidentiary link to the disease, but this link is not usually highlighted, often because the association between the clinical endpoint and the disease is taken for granted. It is also worthwhile noting that both clinical endpoints and biomarkers, including surrogate endpoints, are measurements. For example, in coronary artery disease drug development, myocardial infarction is considered as clinical endpoint and LDL cholesterol is considered as surrogate endpoint. The evidence that associates myocardial infarction with coronary artery disease is strong, by definition, as is the evidence that associates LDL cholesterol with coronary artery disease clinical endpoints (19). Both LDL cholesterol and myocardial infarction are measurements. Assessment of myocardial infarction is not typically considered a measurement, but, in fact, it is a multivariate measurement, involving clinical assessment of symptoms, electrocardiogram findings, and laboratory alterations. These considerations suggest that the distinction between biomarkers, especially surrogate endpoints and clinical endpoints is, at least to some extent, blurred.

APPLICATION OF VALIDATION AND QUALIFICATION TO SELECTED BIOMARKERS

Adiponectin is a 30-kDa protein composed of an N-terminus collagenous domain and a C-terminus globular domain. It exists in the circulation as complex oligomeric forms. Numerous studies have indicated that circulating concentration of adiponectin is closely linked to insulin sensitivity. A gradual decrease in adiponectin concentration is observed from lean to obese to diabetic individuals. Furthermore, PPARγ agonists increase plasma concentration of adiponectin in rodents and humans. Thus, there is a body of evidence that adiponectin is linked to glucose and lipid metabolisms in relation to insulin responsiveness and acts as a biomarker of PPARγ activation. However, in humans, there is discordance between improvements in insulin sensitivity and increases in adiponectin. Although the majority of the patients have increased adiponectin levels in response to PPARγ agonist treatment, only 50–70% of the patients demonstrate clinically improved insulin sensitivity. This suggests that adiponectin increases in any particular individual do not correlate with quantitative improvements in insulin sensitivity. Thus, adiponectin is qualified as a demonstration biomarker for PPARγ agonist activity, associated with adequate preclinical sensitivity and specificity, and linked with insulin sensitivity, but the link has not been reproducibly demonstrated in clinical studies.

Hemoglobin is one of the many proteins that undergo non-enzymatic glycation and Hb_{A1c} represents the most prevalent glycated species. Erythrocytes are freely permeable to glucose, and so the rate of formation of Hb_{A1c} is directly proportional to the ambient glucose concentration in which the erythrocyte circulates and to the duration of exposure. In addition, because of the irreversible nature of the non-enzymatic glycation, Hb_{A1c} represents an integrated measure of the average blood glucose concentration over the life spans of erythrocytes (i.e., 2–3 months). In contrast to a less well-qualified biomarker, such as adiponectin, Hb_{A1c} is associated with an overall database demonstrating that the biomarker can substitute for a clinical endpoint. Qualification of Hb_{A1c} was accomplished primarily in two large, randomized, landmark clinical trials, the U.K. Prospective Diabetes Study (UKPDS) and the Diabetes Control and Complications Trial (DCCT). In addition, regulatory authorities widely consider Hb_{A1c} as the most widely accepted measure of overall, long-term blood glucose control in diabetes and appropriate as a primary endpoint for clinical studies. The assessment is based partly on evidence from the UKPDS and DCCT.

SUMMARY

Method validation is the process of assessing the assay and its measurement performance characteristics, and determining the range of conditions under which the assay will give reproducible data. Qualification is the evidentiary process of linking a biomarker with biological processes and clinical endpoints. For distal or disease-related biomarkers, there are four general categories of increasing levels of qualification: exploration, demonstration, characterization, and surrogacy. A biomarker research plan, like the validation and qualification activities it describes, is a graded, "fit for purpose" process dependent on the intended application. A biomarker research plan can describe activities leading to one or more purposes, or may be iterative in nature, evolving with the use of the biomarker.

REFERENCES

1. Blue JW, Colburn WA. Efficacy measures: surrogates or clinical outcomes. J Clin Pharmacol 1996; 36:767–770.
2. Rolan P. The contribution of clinical pharmacology surrogates and models to drug development: a critical appraisal. Br J Clin Pharmacol 1997; 44:219–225.
3. Biomarkers Definitions Working Group. Biomarkers and surrogate endpoints: preferred definitions and conceptual framework. Clin Pharmacol Ther 2001; 69:89.
4. Lesko LJ, Atkinson AJ. Use of biomarkers and surrogate endpoints in drug development and regulatory decision making: criteria, validation, strategies. Annu Rev Pharmacol Toxicol 2001; 41:347–366.
5. Reichert JM. Trends in development and approval times for new therapeutics in the United States. Nat Rev Drug Discov 2003; 2:695.
6. DiMasi JA. The value of improving the productivity of the drug development process: faster times and better decisions. Pharmacoeconomics 20(suppl 3):1.
7. DiMasi JA, Hansen RW, Grabowski HG. The price of innovation: new estimates of drug development costs. J Health Econom 2003; 22:151.
8. Frank R, Hargreaves R. Clinical biomarkers in drug discovery and development. Nat Rev Drug Discov 2003; 2:566.

9. Kola I, Landis J. Can the pharmaceutical industry reduce attrition rates? Nat Rev Drug Discov 2004; 3:711.
10. Innovation or stagnation? Challenge and opportunity on the critical path to new medical products. United States Food and Drug Administration, 2004.
11. Lee JW, Devanarayan V, Barrett YC, et al. Fit-for-purpose method development and validation for successful biomarker measurment. Pharmaceutical Res 2006; [Epub ahead of print].
12. Zerhouni E. Medicine. The NIH roadmap. Science 2003; 302:63–72. http://nihroadmap.nih.gov.
13. Wagner JA. Overview of biomarkers and surrogate endpoints in drug development. Disease Markers 2002; 18:41–46.
14. Mildvan D, Landay A, De Gruttola V, Machado SG, Kagan J. An approach to the validation of markers for use in AIDS clinical trials. Clin Infect Dis 1997; 24:764–774.
15. Exposure–Response Relationships—Study Design, Data Analysis, and Regulatory Applications. Guidance for Industry, 2003.
16. Sullivan Pepe M, Etzioni R, Feng Z, Potter JD, Thompson ML, Thornquist M, Winget M, Yasui Y. Phases of biomarker development for early detection of cancer. J Natl Cancer Inst 2001; 93:1054–1061.
17. Bjornsson TD. Biomarkers: applications in drug development. Eur Pharmaceut Rev 2005; 1:17–21.
18. Echt DS, Liebon PR, Mitchell B, Peters RW, Obias-Manno D. Mortality and morbidity of patients receiving encainide, flecainide or placebo: the cardiac arrhythmia suppression trial. N Engl J Med 1991; 324:781–788.
19. Scandinavian Simvastatin Survival Study Group. Randomised trial of cholesterol lowering in 4444 patients with coronary heart disease: the Scandinavian Simvastatin Survival Study (4S). Lancet 1994; 344:1383–1389.

4

Dose Selection for First-in-Human (FIH) Trials—Regulatory Perspective

Lois M. Freed

Division of Neurology Products, Center for Drug Evaluation and Research, United States Food and Drug Administration, Silver Spring, Maryland, U.S.A.

INTRODUCTION

One of the most challenging aspects of drug development is the design of the initial clinical protocol, especially the selection of the starting dose for a first-in-human (FIH) trial. For a typical investigational new drug application (IND), selection of the starting dose for the FIH trial, by its very nature, is based solely on non-clinical data (usually in at least two animal species) and, perhaps, in vitro metabolism data in human liver microsomes (or hepatocytes). Although the selection of a safe starting dose is relatively easy, in that one can always pick a very low dose relative to doses used in the animal toxicity studies, the challenge is to select a dose that is safe, but not so low as to result in an unreasonable amount of time being taken to achieve doses that are anticipated to be therapeutically relevant.

The purpose of this chapter is to describe and to provide the basis for the current strategy used by the U.S. Food and Drug Administration's Center for Drug Evaluation and Research (CDER) to select a maximum recommended safe starting dose (MRSD) for FIH trials of new molecular entities (NME) in adult healthy volunteers. Selection of starting doses in FIH trials in patients is not addressed; however, similar principles may apply to selection of starting doses for FIH trials in otherwise healthy patients. Dose escalation is also not addressed. The guidance for industry (*Guidance for Industry and Reviewers: Estimating the Maximum Safe Starting Dose in Clinical Trials for Therapeutics in Adult Healthy Volunteers*, July 2005) has been published.

APPROACH FOR SELECTING THE MRSD FOR FIH TRIALS OF NMEs IN ADULT HEALTHY VOLUNTEERS

The approach most commonly used within CDER for selecting a MRSD for a FIH trial in adult healthy volunteers starts with selection of no observed adverse effect levels (NOAEL) in animals. A NOAEL is defined as the highest dose level that does not produce a significant increase in adverse effects when compared with the control; both statistical and biological significance should be taken into consideration. After NOAELs have been determined in the toxicology studies (typically conducted in rodents and non-rodents), the NOAEL (mg/kg) in each species is normalized by body surface area (mg/m²) using the allometric exponent, 0.67:

$$BSA = BW^{0.67}$$

where BSA is body surface area and BW is body weight (kg). The NOAEL for each species is then converted to human equivalent doses (HED, mg/kg) using the appropriate conversion factor (k_m, Table 1).

$$HED = NOAEL \times k_m$$

Once HEDs are calculated, the most sensitive or appropriate species must be selected. For some classes of drugs, it has been determined from a body of data that one species is more relevant to humans than other species, based on one or more factors. For example, unless data on a specific drug indicate otherwise, monkey is considered the most appropriate animal species for testing the acute toxicity of phosphorothioate oligonucleotides, since potentially life-threatening complement activation is observed in non-human primates (1,2), but not rodents. Also, rodents might be poor animal models for testing the toxicity of antifolate drugs due to differences in tissue folate pools (3,4). If no species is acknowledged to be "the best" model for human, the most sensitive species is defined as the species in which the NOAEL results in the lowest HED.

Once the HED has been selected based on toxicity data in the most sensitive or most appropriate species, a safety factor (SF) is applied to the HED in order to determine the MRSD. The selection of the safety factor is a critical

Table 1   Recommended Species-Specific k_m Values

Species	k_m^a
Human (adult)	37
Mouse	3
Rat	6
Rabbit	12
Dog	20
Cynomolgus monkey	12

$^a k_m$ = body weight (kg)/body surface area (m²).

Table 2   Reasons for Increasing or Decreasing the SF of 10

Increase SF >10
Steep dose–response curve
Severe, non-monitorable, or irreversible toxicity at doses above the NOAEL
Unexplained mortality at doses above the NOAEL
Wide intra- or interspecies variability in PK/ADME or in doses eliciting toxicity
Non-linear PK
Lack of experience with drug class (e.g., novel therapeutic target)
Lack of an appropriate animal model
Data from poorly designed or conducted animal studies
Decrease SF <10[a]
Drug is a member of a well-characterized drug class and animal data have been demonstrated to be predictive for human
Minimal, predictable, monitorable, and reversible toxicities in animals; shallow dose–response
NOAELs based on toxicity studies of substantially longer duration than proposed for humans; must demonstrate that toxicities observed do not increase in severity or that the effect-dose does not decrease with duration of dosing

[a]Animal data must be from well-designed and conducted studies, using drug formulations, dosing regimen similar to those proposed in the FIH trial.
Abbreviations: NOAEL, no observed adverse effect levels; SF, safety factor; PK, pharmacokinetics.

part of the process. The SF selected must provide a reasonable safety margin compared with the proposed clinical start dose (no toxicity should be expected) and must be based on all available non-clinical (including pharmacology, pharmacokinetics–PK/toxicokinetics and metabolism, safety pharmacology, and general toxicity) and in vitro human data. Data in the most sensitive species should not be the sole basis for determining an appropriate SF. The default SF is 10; however, a SF of 10 should not be used automatically. It is simply a starting point. There are many reasons for increasing the SF (Table 2); these include serious, unmonitorable, or unpredictable toxicities observed in animals at doses above the NOAEL, wide intra- or interspecies variability in PK/absorption, distribution, metabolism, and excretion (ADME) and/or toxicity, and deficiencies in study design or conduct. There are cases in which an SF < 10 is acceptable; however, decreasing the safety factor to <10 should be done only with great care (Table 2).

BASIS FOR CDER'S APPROACH FOR SELECTING A MAXIMUM SAFE STARTING DOSE FOR FIH TRIALS IN HEALTHY VOLUNTEERS

Conversion of NOAEL to HED

The best means to extrapolate from animal data to humans has been an area of interest for a number of years. Historically, interspecies extrapolation has been based on the concept of allometric scaling, that is, the process of relating various physiological variables or processes to body weight, using the general equation:

$$Y = \alpha(\text{BW})^\beta$$

where Y is the parameter of interest, BW is body weight in kg, and α and β are scaling parameters [plot of $\log(Y)$ vs. $\log(\text{BW})$, $\log(\alpha)$ is the Y-intercept and β is the slope].

A thorough review of this topic is beyond the scope of this chapter; for discussions of the historical aspects of interspecies extrapolation, the reader is referred to Travis and White (5), Travis (6), and Reilly and Workman (7), among others. Early work in this area demonstrated that a number of physiological variables (e.g., energy metabolism, organ size, and function) increased with body weight; however, the increase was not directly proportional to the body weight, that is, the slope, or β, is <1. As noted by Travis and White (5) in their historical overview, using body surface area (BSA) to make interspecies comparisons was originally based on the early observations that metabolism (i.e., heat loss/production), blood volume, renal parameters (i.e., kidney weight, total number of glomeruli) were proportional to BSA, but not body weight, and that oxygen utilization and caloric expenditure scaled best among the species when normalized based on BSA. The use of dose normalization by BSA for pharmaceuticals was codified in the 1960s in the area of oncology drugs, based primarily on the works of Pinkel (8) and Freireich et al. (9). Pinkel (8) compared the therapeutic doses of five chemotherapeutic agents in humans with doses reported in literature for animals (mouse, hamster, rat), and demonstrated intra- and interspecies similarities in dose when doses were normalized for BSA, but not for body weight.

Freireich et al. (9) addressed interspecies scaling of doses based on data in humans and toxicity data in various animal species (mouse, rat, hamster, dog, monkey) for 18 oncology drugs. The authors demonstrated that the LD_{10} or maximum tolerated dose (MTD) (considered to be equivalent) was similar among a variety of animal species (mouse, rat, dog, monkey) and humans when normalized by BSA. The data used by Freireich et al. (9) and data on 25 oncology drugs published by Schein et al. (10) were subsequently re-examined by others [including Travis and White (5); Watanabe et al. (11)]. Based on their reanalysis, Travis and White (5) concluded that an interspecies scaling power (β) of 0.75 was more appropriate than the 0.67 power recommended by Freireich et al. (1966). When data for 14 oncology drugs from the Freireich et al. (9) database were examined, the best estimate of β was 0.72, with 95% confidence limits of 0.67 and 0.77; reanalysis of 13 oncology drugs from the Schein et al. (10) database resulted in a best estimate of β as 0.74, with 95% confidence limits of 0.67 to 0.82. Neither result excluded a β of 0.67. However, when the combined dataset was analyzed, the best overall estimate of β was 0.73, with 95% confidence limits of 0.69 and 0.77, thus, excluding 0.67 (BSA correction).

Watanabe et al. (11) confirmed the overall results of Travis and White (5), concluding that the "best case" estimate of 0.75 is the most appropriate scaling factor; however, when the data were analyzed assuming greater variability (based on the degree of uncertainty regarding quality of the data, particularly in humans), they concluded that scaling by either factor is acceptable. While Travis and Morris (12) acknowledged the validity of the analyses performed by Watanabe et al. (11), they concluded that 0.75 was the most appropriate interspecies scaling factor based on the work of Travis and White (5) and published reports demonstrating that a number of physiological processes (i.e., metabolic rate, cardiac output, alveolar ventilation volume, renal clearance, energy utilization) scale best across species when body weight is raised to the 0.75 power. Travis and White (5) noted that an early report in which Rubner (in 1883) stated that heat production was proportional to BSA (i.e., $\beta = 0.67$, not 0.75) was based on intraspecies (i.e., dog), not interspecies, comparisons. Reilly et al. (7), in their discussion of the historical aspects of interspecies comparisons, noted that, as early as 1932, Kleiber demonstrated in animals (ranging in size from rat to cow) that basal metabolic rate increased with body weight to the power of 0.75.

Thus, the available body of data suggests that interspecies comparisons are best made by normalizing dose by body weight to the 0.75 power. However, it is important to note certain considerations that may limit the conclusions based on the analyses of the Freireich et al. (9) and the Schein et al. (10) datasets. Both datasets were based on evaluation of data only on oncology drugs, and using various routes of administration and dosing schedules. The toxicity data reported by Freireich et al. (9) were collected using IP, IV, and PO dosing. Of the 25 oncology drugs included in the Schein et al. (10) database, data for only three drugs were from oral studies; the remaining drugs were from IV studies. Routes of drug metabolism may vary widely and unpredictably among animal species, and drug metabolism (as opposed to energy metabolism) may not scale proportionate to either BSA (i.e., $\beta = 0.67$) or basal metabolic rate (i.e., $\beta = 0.75$) (13). These factors may limit the applicability of the conclusions based on analysis of these datasets to dose selection in drugs for other therapeutic areas. At present, it does not appear that there are sufficient data to select one interspecies scaling approach over another.

In order to determine the impact of using either approach on calculating a HED, conversion factors (k_ms) calculated using $BW^{0.67}$ and $BW^{0.75}$ were compared for various animal species (mouse, rat, rabbit, dog, monkey) and humans averaged over wide body weight ranges. In all cases, the mean HED calculated using $BW^{0.75}$ was higher than the mean HED calculated using $BW^{0.67}$. The greatest difference was in the smaller animal species (ratio of 0.75–0.67 was 1.88 in mouse and 1.57 in rat). In monkey and dog, the mean HED based on 0.75 was only 27% and 17% higher, respectively, than the mean HED based on 0.67. Therefore, this analysis indicated that, although using $BW^{0.67}$ would always be a more conservative approach, it would not result in a markedly lower MRSD compared with the start doses calculated using $BW^{0.75}$. Watanabe et al. (11) used LD_{10} data in mouse to predict MTD values in humans for 25 compounds [from the Freireich et al. (9) and Schein et al. (10) datasets], using either BSA (0.67) or metabolic rate (0.737) corrections. For 14 of the 25 compounds, the actual MTD identified in clinical trials was greater than the MTD predicted using either 0.67 or 0.737 (i.e., successful predictions). For seven compounds, the actual MTD was less than the MTD predicted using either scaling power (i.e., failures of prediction). For four compounds, the actual MTD was greater than the MTD predicted using 0.67, but less than the MTD predicted using 0.737. Watanabe et al. (11) noted that, although BSA correction always resulted in lower doses, it should not be considered as a conservative approach.

This discussion is certainly not intended to be a thorough review of the available literature on interspecies scaling of doses for pharmaceuticals. It is, instead, intended to provide a basis for the use of BSA (0.67) normalization to calculate a maximum safe starting dose for FIH trials in healthy adult volunteers. BSA normalization has been selected for interspecies scaling since (*i*) there is no body of literature that clearly establishes "the best" interspecies scaling approach, (*ii*) BSA (0.67) correction provides a more conservative estimate of HED than does correction based on basal metabolic rate (0.75), and (*iii*) reviewers in CDER have a great deal of experience using BSA correction for selecting safe starting doses and for other interspecies comparisons (e.g., comparison of effect- and no-effect doses). However, the results of Watanabe et al. (11) certainly suggest that simple conversion of a NOAEL in animals to a HED is alone not sufficient to ensure a safe starting dose in humans.

Use of Standard Conversion Factors to Calculate HEDs

Calculation of HEDs requires stepwise conversion of doses in mg/kg in animals to mg/m^2 in animals, followed by conversion to mg/m^2 in humans and, finally, mg/kg in humans. Conversion of mg/kg to mg/m^2 in animals is accomplished using the equation, $Dose^2_{mg/m} = k_m (Dose_{mg/kg})$. The term, k_m, is a conversion factor unique to each species and, within each species, it varies according to body weight. Since it is impractical to calculate HED taking into account body weight variations in individual animals and humans, a standard factor is used for each species (Table 1). To determine the effect of using a standard factor on calculation of HED, k_ms were calculated over a range of body weights in rats (0.090–0.460 kg) and humans (50–80 kg). The results indicated that using a standard k_m provided reasonable estimates of the HED (i.e., within 20%) over a fairly wide range of body weights.

Selection of Safety Factors (SFs)

A default SF of at least 10 is recommended. This recommendation has no scientific basis, but does take into consideration that interspecies differences have, in part, been addressed by normalization of dose by BSA.

A range of SFs has been suggested in published literature (9,11,14); however, comparing values among publications is difficult since the safety factors are often applied to different endpoints and for different purposes (e.g., estimate of safe lifetime environmental exposure in humans). Bonate and Howard (15) note that, according to an early method outlined by the Association of Food and Drug Officials of the United States, the maximum starting dose for a FIH trial should be 1/10 of the highest no-observed-effect level in a chronic toxicity study in rodent, 1/6 of the no-observed-toxic-effect level in a chronic study in dog, or 1/3 of the highest no-observed-toxic-effect level in monkey, whichever results in the lowest dose. For oncology drugs, starting doses of 1/10 of the rodent LD_{10} or the STD_{10} (i.e., dose, expressed in mg/m^2, producing severe toxicity or death in 10% of the animals), or 1/3 the estimated MTD in humans (mg/m^2) have been recommended (9,16); however, Freireich et al. (9) cautioned that data from multiple species should be taken into consideration in selecting a safe starting dose. Hertzberg (17) described the approach used by the U.S. Environmental Protection Agency for cancer risk assessment; NOAELs (mg/kg) from chronic animal studies are divided by 100 (a factor of 10 for species differences and another factor of 10 for differences in sensitivity among different human subpopulations).

Dourson and Stara (18) reviewed the regulatory history of SFs and conducted an analysis of SFs used to estimate acceptable daily intakes (i.e., lifetime exposure to, e.g., food additives) in humans. They noted that an SF of 100, applied to an animal NOAEL (expressed as mg/kg of diet or mg/kg body weight), was recommended by various agencies (including the U.S. FDA). Although the reasons given for the 100-fold SF differed somewhat among agencies, they generally addressed two basic concerns: intraspecies (10-fold) and interspecies (10-fold) variability. Recommendations to increase the safety margin are generally based on increased uncertainty (e.g., lack of animal data) or the use of a low-effect level instead of a NOAEL in animals, whereas recommendations to decrease the safety margin are based on decreased uncertainty (e.g., availability of human data). Based on their evaluation of published data, Dourson and Stara (18) concluded that there was support for using 10-fold safety margins to address intra- and interspecies differences, and further noted that a 10-fold safety margin would appear reasonable if interspecies differences in sensitivity were adequately addressed by normalizing doses to BSA, as proposed.

However, as previously noted, SF recommendations have no firm scientific basis. The 10-fold safety margin recommendation should be considered as a reasonable starting point, considering that interspecies differences in sensitivity have been (at least in part) addressed by normalization of dose to BSA. It should be increased in cases where there is greater uncertainty or concern (Table 2), and decreased (with caution) when warranted. This issue is further discussed in the following section.

VALIDATION

Chan et al. (19) evaluated CDER's approach to selection of the MRSD, using data from 35–36 non-cytotoxic drugs tested in humans during the years 1996–2002. Although not stated, it is assumed that the SF used in each case was the default factor of 10, since there was no discussion of a range of SFs. For all 35–36 drugs, the cardiovascular, gastrointestinal, and nervous systems were the most frequent sites of adverse effects. For 20–21 drugs, a no-effect or minimal-effect dose was identified. The calculated MRSD was lower than the no- or minimal-effect clinical dose in 11 of the 21 cases (52%). In the worst case, the calculated MRSD was 20 times higher than the no- or minimal-effect clinical dose. For 15 drugs, the lowest dose associated with what were considered significant adverse effects was identified. The calculated MRSD was lower than the clinical dose associated with significant adverse effects in 12 of the 15 cases (80%). In the worst case, the calculated MRSD was approximately six times higher than the clinical dose associated with significant adverse effects.

An internal effort has been initiated in order to validate CDER's approach described in the guidance for industry. The first step in this validation was to identify a number of drugs for which sufficient data were available to determine whether or not selection of the MRSD according to CDER's algorithm would have been successful, that is, starting dose associated with no (or minimal) toxicity. The analysis was based on data for 69 drugs, representing all review divisions. Reviewers were asked to provide the following information for each case: (*i*) therapeutic indication, (*ii*) the route of administration used and the duration of the toxicity studies used to determine NOAELs in animals, (*iii*) the NOAEL in the most sensitive species, (*iv*) the start dose and the route of administration used in the FIH trial, (*v*) the findings in humans at the start dose, (*vi*) the highest dose tested in the FIH trial, if known, and (*vii*) the human dose associated with significant toxicity, if identified.

For six drugs, there were insufficient data in humans to be included in the analysis. Therefore, the overall analysis included data from 63 drugs. For 20 of the 63 drugs, a toxic dose was identified in humans. For 35 drugs, data at doses above the starting dose were available; however, no toxic dose was identified. For eight drugs, human data were only available at the starting dose. For one drug, the route of administration differed between animals (subcutaneous) and humans (sublingual). In the majority of the cases, NOAELs in animals were based on toxicity studies of up to 3 months in duration; for two drugs, NOAELs were based on 6-month studies; for one drug, NOAELs were based on data from 13- to 26-week studies. It is not known how the actual starting dose used was selected in each case. Generally, the reviewer calculates a MRSD, using the method described, and compares that with the start dose proposed by the sponsor. However, reviewers do not routinely recommend adjusting the starting dose proposed by the sponsor unless a safety concern is raised.

In all but two of the 63 cases, the starting dose was successful, in that it was not associated with adverse effects. However, an important factor in some cases was selection of the safety margin. For the cases in which a toxic dose had been identified, the safety margins selected (i.e., HED/HSD) ranged from 0.7 to 300. Overall, safety margins used ranged from 0.4 to 2700. By category, 25/63 cases used a safety margin of < 10, 3/63 cases used a safety margin of 10, 24/63 used a safety margin between 10 and 100, and 11/63 used a safety margin of > 100. For the cases in which a toxic dose in humans had been identified, use of a 10-fold safety margin would have resulted in a HSD greater than the toxic dose in two cases. In 12 of the 20 cases, the toxic dose:HSD ratio would have been < 10. Therefore, the selection of a sufficient safety margin would appear to be critical.

The conclusions of CDER's preliminary analysis are limited by the fact that the cases examined were not random samples of relevant cases, that in some instances selection of the starting dose was based on human data, and by the lack of sufficient data from the initial clinical trial. Cases are continuing to be collected in order to complete the evaluation of CDER's approach to selection of the MRSD. However, the results of Chan et al. (19) and the preliminary internal analysis both indicate that serious consideration should be given to selection of an appropriate safety margin, and that a 10-fold SF may not be sufficient in some cases.

ALTERNATIVE APPROACHES TO ESTIMATION OF MRSD FOR FIH TRIAL IN HEALTHY VOLUNTEERS

Although dose normalization by BSA is currently the approach routinely used in CDER, it is acknowledged that a variety of other strategies may be acceptable. These include, but are not necessarily limited to, dose based directly on body weight, physiological-based modeling, allometric scaling of various PK parameters, and allometric scaling based on pharmacologically active dose (instead of doses associated with toxicities).

Physiological-Based Modeling

Physiological-based modeling is complex and is not commonly used in determining start doses for FIH trials. Therefore, this approach will not be discussed further. A publication by Dedrick (13) provides an early discussion of the use of physiological-based modeling applied to interspecies scaling. More recent discussions of physiological-based modeling applied to interspecies scaling of PK data have been reported by Ings (20), Iwatsubo et al. (21), Kawai et al. (22), Kirman et al. (23), Suzuki et al. (24), and others.

Interspecies Comparisons Based on mg/kg

There may be circumstances in which dose extrapolation among species is linear, that is, the most appropriate interspecies comparison is based on scaling directly to body weight, i.e., NOAEL (mg/kg) = HED (mg/kg). For example, if the NOAEL in each animal species is similar on an mg/kg basis, then extrapolation to humans based on mg/kg may be acceptable. However, since such a similarity could result from factors unrelated to drug sensitivity (e.g., differences in absolute oral bioavailability), if data from only two animal species are available, then additional information is needed. It would need to be demonstrated that: (*i*) NOAELs in the two animal species are defined by local toxicity (e.g., gastrointestinal) that directly scale by body weight across species, (*ii*) other drugs in the class exhibit similar toxicity in humans and animals at doses that correlate across species on an mg/kg basis, (*iii*) other pharmacological (e.g., pharmacologically active dose) and toxicological (e.g., MTD) endpoints also scale by mg/kg across species, or (*iv*) there is good correlation between plasma exposure (C_{max} and AUC) and mg/kg dose among species.

Since this approach results in a higher MRSD than when dose is normalized by BSA, it should be used with caution. Published studies indicate that such an approach has led, in a number of cases, to most unfortunate results (including death), at least in animals (25,26). Based on their examination of data from Freireich et al. (9) and Schein et al. (10), Watanabe et al. (11) concluded that interspecies scaling based on mg/kg would have overpredicted the MTD in humans in every case examined.

Allometric Scaling of PK Parameters

Allometric scaling of various PK parameters has received particular interest since Boxenbaum (27) [based, in part, on the work of Dedrick et al. (28)] proposed that PK parameters, such as volume of distribution and clearance, are related to body size or mass, since various physiological parameters (e.g., renal clearance, cardiac output) determining the PK parameters are also related to body size or mass, using interspecies allometric scaling. It is an empirical approach to interspecies scaling (as is interspecies extrapolation of dose), and may require knowledge of toxicity in animals in order to determine a starting dose (depending upon whether the PK parameter of interest is being related to some measure of toxicity, e.g., LD_{10}).

As noted by Bonate and Howard (15), there are limitations to predict the start dose based on allometric scaling of PK parameters. Selection of the "best" allometric exponent(s) may depend upon the specific parameter under consideration, may require information that is not available at the time of initial dose selection, for example, primary route of elimination (renal, hepatic) in humans, and may require a larger body of data in animals (e.g., data in a greater number of species) than is usually available. Interspecies differences in metabolism may be particularly problematic. Lave et al. (29) summarized the results of a number of published studies examining interspecies scaling of clearance for drugs from various therapeutic classes for which clearance data were available in humans. The authors noted that while prediction of total clearance was good for some drugs, it was poor for others. For certain drugs (i.e., triazolam, nordiazepam, diazepam), poor prediction of total clearance resulted from species differences in metabolism. Ward et al. (30) described the challenges in conducting interspecies scaling of clearance for drugs that are metabolized slowly and/or primarily by phase II metabolism. Lave et al. (31) reported the failure of allometric scaling to predict the PKs of napasagatran (a low molecular weight thrombin inhibitor) in humans. Napasagatran is actively excreted intact by the liver (into bile) and kidney, and it demonstrated wide interspecies variability in excretion based on PK data in rat, rabbit, dog, and monkey. Lave et al. (31) concluded that data on the transporters involved in the elimination of napasagatran might allow for more successful interspecies extrapolation. Chiou et al. (32) examined differences between rat and human in plasma clearance of 54 extensively metabolized drugs. While rat was considered to be, in general, a good model for predicting clearance in humans, Choiu et al. (32) also noted that there was large variability among drugs in the rat-to-human clearance ratio. Therefore, they recommended caution in attempting to use clearance in rat to predict clearance in human for FIH trials.

Numerous published studies have mostly conducted retrospective analyses of interspecies scaling of PK parameters for drugs for different therapeutic indications (e.g., 33). In reviewing the use of allometric scaling techniques in drug development, Mahmood (34) emphasized the potential importance of allometric scaling of PK parameters in selecting a safe starting dose for FIH trials, but concluded that failures of prediction are sufficiently common to warrant caution in making such predictions. A number of investigators have considered various approaches in an attempt to improve predictive ability, such as using in vitro metabolism data or incorporating factors such as brain weight or maximum life span. However, there is a question as to how successfully one or more of these approaches can predict a MRSD prior to a FIH trial, that is, before data in humans are available.

Pharmacologically Active Dose

There may be circumstances in which selection of MRSD may more appropriately be based on allometric scaling of a pharmacologically active dose (PAD) rather than a NOAEL. One example of this would be a drug for which dose-limiting toxicities in animals solely reflect exaggerated pharmacological effects. Selection of a PAD may be complex, since most drugs exert effects on more than one receptor system or biological process, and would certainly involve different factors depending upon the pharmacological class. Once a PAD is selected, based on in vivo studies in the most sensitive or most appropriate animal species, a HED can be calculated using BSA normalization.

SURVEY OF INDUSTRY APPROACHES

Some attempt has been made to document "current" practices for selection of starting doses in FIH trials within pharmaceutical companies. Reigner et al.

(35) conducted a survey within one pharmaceutical company to determine the extent and outcome of using PK and/or pharmacodynamic (PD) data to design clinical trials. A total of 18 projects were identified; in 13 of these, PK/PD data were considered to have had an important impact on drug development. Of these 13, five involved the use of PK and/or PD data to select a starting dose for a FIH trial. Although no details were provided, the selection of the start dose was based on allometric scaling of PK data in animals and previous pharmacodynamic data on other compounds of the same pharmacological class. Reigner et al. (35) noted that the starting dose, safely administered in all cases, was generally higher using the PK/PD approach than if based on animal toxicity data, and that smaller SFs were used. In a more recent review, Reigner and Blesch (36) described various approaches to selection of a starting dose for a FIH trial of cytotoxic and non-cytotoxic compounds. In selecting a starting dose for FIH trials of cytotoxic compounds, greater toxicity is tolerated due to the need to quickly achieve predicted therapeutic doses in patients, which is not appropriate for selection of a starting dose in FIH trials in healthy volunteers. Reigner and Blesch (36) identified four general approaches to select a starting dose for a FIH trial of a non-cytotoxic compound: (*i*) dose by factor, that is, dose identified in animals, expressed in mg/kg and multiplied by an SF, (*ii*) similar drug approach, that is, dose selection based on safety data (in humans and animals) available for a drug "similar" to the one being investigated and adjustment by some SF, (*iii*) pharmacokinetically guided approach, that is, use of systemic exposure (AUC or C_{max}) at the NOAEL in animals and prediction of clearance in humans based on allometric scaling of animal PK, and (*iv*) the comparative approach, that is, calculation of the starting dose using two or more approaches. Reigner and Blesch (36) also updated the results of the internal survey conducted within their pharmaceutical company in 1995 (35). In the more recent survey, 15 projects (conducted between 1996 and 2000) were identified. The results of both the 1995 and the 2000 surveys indicate that the PK-guided approach was the most commonly used approach (being used in eight of the 15 projects in both survey years) and the comparative approach being the most rarely used (no projects in 1995 and only one in 2000). The dose by factor approach was used in 3/15 and 5/15 projects in 1995 and 2000, respectively, and the similar drug approach was used in 4/15 and 1/15 projects in 1995 and in 2000, respectively.

CONCLUSIONS

CDER's current approach in the selection of a MRSD for FIH trials in healthy volunteers has been described. CDER's approach does not apply to FIH trials to be conducted in patients, since, in most cases, FIH trials in patients assume greater risk (and may require more aggressive dosing) due to the nature of the therapeutic indication being investigated (e.g., cancer chemotherapy, certain classes of antibiotics). It may, however, be applicable to otherwise healthy patients, in which rapid escalation to predicted therapeutic doses is not critical.

Justification for the use of this approach has also been provided, although a comprehensive review of relevant literature was beyond the scope of this paper.

NOAEL in a sensitive animal species by BSA, with subsequent application of an SF, provides a more conservative MRSD (compared with normalization based on basal metabolic rate). This is a fairly straightforward process using standard conversion factors, and takes into account all available data (including in vitro/in vivo animal data and in vitro human data). However, it is acknowledged that other approaches for selecting a MRSD may be acceptable. There are reports of successful interspecies scaling of PK parameters. However, the use of this approach may require more data than are routinely available to support an FIH trial and may be based on assumptions of interspecies similarities (e.g., in metabolism) that are unfounded. There are cases in which dose appears to scale linearly with body weight; however, extrapolating animal data to a human on an mg/kg basis is a less conservative approach than normalization based on either BSA or basal metabolic rate, and has been reported to result in unexpected and unacceptable toxicities. Therefore, additional justification is needed if this approach is used.

It must be emphasized that data that clearly demonstrate the validity of one interspecies scaling approach over another do not exist. In fact, it is clear that no one approach is "best" for all drugs. Ideally, one would have sufficient data on a drug to compare the various approaches. However, this is generally not feasible and certainly not required. Whatever approach is used to select an MRSD needs to be adequately justified. An alternative approach that results in an MRSD lower than the MRSD obtained using CDER's approach requires less justification, whereas one that results in a higher MRSD would require greater justification. Other approaches, such as allometric scaling of PK parameters, have been successfully, although not commonly, used to support dose selection for an FIH trial. The challenges faced in selecting a safe starting dose that is not unacceptably low (compared with the anticipated therapeutic dose range) are illustrated by the current lack of general regulatory guidance on this process. The guidance developed by CDER is an attempt to provide some regulatory framework for, and standardization to, this process. Hopefully, future work in this area will provide data to refine or revise CDER's thinking.

REFERENCES

1. Black LE, Farrelly JG, Cavagnaro JA, et al. Regulatory considerations for oligonucleotides drugs: updated recommendations for pharmacology and toxicology studies. Antisense Res Develop 1994; 4:299–301.
2. Henry SP, Beattie G, Yeh G, et al. Complement activation is responsible for acute toxicities in Rhesus monkeys treated with a phosphorothioate oligodeoxynucleotide. Int Immunopharm 2002; 2:1657–1666.
3. Habeck LL, Chay SH, Poland RC, Worzalla JF, Shih C, Mendelsohn LG. Whole-body disposition and polyglutamate distribution of the GAR formyltransferase

inhibitors LY309887 and lometrexol in mice. Cancer Hemother Pharmacol 1998; 41:201–209.

4. Gates SB, Worzalla JF, Shih C, Grindey GB, Mendelsohn LG. Dietary folate and folylpolyglutamate synthetase activity in normal and neoplastic murine tissues and human tumor xenografts. Biochem Pharmacol 1996; 52:1477–1479.

5. Travis CC, White RK. Interspecies scaling of toxicity data. Risk Anal 1988; 8(1):119–125.

6. Travis CC. Interspecies extrapolation in risk analysis. Ann 1st Super Sanita 1991; 27(4):581–593.

7. Reilly JJ, Workman P. Normalisation of anti-cancer drug dosage using body weight and surface area: is it worthwhile? Cancer Chemother Pharmacol 1993; 32:411–418.

8. Pinkel D. The use of body surface area as a criterion of drug dosage in cancer chemotherapy. Cancer Res 1958; 18:853–856.

9. Freireich EJ, Gehan EA, Rall DP, Schmidt LH, Skipper HE. Quantitative comparison of toxicity of anticancer agents in mouse, rat, hamster, dog, monkey, and man. Cancer Chemother Rep 1966; 50(4):219–244.

10. Schein PS, Davis RD, Carter S, Newman J, Schein DR, Rall DP. Commentary: the evaluation of anticancer drugs in dogs and monkeys for the prediction of qualitative toxicities in man. Clin Pharmacol Therap 1979; 11(1):3–40.

11. Watanabe K, Bois FY, Zeise L. Interspecies extrapolation: a reexamination of acute toxicity data. Risk Anal 1992; 12(2):301–310.

12. Travis CC, Morris JM. On the use of 0.75 as an interspecies scaling factor. Risk Anal 1992; 12(2):311–313.

13. Dedrick RL. Animal scale-up. J Pharmacokinet Biopharm 1973; 1(5):435–461.

14. Posvar EL, Sedman AJ. New drugs: first time in man. J Clin Pharmacol 1989; 29: 961–966.

15. Bonate PL, Howard D. Prospective allometric scaling: does the emperor have clothes? J Clin Pharmacol 2000; 40(4):335–340.

16. DeGeorge JJ, Ahn C-H, Andrews PA, et al. Regulatory considerations for preclinical development of anticancer drugs. Cancer Chemother Pharmacol 1998; 41:173–185.

17. Hertzberg RC. Fitting a model to categorical response data with application to species extrapolation of toxicity. Health Physics 1989; 57(suppl 1):405–409.

18. Dourson MI, Stara JF. Regulatory history and experimental support of uncertainty (safety) factors. Reg Toxicol Pharmacol 1983; 3:224–238.

19. Chan G, Gray P, Glue P. An evaluation of the FDA draft guidance for estimating the maximum recommended starting dose (MRSD) for first-in-human (FIH) studies. Clin Pharmacol Therap 2004; P8:PI–P19.

20. Ings RMJ. Interspecies scaling and comparisons in drug development and toxicokinetics. Xenobiotica 1990; 20(11):1201–1231.

21. Iwatsubo T, Hirota N, Ooie T, et al. Prediction of in vivo drug metabolism in the human liver from in vitro metabolism data. Pharmacol Ther 1997; 73(2):147–171.

22. Kawai R, Mathew D, Tanaka C, Rowland M. Physiologically based pharmacokinetics of cyclosporine A: extension to tissue distribution kinetics in rats and scale-up to human. J Pharm Exp Therap 1998; 287(2):457–468.

23. Kirman CR, Sweeney LM, Meek ME, Gargas ML. Assessing the dose-dependency of allometric scaling performance using physiologically based pharmacokinetic modeling. Reg Toxicol Pharmacol 2003; 38:345–367.

24. Suzuki T, Iwatsubo T, Sugiyama Y. Applications and prospects for physiologically based pharmacokinetic (PB-PK) models involving pharmaceutical agents. Toxicol Letts 1995; 82/83:349–355.
25. Boxenbaum H, DiLea C. First-time-in-human dose selection: allometric thoughts and perspectives. J Clin Pharmacol 1995; 35:957–966.
26. Van Miert ASJPAM. Extrapolation of pharmacological and toxicological data based on metabolic weight. Arch Exper Vet Med 1989; 43:S481–S488.
27. Boxenbaum H. Interspecies scaling, allometry, physiological time, and the ground plan of pharmacokinetics. J Pharmacokinet Biopharm 1982; 10(2):201–227.
28. Dedrick RL, Bischoff, KB, Zaharko DZ. Interspecies correlation of plasma concentration history of methotrexate (NSC-740). Cancer Chemother Rep Part 1 1970; 54:95–101.
29. Lave T, Coassolo P, Reigner B. Prediction of hepatic metabolic clearance based on interspecies allometric scaling techniques and in vitro–in vivo correlations. Clin Pharmacokinet 1999; 36(3):211–231.
30. Ward KW, Azzarano LM, Bondinell WE, et al. Preclinical pharmacokinetics and interspecies scaling of a novel vitronectin receptor antagonist. Drug Met Disp 1999; 27(11):1232–1241.
31. Lave T, Portmann R, Schenker G, Gianni A, Guenzi A, Girometta M-A, Schmitt M. Interspecies pharmacokinetic comparisons and allometric scaling of napsagatran, a low molecular weight thrombin inhibitor. J Pharm Pharmacol 1999; 51:85–91.
32. Chiou WL, Robbie G, Chung SM, Wu T-C, Ma C. Correlation of plasma clearance of 54 extensively metabolized drugs between humans and rats: mean allometric coefficient of 0.66. Pharmaceutical Res 1998; 15(9):1474–1479.
33. Obach RS, Baxter JG, Liston TE, et al. The prediction of human pharmacokinetic parameters from preclinical and in vitro metabolism data. J Pharmacol Exp Therap 1997; 283:46–58.
34. Mahmood I. Allometric issues in drug development. J Pharmaceutical Sci 1999; 88(11):1101–1106.
35. Reigner BG, Williams PEO, Patel IH, Steimer J-L, Peck C, van Brummelen P. An evaluation of the integration of pharmacokinetic and pharmacodynamic principles in clinical drug development: experience within Hoffman La Roche. Clin Pharmacokinet 1997; 33(2):142–152.
36. Reigner BG, Blesch KS. Estimating the starting dose for entry into humans: principles and practice. Eur J Clin Pharmacol 2002; 57:835–845.

5

Novel Clinical Trial Designs in Clinical Pharmacology and Experimental Medicine

Rajesh Krishna

*Department of Clinical Pharmacology, Merck Research Laboratories,
Merck & Co., Inc., Rahway, New Jersey, U.S.A.*

James Bolognese

*Departments of Clinical Pharmacology and Biostatistics and Research Decision
Sciences, Merck Research Laboratories, Merck & Co., Inc., Rahway,
New Jersey, U.S.A.*

INTRODUCTION

With the increased emphasis of model-based drug development through the FDA critical path initiative (1), it is increasingly apparent that in addition to gaining a quantitative understanding of the relationship between dose (exposure or concentration) and response, it is equally important to be able to predict and simulate the effect of a drug on disease pathophysiology to an extent greater than has been accomplished in the past. It is assumed that through these novel processes, a more informed understanding of the appropriate selection of doses is achieved. To consider the potential benefits of model-based drug development, it is perhaps necessary to review whether the current commonly employed designs for Phase I/II studies are adequate approaches to the desired goals and consider the advantages and disadvantages of some newer designs in the realm of clinical pharmacology and experimental medicine.

Drug development statistics reveal that both the length of the new chemical entity compound progression time and increased attrition rates are impediments to the desire to bring key medical and pharmaceutical breakthroughs to satisfy many unmet medical needs (2). As increased emphasis is put on shortening drug development timelines and reducing attrition rates, it is important to insure the quality of new chemical entities (NCEs) through concept- and hypothesis-based clinical investigation, such that the risk/benefit is more accurately and quantitatively understood.

To meet these increased demands, the discipline of clinical pharmacology and experimental medicine in early drug development is appropriately poised to develop a key understanding of the following aspects of drug development that profile the risk/benefit for a given NCE: initial safety, tolerability, pharmacokinetics (PK), pharmacodynamics (PD), preliminary efficacy and the maximum tolerated dose (MTD); the dose or exposure/response relationships (e.g., minimum effective dose); and determination of the PK and PD variability in drug response (e.g., formulation, food, age, gender, renal/hepatic impairment, disease, pediatrics, pregnancy, concomitant medication, etc.). These assessments will ultimately guide the selection of doses and dosing regimen to be evaluated in further efficacy trials and also lead to better understanding of the mechanism of action and clinical validation of the target through proof of mechanism, proof of concept, and proof of principle clinical trials. Consequently, it is imperative to explore proof of concept as soon as possible in early clinical development, such that informed decisions could be made for long-term clinical efficacy studies. These considerations encourage the widespread application of biomarkers, and surrogate and clinical endpoints in early development to gain an understanding of the mechanism of action and also key responses related to safety and/or efficacy. More recently, complex computational tools have been utilized that mathematically chart the course of disease progression while factoring in the PK and PD properties of a given new molecule.

The primary focus of this chapter is on the clinical trial designs used in clinical pharmacology and experimental designs to enable proof of mechanism and/or concept as they relate to early clinical development. The chapter will review the current commonly employed designs, provide discussion on newer clinical designs as they relate to adaptive dosing or stopping, and provide pros and cons to each approach as they relate to dose optimization. Studies that are commonly performed to understand the PK and PD variability, which is also a scope for the discipline of clinical pharmacology, are covered in Chapter 7 in this book.

Many of the approaches discussed in this chapter pertain to study designs that employ relatively smaller sample sizes as compared with Phase IIB/III studies; nonetheless, some of the concepts could be extended to large populations although not a focus here. Furthermore, additional considerations for trial designs are also presented in Chapter 9.

CONVENTIONAL DESIGNS

Phase I Studies

Phase I studies are hypothesis-driven, placebo-controlled, learning-type clinical investigations, which are typically performed in healthy human volunteers and commonly use single or multiple dosing of the study drug.

The primary objective of initial clinical pharmacology studies is to define the dose of a new molecule that results in unacceptable adverse events, which aids in the definition of dose-limiting toxicity and MTD. Secondary objectives may encompass a preliminary understanding of exposure/response relationships and also an understanding of common factors that result in PK variability. Consistent with a learning paradigm, the PD response is typically an exploratory or cataloged biomarker, which may be subsequently bridged to a surrogate or a clinical endpoint in the confirmatory clinical investigation. An early determination of the MTD enables later trials to provide dose focus and refinement for risk/benefit assessments.

First Introduction to Human

The first introduction to human study is typically a double-blind, placebo-controlled, randomized trial in healthy subjects. A healthy subject population enables a good assessment of drug properties in the absence of confounding variables of disease and other intrinsic and extrinsic factors, and also presents a fair assessment of risk, depending on preclinical safety profile and target organ toxicities (3–7). This initial study is limited in sample size (usually six active and two placebo), is somewhat inflexible in inclusion/exclusion criteria, and involves administration of rising single doses of the treatment until a dose-limiting safety/tolerability is attained or PK exposures result in non-linear plateau on exposure at a certain dose beyond which no appreciable increase is observed, or that a maximum feasible dose is reached in the absence of safety or tolerability finding. The study is also carefully monitored for any apparent safety issues via a battery of clinical safety assessment panels. The selection of doses is based on an understanding of safety margins and multiples of exposure from toxicological species, preclinical PK and PD data, and prediction of human PK and drug response considerations. For a detailed review on how these doses are selected, the reader is referred to the chapter by Freed (Chap. 4). Dose escalation may proceed such that an MTD is identified, but done carefully as more information on the safety, tolerability, and PK/PD is gained from the preceding doses. Data from this initial study would inform subsequent studies in terms of either additional preclinical toxicology studies, or inclusion of appropriate additional safety tests for monitorable toxicology events.

Although the key objective of a first-in-human (FIM) study is identification of the MTD and understanding of the common adverse experiences made possible via a battery of laboratory safety, AEs, vital signs, and ECG profiles, this is the first opportune time to learn the preliminary effect on desired response. Whenever possible, both validated and non-validated exploratory biomarkers are incorporated into these studies, and, in the event, a single dose of a given molecule in a healthy volunteer population is sufficient to elicit a desired pharmacological response. For a greater understanding of biomarker validation, the reader is referred to the chapter by Wagner (Chap. 3). In many therapeutic areas, human healthy volunteers often do not predict the response typically seen in the target patient population. This is commonly encountered in drugs for central nervous system disorders, such as Alzheimer's disease, multiple sclerosis, or Parkinson's disease. Certain variations of the FIM designs have also been performed.

Commonly employed FIM designs are either serial panel rising doses or an alternating panel design, wherein two or maybe even three panels of subjects receive the treatments in three or four treatment periods. The alternating panel design allows for greater flexibility in dose selection while providing an intra-subject evaluation. Depending on whether a given molecule is favorably or adversely influenced by food or whether a given molecule is a substrate and/or inhibitor of a drug metabolizing enzyme (e.g., a CYP 3A4), the design is modified to incorporate a food-effect arm either as a returning cohort at an identical dose or as a cross-over design at a dose well below the anticipated MTD. It is also not uncommon to enroll a panel of patients once an MTD is identified to determine comparability in performance in both the populations.

Multiple Dose Study

The multiple dose study is typically a second Phase I study performed after completion of the FIM study to evaluate the safety, tolerability, PK, and PD of multiple doses of the new molecule. Depending on the anticipated PK and PD properties, and depending on the turnover rates for the biomarker response, the duration of the study can range from one to four weeks, or to the extent that there is comparable duration of preclinical safety coverage that allows it. This is usually the first instance when the performance of the new molecule on multiple dosing is gained. This type of study will yield crucial information on whether the new molecule exhibits desirable safety profile in a multiple dose setting, whether the safety finding is more likely to manifest itself after repeat dosing than a single time (e.g., a delayed-type hypersensitivity), whether single dose PK reasonably predict multiple dose PK, degree of accumulation, and magnitude of PD response, among other data.

Similar to the FIM study, the sample size is typically small (e.g., six active and two placebo per dose level), and somewhat limited in scope in terms of power needed to detect small changes in safety and/or response. Although the multiple dose study is commonly performed in healthy volunteers, it can also incorporate patients. If the biomarker or PD response is simple and can be discerned within the framework of this type of study, it is not uncommon to consider a test of concept in such a study, provided additional elements of statistical power and design are appropriately addressed.

For a detailed description of Phase I clinical designs, the reader is referred to some authoritative reviews in this area (8–14). Innovation in Phase I clinical trials have provided ample opportunities in discerning early readout of drug activity and mechanism of action. These include, though are not limited to, biomarkers, pharmacogenomics, and non-invasive imaging probes (15,16).

PD Studies

In addition to the studies described previously, the third type of study commonly performed in clinical pharmacology includes studies designed to evaluate and validate certain types of experimental medicine methodology or concepts (6,10,11,14,17–20). These studies may be used for preliminary indication on efficacy (e.g., pain model), or for developing a certain type of approach that could be customized for a desired outcome across a therapeutic area (e.g., food intake or energy expenditure study, positron emission tomography study for receptor occupancy, and so on). Before a wider use is implicated, studies exploring these concepts or tools may be needed to build an experience database or simply to evaluate whether these methodologies are safe. Most often, the types of studies used to assess PD are geared to demonstrate a desired degree of biologic/pharmacologic activity that may be reminiscent of subsequent clinical success or failure, such that adequate refining of the concept or study is warranted. The study may also enable dose or concentration versus effect relationships and provide insight into the duration of effect. For example, compounds for Alzheimer's disease would generally need more than 6–12 months of treatment to discern a treatment-related effect on cognitive endpoints. An experimental medicine model would probably be a clinical investigation for a shorter treatment duration, which may discern beneficial effects on biomarkers that relate to the long-term treatment effects on cognition. Another example would be to understand the influence of formulation on the peak/trough ratio for an antihypertensive medication to overcome deficiencies in short terminal half-life.

The key attributes of experimental medicine studies are that the study sample size is generally small and the level of statistical significance in order to discern a desired trend in treatment effect may be higher than the normal α of 0.05 for decision-making purposes regarding future definitive trials. The experimental medicine studies are also characterized as being driven by the disease pathophysiology and drug pharmacology considerations. They are in most cases methodologically and statistically flexible. They are particularly useful to determine response in specific subpopulations that likely to more favorably respond to a treatment effect, which may yield an understanding of the magnitude of an effect and ascertain the benefit of the new molecule under investigation.

As an example of a preliminary proof-of-concept, double-blind, placebo-controlled test of concept, Haringman et al. evaluated an oral CCR1 antagonist in a small number of patients with rheumatoid arthritis (21). Specifically, they performed synovial biopsies on days one and 15 of the two-week treatment period to evaluate chemokine blockade. A statistically significant reduction in the number of macrophages and CCR1+ cells for the active treatment, compared with the placebo group, provided a simple test of concept for the new molecule (Fig. 1). Another example of a novel Phase I study which encompassed safety and preliminary proof of concept was described in 2003 by Rustin et al. (22,23).

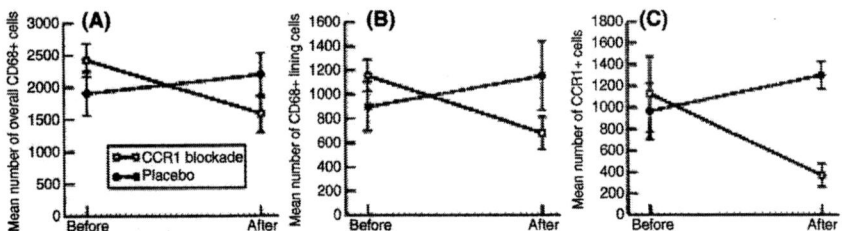

Figure 1   Proof-of-concept for a CCR1 antagonist. *Source*: From Ref. 21. Courtesy of BMJ Publishing Group.

The Phase I trial was performed with combretastatin A4 phosphate (CA4P), a novel antivascular agent, wherein 167 patients received 10-minute weekly infusion for three weeks followed by a week gap, with intrapatient dose escalation until grade 2 toxicity was observed. Positron emission tomography (PET) was used to measure the effects of this vascular targeting agent on tumor and normal tissue perfusion and blood volume. Significant dose-dependent reductions in tumor perfusion and tumor blood volume after CA4P administration were observed.

Phase IIa Studies (Proof-of-Concept)

A Phase IIa study designed to evaluate clinical concept is a study that is further on in the early development value chain; it serves to provide a more "definitive" read on the proof-of-concept for a given indication for which a new molecule is being developed (24–26). These double-blind, randomized, placebo-controlled trials intend to measure effect on a predetermined surrogate and/or clinical endpoint in a larger sample of patients and generally longer duration of therapy ($\sim$ up to 12 weeks). These studies provide the best opportunity in early drug development to more accurately refine dose and dosing regimen focus for definitive dose–response Phase IIb investigations. Furthermore, these studies provide a greater understanding of the common adverse experiences and/or target organ toxicity. Key compound development progression decisions are generally predicated on the outcome of these trials; consequently, the studies are often designed more ruggedly than the previously described experimental medicine studies, such that sound scientific rationale is presented for the target patient population going forward.

IMPETUS FOR NOVEL DESIGNS

The historical focus of clinical development was on hypothesis-driven, adequately powered clinical trials where fixed sample size designs were generally the norm. Recent years witnessed a number of key regulatory initiatives, which add fuel to the thoughts on considering dose optimization more broadly and also making quantitative assessments of risk/benefit. These include:

- End of Phase IIa meeting concept by the U.S. Food and Drug Administration (FDA) as a means to evaluate exposure/response relationships, such that doses and dosing regimens are appropriately selected (27);
- Critical path initiative by the U.S. FDA, which reinforces model-based drug development as a learning/confirming paradigm (1);
- European Medicines Agency's release of a guideline on clinical trials in small populations (28).

Probably all of these activities have a vested interest in making drug development successful by reducing late stage attrition rates, particularly at the key interface between end of Phase I and start of Phase II/III, at which time the need to predict the risk/benefit is a key consideration. Traditionally, Phase II and III trials have been fixed allocation clinical investigations, with the exception of some newer oncology trials, which have incorporated stopping rules in the event there is failure of the treatment. While the latter of the three initiatives is aimed at efficacy trials performed in smaller trial sets, the common principles lend themselves to broader applications of hypothesis-based drug development. These proposals are timely, given the advances in the field of pharmacogenetics and pharmacogenomics (Chap. 8) that permit unique approaches to individualizing drug therapy, and thus are fundamentally amenable to novel approaches to clinical design.

The seminal work of Donald Berry provides adequate thought to the fundamental basis of clinical investigations (19,25,29–31). Whereas his work bears importance to the so-called late stage clinical trials (Phase IIb/III), the philosophy of his work has important relevance to early clinical investigations, particularly Phase Ib or IIa. Berry's work on adaptive designs provides insight into the nature and design of clinical trials by creating flexibility in investigation, such that a dynamic environment is created, in which a trial can either be stopped or continued, depending on responses at the previous treatment or doses. The flexibility also is shaped by adding or rearranging treatment options, such that one can maximize the amount of useful information generated in the trial.

Needless to say, the ultimate utility and value of novel study designs is contingent upon a thorough understanding of the disease pathophysiology. Here, advances in the field of biomarkers will provide a disease fingerprint for the scope of efficacy for a new molecule by ascertaining the selection and validity of endpoints.

With the advent of complex computational tools to mathematically model the rate and magnitude of disease progression and effectively integrate PK with disease progression, it has become possible to simulate "what-if" scenarios to conveniently guide not only dose selection but also the clinical trial design. For a discussion of disease progression modeling, the reader is referred to Chapter 2. These advanced biodynamic simulation models can quantify the degree of uncertainty in a given response while discerning the probability of success in attaining a desired trial outcome.

Adaptive Dose Designs

The premise of adaptive dosing design is in minimizing failure in treatment effects at doses due to safety on the upper end and efficacy on the lower end of the underlying respective dose–response relationship, as compared to randomized study designs with fixed sample size allocated to fixed treatments or doses (32–34). The simplest form of an adaptive dose design is the classical up and down design (35,36). In this design, subjects enter into the trial sequentially and a binary response is monitored for each subject. The dose for the first subject is determined based on prior knowledge about effectiveness and toxicity. The dose for each subsequent subject is either the next dose lower in the sequence of doses being evaluated (if positive outcome for the previous subject), or the next higher dose (if negative outcome for the previous subject).

An example of a group-sequential, adaptive, placebo-controlled up and down designs was published by Hall et al. in 2005 (37), wherein the objective was to test mechanism of action for a drug for migraine headache and to select a dose range for later clinical trials. This design (Fig. 2A) was used, given a lack of information across a desired target dose range, small sample size, and to reduce exposure of patients to ineffective treatment. Adaptive dose selection was based on response rate of 60% that is observed with other drugs. If more than 60% of the treated patients in each sequential group responded favorably to the drug, a next lower dose was evaluated in the next sequential group and a next higher dose was tested if unfavorable. An adaptive stopping rule was

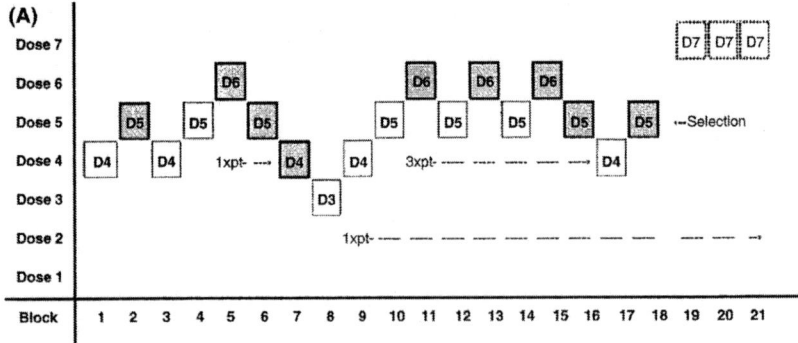

xpt denotes patients who had to be randomized before the complete information from the previous group was available at the randomization center (the next lower dose level was to be chosen in these cases)

Figure 2 (A) An example of an up and down design. (B) Similar dose–response relationship yielded by dose-adaptive (*up and down*) design as for the conventional design. *Abbreviation*: CI, confidence interval. *Source*: From Ref. 35. Courtesy of Elsevier.   (*Continued*)

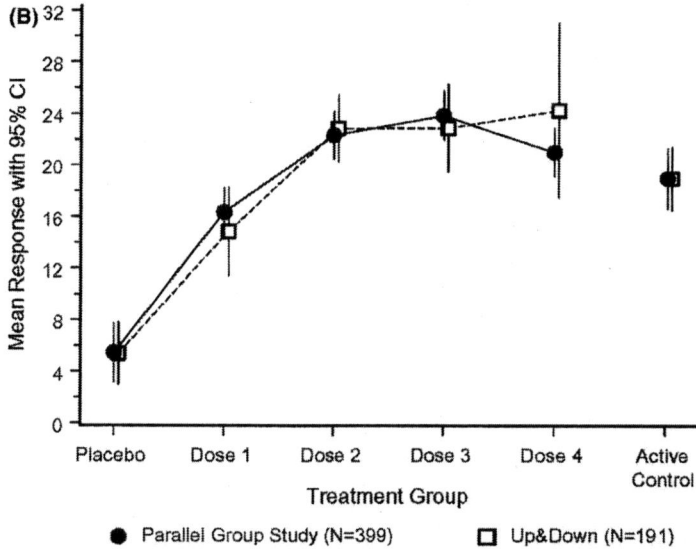

Figure 2 (*Continued*).

used to stop the trial once a selected dose level attained a statistically significant (controlling experiment-wise error) effect over the placebo.

Case Study

Data from a completed dose–response study were used to demonstrate the usefulness of the simple up and down design. This was a parallel group study comparing four doses of test drug versus placebo and an active control. In order to simulate what an adaptive dosing scheme would have yielded, the patients were sorted in ascending order of allocation number (AN) within a treatment group. Sequential groups of patients (three placebos, six test drugs, three active controls) were entered into an up and down design according to the following algorithm based on whether the group demonstrated response or non-response.

Response was defined as test drug mean minus placebo mean ≥ 15 units, and test drug mean minus active control mean > 0. The dose-adaptive algorithm was:

- First group is comprised of three placebos, six at dose 2, three active control patients.
- The mean response for each treatment within the group was computed.
- Dose for the next group was decreased by one dose level if the test drug group demonstrated "response," or increased by one dose level if the test drug group demonstrated "non-response."

- Test drug dose level for each subsequent group was determined similarly based on the previous group's response/non-response.
- Patients were chosen in sequence by increasing AN within the treatment group.
- Sampling continued until all active control patient data was used; the aim was to generate comparator datasets for placebos and active controls of similar size to those planned for the original study, and about twice those sizes for the test drug doses combined, since test drug observations will cluster around the dose, which yields the defined level of response, OR, if available doses are too low, around the maximum dose.

Rationale for these choices regarding this design is as follows:

- Patients are plentiful and enter rapidly; thus, a group sequential approach seems preferable to entering patients one at a time.
- Both active and placebo control treatments are needed; therefore, three treatments per sequence group are used for each.
- To maximize information in the test treatment group, yet to provide information on placebo and comparator, a 1:2:1 allocation ratio was used.
- A sufficient number of sequence groups is needed to allow the design to span the space of doses, so $\sim 8-20$ seems reasonable. The example trial had 47 control patients and 51 placebo patients; therefore, to match that sample size, 16 groups of 12 (3:6:3) were used. The last group will have only two comparator patients to avoid re-sampling.
- The definition of response was derived from meta-analyses of prior studies.

Note that the treatment response means yielded by the up and down designs are similar (Fig. 2B) to those yielded by the entire study, and that the up and down designs spare a substantial number (greater than half) of observations at doses not near the dose that yields the prescribed level of response according to the definition. However, the fixed sample design yielded more precise (tighter) confidence intervals (CIs) for mean response. In spite of the loss of precision with the up and down designs, the 95% CIs for the placebo and dose 1 groups do not overlap with those from doses 2 and 3. Thus, the conclusions from both designs are the same.

An extension of the up and down designs is the biased coin designs, which can adapt to any level of response. These and the up and down designs enable the assignment of doses for each subject based on the response of the previous subject or group of subjects. A hallmark of Bayesian adaptive designs is leveraging prior information on responses from all prior subjects to enable dose assignment for each new subject. The approach provides adequate flexibility in modeling safety and efficacy responses by calculating a joint posterior

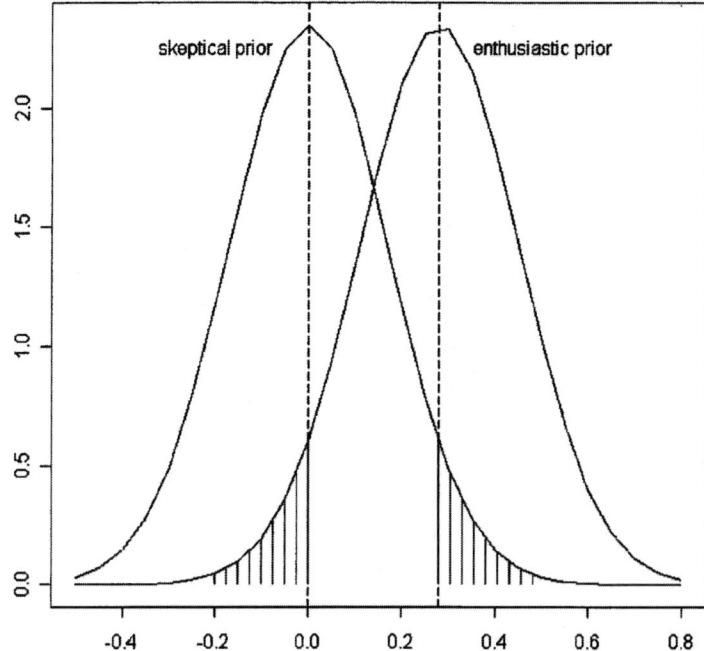

Figure 3 Skeptical and enthusiastic priors for Bayesian analysis.

distribution of a biomarker endpoint for efficacy and an endpoint for safety. Acceptable doses can then be defined as those with posterior probability that efficacy is above a given threshold value and posterior probability of toxicity being lower than some chosen value. Each successive dose is then assigned from the set of possible doses as that dose with posterior probability of response closest to the target level. Speigelhalter et al. have proposed a framework for Bayesian clinical trials in the early 1990s that leverages the range of equivalence, the community of priors, and monitoring and stopping rules. Selecting a priori is a crucial element in Bayesian analysis, for which Speigelhalter et al. proposed a variety of priors, including reference priors, clinical priors, skeptical priors, and enthusiastic priors (38). Skeptical and enthusiastic priors reflect skepticism or enthusiasm about a given treatment (Fig. 3). An example of this application to a clinical Phase II trial of gemcitabine in metastatic nasopharyngeal cancer is illustrated in Figure 4 (39–42).

Response and Covariate-Adaptive Designs

The study design methodology can be made sufficiently flexible, such that for a given set of treatment conditions (or dose groups), patients can be allocated to those treatments to which patients best respond (33). These response-adaptive

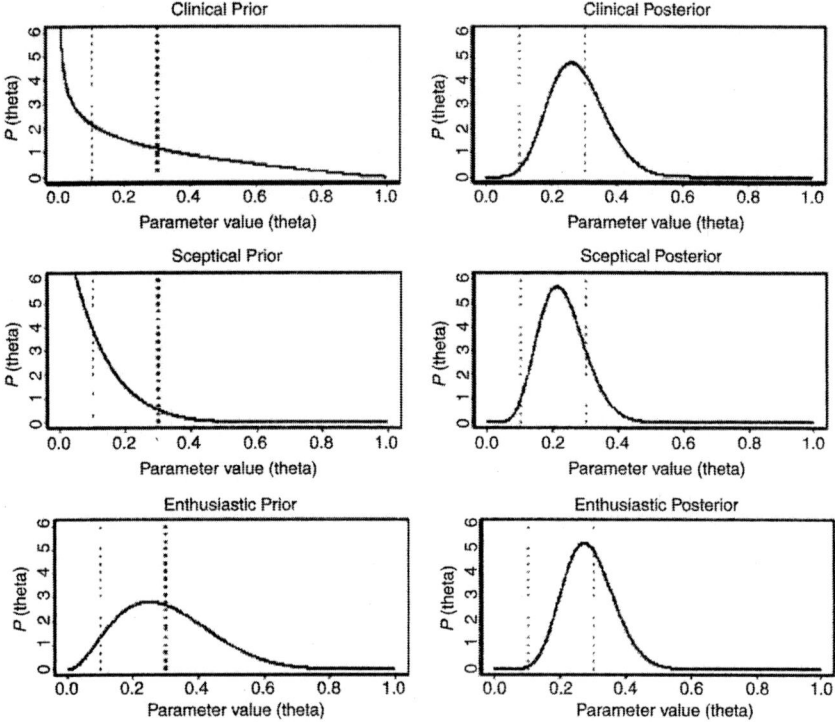

Figure 4 Prior and posterior distributions. *Source*: From Ref. 37. Courtesy of Macmillan Publishers Ltd.

designs are biased towards those treatment(s) that are successful and are predicated on prompt availability of endpoint effect. These designs are also referred to as continual reassessment methods used for dose selection. These methods are, in principle, better than the conventional "up and down" dose-finding designs in that they determine the optimal dose sooner while treating a greater proportion of patients with an optimal dose. However, they tend to focus on allocated doses very close to optimal and yield little information at other doses of the underlying dose–response curve. Since the up and down designs are less efficient than the Bayesian dose-adaptive designs, they tend to provide more information at more doses across the dose–response range of interest. Hence, if the only objective is to estimate a particular quantile of the dose–response curve, Bayesian designs would be preferred; however, if study objectives include yielding information on dose–response curve, and also estimating a particular quantile, then biased coin designs may be preferable. An area for further development is extending Bayesian dose-adaptive designs with criteria for dose selection that includes providing information across the dose–response range of interest.

There is another type of method that depends on the covariates used, and thus called covariate-adaptive method. Covariate-adaptive methods are particularly useful when there are several stratification options available for which stratification per se may not be entirely useful (43,44). Such a method corrects for any apparent imbalance with respect to measure covariates made possible via allocation to the designated treatments. This approach is more commonly applied in oncology, where patients may respond differentially to chemotherapeutic regimens administered in various stages for variable durations (45–50). If, after randomization, each patient were to receive up to certain stages of chemotherapy, the patient's disease condition would be evaluated after the completion of each stage and treatment continued if disease is stable or treatment discontinued if treatment fails. A probability model accounts for baseline covariates and the treatment/evaluation structure. Covariate-adjusted adaptive randomization is achieved based on a score that represents the patient's cumulative probabilities of treatment success or failure.

The Bayesian approach to clinical study design stems from leveraging prior information or trial evidence to inform continuance or termination (11,29,31,38,51–53). As new information becomes available, a Bayesian prior estimate of the probability for a particular event to occur is updated, using Bayes Theorem to calculate the posterior probability. This has particular benefits in drug development as they relate to dose selection and effective management of study outcomes. Bayesian applications are widespread in medical device development and clinical trials using these approaches are on the rise, particularly in oncology where therapeutic benefits to the patient are vital. This approach was successfully applied by Krams et al. for a stroke trial (25). Krams, Lees, and Berry using the ASTIN (acute stroke therapy by inhibition of neutrophils) approach exemplify the value of adaptive treatment allocation in a sequential design using an algorithm based on Bayesian principles of prior knowledge. The assignment of doses was based on prior dose–response knowledge and the requirement that data are available in real time, with the objective of identifying the minimal dose that will provide optimal efficacy. Krams et al. developed a decision algorithm for response-adaptive learning about dose–response in a single subject. Decision analysis is performed throughout the cycle but, more importantly, the algorithm calls for study termination due to futility or two types of continuance, whether clinical significance has been attained so that it is no longer necessary to continue the trial, or that the dose finding should continue. The decision to stop due to clinically significant effects is based on posterior probability that treatment effect size is larger than expected.

The value of Bayesian sequential design and continuous re-assessment of dose–response is exemplified in the ASTIN study with UK-279276 by the same authors (54,55). UK-279276 was a neutrophil inhibitory factor which showed good preclinical efficacy for stroke in the MCAO model. A novel Phase II proof-of-concept in patients with acute stroke was designed, such that adaptive allocation to one of the 15 doses ranging from 10 to 120 mg or placebo was achieved with early termination for treatment success or failure. There was no treatment effect with a posterior probability of failure at 0.89, which allowed early termination of the trial due to failure. The dose effect curve of the change in the Scandinavian Stroke Scale effect over placebo confirms a flat dose response in the population with no meaningful difference in tPA-treated and non-treated patients.

Dragalin and Fedorov (56) have developed a continual reassessment method, which incorporates criteria for determining both a quantile of the efficacy of the dose–response curve and MTD. It is based on updating the joint likelihood function after each observation and choosing the dose for the next subject, as that will maximize the joint likelihood function at the next stage.

Dose-adaptive designs are generally more difficult to implement than conventional fixed sample/fixed dose designs. Up-front statistical computations of study precision generally require extensive computer simulations to justify the proposed dose-adaptive scheme; this requires substantial computer programming effort, and also clinical and statistical expertise to interpret the simulation study results. During the trial, an on-call unblinded person(s) is needed to assess previous response data and generate the resultant dose for the next subject or group of subjects. This step could be automated, but that could require substantial computer programming resources. Finally, there is need for an unblinded pharmacist at the study site to package/select the dose for each patient. However, this could be overcome by labeling all the drug supplies via kit numbers and having the unblinded analytical persons or the computer program that computes the dose for next subject identify the associated kit number to be assigned.

Sequential Designs

Sequential designs offer the flexibility of reducing sample size by demonstrating statistically significant effect when a treatment is better relative to control (57). These designs can be sufficiently flexible to enable assigning patients until a reliable positive or negative conclusion about the treatments is possible. An adaptive group-sequential design was tested in a study for knee osteoarthritis with a stopping criterion for efficacy if the p value was <0.0041 at first interim analysis (58). The sample size was revised based on the negative outcome at first interim analysis, at which point, the second interim analysis revealed a statistically significant effect at a revised significance level.

N = 1 Trials

A relatively new concept of n-of-1 trials has emerged and it has potential value for experimental medicine designs (59–61). The design focuses on the treatment and not on the patient, and so trials are performed with one patient, and with active versus control treatments, the sequence of which is randomized.

The patient is randomly assigned to the first treatment and randomized again at the end of the treatment period. A series of *n*-of-1 trials can also be performed, such that a trend for a consistent preference to a particular treatment is discerned. This type of design is particularly useful in those disease areas in which the end-point returns to baseline post-treatment and in patients with chronic conditions. For example, Pope et al. (59) used the *n*-of-1 trial to compare the effect observed in a placebo-controlled trial with conventional NSAID treatment. Fifty-one patients with osteoarthritis were randomized either to a conventional treatment group (*n* = 25) or to an *n*-of-1 group (*n* = 24). The *n*-of-1 group received, in a random, double-blind manner, the NSAID or placebo for two weeks over a total study period of three months. All patients in the control group received NSAID as a conventional treatment. NSAID was found to be effective in 81% of the *n*-of-1 group and in 79% of the "conventional" group, whereas, none in the placebo group preferred placebo. Although the authors positioned the latter group as "*n*-of-1" group, it is really a 24-patient period-period cross-over study. Wegman et al. (60) selected 13 patients and randomized them to five sequences of two weeks of NSAID and two weeks of paracetamol. Only five patients completed the study and a modest difference was seen between the two treatment regimens. These examples highlight the complexity of these types of designs and the issue of statistical power versus lack of a treatment effect.

Clinical data with quinine sulfate indicates lack of efficacy in nocturnal cramps until Woodfield et al. (61) enrolled 13 patients for three four-week blocks (two weeks of active treatment and two weeks of placebo). Treatment allocation was random. The primary outcome was the mean difference in the self-reported number of cramps. Compliance was measured by plasma quinine concentrations. Of the 10 patients who completed the trials, three showed significant reductions in the frequency of cramps, while six had non-significant reductions, with one patient showing no effect.

MODELING AND SIMULATIONS FOR CLINICAL TRIAL DESIGNS

The past decade or two have witnessed considerable scientific and technological advances in computational modeling and simulations of complex biological systems and disease processes (62–65). It is important to note that these funda-mental technologies have been in existence and application in a number of fields, most commonly in aeronautics, business, weather forecasting, and engineering; however, their assimilation and integration in drug development is recent. The concerted efforts of regulatory authorities in model-based drug development have also fueled this integration (see Chap. 9 for discussion). Empirical PK/PD analyses are now routinely supplemented with complex mechanistic models that effectively integrate population PK with disease pathophysiology and response, thereby enabling a greater understanding of drug effects and influence of covariates in the target population, and predicting the probability of clinical success for a desired therapeutic endpoint.

The technique of population PK and PD modeling is assumption-dense and depends on a clear understanding of the known PK behavior of a drug, the disease pathophysiology and biological framework within the context of drug action, and sound computational and statistical principles. The process of model building starts from pooling all available PK information from clinical studies to develop a structural population PK model. This would encompass, for example, all Phase I/IIa studies to support dose/regimen and trial design for Phase IIb. The next step, usually, is to determine which covariates of interest (e.g., age, gender, food, formulation, disease, creatinine clearance, BMI, and so on) may influence PK parameters of interest, for example, the clearance and/or volume of distribution, such that a covariate-adjusted model is developed. Integration of the structural PK model with PD endpoint is then performed, wherein the endpoint may be a biomarker or surrogate for efficacy or for safety or a combination of both. Appropriate validation of the integrated model will inform the predictive performance of the developed model.

Clinical trial simulations (Monte-Carlo simulations) represent an area of current interest in drug development, which allow for dose optimization by posing "what-if" scenarios for clinical trial outcome likelihood, and quantifying degree of uncertainty in achieving a desired safety and/or efficacy endpoint, and thus developing a clinical utility index using a decision analytic approach (63–68). Once a population PK and/or PD model is developed, the next step in the process is to predict the response (or the desired endpoint) in a hypothetical subject or a cohort of subjects for a given clinical trial design(s), known disease pathophysiology and physiology, and known PK and PD properties of a drug. This virtual simulation of a clinical trial includes data associated with an actual trial, such as subject demographics, inclusion/exclusion criteria, accrual and allocation process, drug administration, and subject compliance/missing data. At the end of the virtual trial, valuable information is generated on the probability of success of attaining a desired therapeutic endpoint. This information can be used prospectively to design an actual trial, determine what adaptive designs best inform the effectiveness of a given drug, provide dose focus and guidance for late stage large efficacy trials, and also provide a quantitative risk/benefit assessment. As an example, the probability of attaining a specific PD target, in this case, target angiotensin-converting enzyme (ACE) inhibition at 24 hours, at several doses or dosing regimens, can be simulated in a virtual manner (69). Simulations reveal desired extent of ACE inhibition in a proportion of subjects at various doses and provide valuable guidance on selection of dosing regimens. This type of information can inform the design of a clinical trial by determining an appropriate effect size and sample size needed to meet a desired therapeutic target.

As much as the advantages appear appealing for drug development, the success of this approach is predicated on prior available data on the drug, the disease, and factors or conditions that influence a response. It also depends on the question being asked and whether there is sufficient scientific evidence to support the hypothesis. Despite these advantages and implications for drug development, there are only limited case examples in the published domain that maximize the potential which this new science has to offer. This could be due in part to the highly specialized and limited talent pool available, limited didactic training, and cost, resource, time, and infrastructure considerations. Even with these apparent drawbacks, the incorporation of these technologies into pharmaceutical research and development as they relate to clinical pharmacology will make quantitative clinical pharmacology a near-term reality.

Disease Progression Modeling

A relatively underutilized form of modeling in drug development is disease progression modeling, which models the rate of natural progression of a disease and effect of drug treatment. The seminal work of Holford et al. has illustrated the profound advantages of this approach in determining the time course of symptomatic or protective treatment effects on disease progression, particularly in the realm of neurodegenerative diseases (70–74). Holford et al. have leveraged exposure/response relationships and stochastic simulation tools to predict the long-term consequences of drug effects.

Disease progress models can either be linear or asymptotic, depending on the nature of the deterioration (Fig. 5). A given drug can influence the disease by delaying the rate or rate and extent of progression, which, upon discontinuation, may either result in the regaining of disease status or reduced slope of recovery. Key considerations for a disease progression model include slope of the model, the disease progression half-life (TP), the maximum burnt-out disease status (S_{ss}), and baseline disease state parameter, S_0. Any of these parameters may be influenced by the type of model process employed, that is, linear or asymptotic (70).

There is greater utility of disease progression modeling in late stage clinical development as long-term longitudinal assessment will aid in the time course of the progression. Epidemiological data can be leveraged for this purpose. Disease progression models can aid in the design of clinical trials using simulation approaches. One good example of the time course of disease progression was highlighted by Holford and Peace, who showed that the rate of Alzheimer disease progression was significantly influenced by treatment with tacrine by using a population PD approach. Specifically, the rate of disease progression was 6.17 ADASC units per year and the effect of tacrine was a delay in the disease progress curve by -2.99 ADASC units or 177.6 days at a dose of 80 mg/day (73).

The effective integration of PK and PD data including the disease progression component was reflected in a recent publication by Frey et al. (74), wherein a large database of type 2 diabetic patients was used to develop a PK/PD model by using a non-linear mixed-effect analysis. Responders to treatment were identified using a mixture model and reduction in fasting plasma

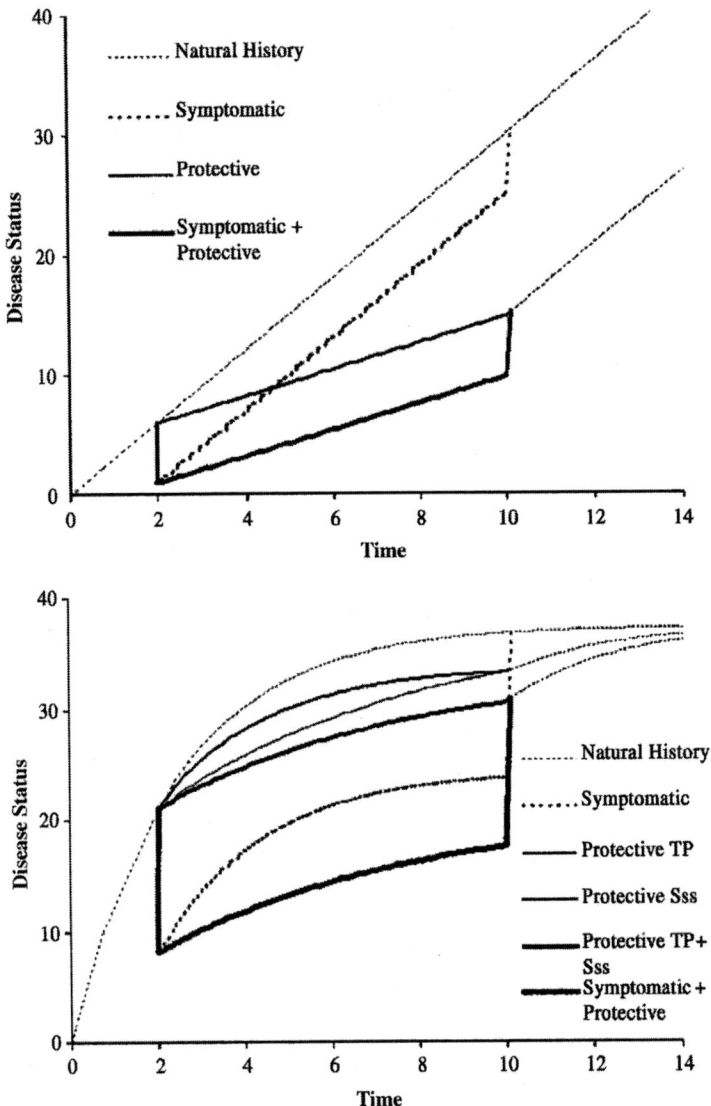

Figure 5 An illustration of linear and asymptotic disease progression model. The rectangular box represents the treatment start and stop times. *Source*: From Ref. 67. Courtesy of Annual Reviews.

glucose was linked to drug exposure by E_{max} relationship. The large database enabled a development of a linear disease-progression model to evaluate glycemic deterioration longitudinally, which revealed that the constant rate of the disease progression was 0.84 mmol/L per year. Simulations defined the time course of the antidiabetic effect of gliclazide MR and revealed the dose needed to elicit a meaningful influence on glycemic control at 12 months of treatment.

These modeling and simulation technologies can be used prospectively to design clinical trial designs more optimally than conventionally used approaches. As illustrated previously, many elements of trial design can be evaluated, and these include power, estimation, pros and cons for competing designs, sampling considerations for PKs or response measures, and also determining the impact of disease progression.

SUMMARY

The integration of new technologies in biomarkers and experimental medicine has improved our ability to understand the effect of a given drug on a given disease more informatively than has been done in the past. Dose selection and focus is critically dependent on informative clinical trial designs and our ability to define treatment effects in a clinically meaningful manner. Novel experimental clinical designs provide greater flexibility for adaptive stopping or dosing in generating meaningful information on the effectiveness of a given treatment based on prior valuable information, such that patient exposure is limited for an ineffective treatment or continued if treatment course meets a certain desired therapeutic target. Ultimately, it is hoped that these approaches will have a positive impact on drug development by selecting the winners, and reducing attrition rates of drugs from later stages of development by terminating drugs with negligible benefit, while shortening the drug development time.

REFERENCES

1. Challenge and opportunity on the critical path to new medical products. US Food and Drug Administration, 2004.
2. Tufts Center for the Study of Drug Development. Backgrounder: How New Drugs Move Through the Development and Approval Process. Boston: November 2001.
3. Posvar EL, Sedman AJ. New drugs: first time in man. J Clin Pharmacol 1989; 29(11):961–966.
4. Colburn WA. Controversy V: phase I, first time in man studies. J Clin Pharmacol 1990; 30(3):210–222.
5. Bolognese JA. Statistical issues for the initial human safety study. Proc Biopharm Am Stat Assoc 1991; 274.
6. Collins JM, Grieshaber CK, Chabner BA. Pharmacologically guided Phase I clinical trials based upon preclinical drug development. J Natl Cancer Inst 1990; 82:1321–1326.
7. Collins JM, Zaharko DS, Dedrick RL, Chabner BA. Potential roles for preclinical pharmacology in Phase I clinical trials. Cancer Treat Rep 1986; 70:73–80.
8. Simon R, Freidlin B, Rubinstein L, Arbuck SG, Collins J, Christian MC. Accelerated titration designs for Phase I clinical trials in oncology. J Natl Cancer Inst 1997; 89(15):1138–1147.

9. Newell DR. Pharmacologically based Phase I trials in cancer chemotherapy. Hematol Oncol Clin N Am 1994; 8:257–275.

10. Eisenhauer EA, O'Dwyer PJ, Christian M, Humphrey JS. Phase I clinical trial design in cancer drug development. J Clin Oncol 2000; 18:684–692.

11. Haines LM, Perevozskaya I, Rosenberger WF. Bayesian optimal designs for Phase I clinical trials. Biometrics 2003; 59(3):591–600.

12. Rosenberger WF, Haines LM. Competing designs for Phase I clinical trials: a review. Stat Med 2002; 21(18):2757–2770.

13. Peace K. Biopharmaceutical statistics for drug development. New York: Marcel Dekker, Inc, 1988.

14. Sheiner LB, Beal SL, Sambol NC. Study designs for dose-ranging. Clin Pharmacol Ther 1989; 46(1):63–77.

15. Collins JM. Functional imaging in Phase I studies: decorations or decision making? J Clin Oncol 2003; 21(15):2807.

16. Lesko LJ, Atkinson AJ. Use of biomarkers and surrogate endpoints in drug development and regulatory decision making: criteria, validation, strategies. Annu Rev Pharmacol Toxicol 2001; 41:347–366.

17. Sheiner LB, Holford NH. Determination of maximum effect. Clin Pharmacol Ther 2002; 71(4):304 (author reply 304–305).

18. Holford NH, Sheiner LB. Understanding the dose–effect relationship: clinical application of pharmacokinetic-pharmacodynamic models. Clin Pharmacokinet 1981; 6(6):429–453.

19. Berry DA. General keynote: clinical trial design. Gynecol Oncol 2003; 88:S114-S116.

20. Sheiner LB. Learning versus confirming in clinical drug development. Clin Pharmacol Ther 1997; 61(3):275–291.

21. Haringman JJ, Kraan MC, Smeets TJ, Zwinderman KH, Tak PP. Chemokine blockade and chronic inflammatory disease: proof of concept in patients with rheumatoid arthritis. Ann Rheum Dis 2003; 62(8):715–721.

22. Rustin GSJ, Galbraith SM, Anderson H, et al. Phase I clinical trial of weekly combretastatin A4 phosphate (CA4P): clinical and pharmacokinetic results. J Clin Oncol 2003; 21:2815–2822.

23. Anderson HJ, Yap JT, Miller MP, et al. Assessment of pharmacodynamic vascular response in a phase I trial of combretastatin A4 phosphate. J Clin Oncol 2003; 21:2823–2830.

24. Simon R. Optimal two-stage designs for Phase II clinical trials. Control Clin Trials 1989; 10:1–10.

25. Krams M, Lees KR, Berry DA. The past is the future: innovative designs in acute stroke therapy trials. Stroke 2005; 36(6):1341–1347.

26. Estey EH, Thall PF. New designs for Phase II clinical trials. Blood 2003; 102(2):442–448.

27. US Food and Drug Administration. Advisory Committee for Pharmaceutical Sciences, Clinical Pharmacology Subcommittee. Proposal for End-of-Phase IIA meetings. Lesko L, November 17–28, 2003.

28. European Medicines Agency. CHMP Draft guideline on clinical trials in small populations, 17 March 2005.

29. Berry DA, Mueller P, Grieve AP, Smith MK, Parke T, Krams M. Bayesian designs for dose-ranging drug trials. In: Gatsonis C, Kass RE, Carlin B, Carriquiry A, Gelman A,

Verdinelli I, West M, eds. Case Studies in Bayesian Statistics. Vol 5. New York, NY: Springer-Verlag, 2002:99–181.

30. Giles FJ, Kantarjin HM, Cortes JE, et al. Adaptive randomized study of idarubicin and cytarabine versus troxacitabine and cytarabine versus troxacitabine and idarubicin in untreated patients 50 years or older with adverse karyotype acute myeloid leukemia. J Clin Oncol 2003; 21:1722–1727.

31. Berry DA, Stangl DK. Bayesian methods in health-related research. In: Berry DA, Stangl DK, eds. Bayesian Biostatistics. New York: Marcel Dekker Inc., 1996:3–66.

32. Potter DM. Adaptive dose finding for Phase I clinical trials of drugs used for chemotherapy of cancer. Stat Med 2002; 21(13):1805–1823.

33. Rosenberger WF, Lachin JM. The use of response-adaptive designs in clinical trials. Control Clin Trials 1993; 14(6):471–484.

34. Durham SD, Flournoy N, Rosenberger WF. A random walk rule for Phase I clinical trials. Biometrics 1997; 53(2):745–760.

35. Hsi BP. The multiple sample up-and-down method in bioassay. J Am Statist Assoc 1969; 64:147–162.

36. Bolognese JA. A Monte Carlo comparison of three up-and-down designs for dose ranging. Contr Clin Trials 1983; 4:187–196.

37. Hall DB, Meier U, Diener HC. A group sequential adaptive treatment assignment design for proof of concept and dose selection in headache trials. Contemp Clin Trials 2005; 26(3):349–364.

38. Speigelhalter DJ, Freedman LS, Parmar MKB. Bayesian approaches to randomized trials (with discussion). J Roy Statist Soc Ser A 1994; 157:357–416.

39. Stallard N. Sample size determination for Phase II clinical trials based on Bayesian decision theory. Biometrics 1998; 54:279–294.

40. Tan SB, Machin D, Tai BC, Foo KF, Tan EH. A Bayesian re-assessment of two Phase II trials in gemcitabine in metastatic nasopharyngeal cancer. Brit J Cancer 2002; 86:843–850.

41. Carmichael J, Possinger K, Phillip P, et al. Advanced breast cancer: a Phase II trial with gemcitabine. J Clin Oncol 1995; 13:2731–2736.

42. Foo KF, Tan EH, Leong SS, et al. Gemcitabine in metastatic nasopharyngeal carcinoma of the undifferentiated type. Ann Oncol 2002; 13:150–156.

43. Thall PF, Wathen JK. Covariate-adjusted adaptive randomization in a sarcoma trial with multi-stage treatments. Stat Med 2005; 24(13):1947–1964.

44. Thall PF, Cook JD. Dose-finding based on efficacy-toxicity trade-offs. Biometrics 2004; 60(3):684–693.

45. Heitjan DF. Bayesian interim analysis of Phase II cancer clinical trials. Stat Med 1997; 16:1791–1802.

46. Lund B, Ryberg M, Petersen PM, Anderson H, Thatcher N, Dombernowsky P. Phase II study of gemcitabine (2′,2′-difluorodeoxycytidine) given as a twice weekly schedule to previously untreated patients with non-small cell lung cancer. Ann Oncol 1994; 5:852–853.

47. Possinger K, Kaufmann M, Coleman R, et al. Phase II study of gemcitabine as first-line chemotherapy in patients with advanced breast cancer. Anticancer Drugs 1999; 10:155–162.

48. Scheithauer W, Kornek GV, Raderer M, et al. Phase II trial of gemcitabine, epirubicin and granulocyte colony-stimulating factor in patients with advanced pancreatic adenocarcinoma. Br J Cancer 1999; 80:1797–1802.

49. Giles FJ, Kantarjian HM, Cortes JE, et al. Adaptive randomized study of idarubicin and cytarabine alone or with interleukin-11 as induction therapy in patients aged 50 or above with acute myeloid leukemia or high-risk myelodysplastic syndromes. Leuk Res 2005; 29(6):649–652.

50. Citron ML, Berry DA, Cirrincione C, et al. Randomized trial of dose-dense versus conventionally scheduled and sequential versus concurrent combination chemotherapy as postoperative adjuvant treatment of node-positive primary breast cancer: first report of Intergroup Trial C9741/Cancer and Leukemia Group B Trial 9741. J Clin Oncol 2003; 21(8):1431–1439.

51. Parmar MKB, Spiegelhalter DJ, Freedman LS, CHART Steering Committee. The CHART trials: Bayesian design and monitoring in practice. Stat Med 1994; 13:1297–1312.

52. Spiegelhalter DJ, Freedman LS, Parmar MKB. Bayesian approaches to randomised trials. J Roy Statist Soc A 1994; 157:357–387.

53. Thall PF, Simon R. Practical Bayesian guidelines for Phase IIB clinical trials. Biometrics 1994; 50:337–349.

54. Krams M, Lees KR, Hacke W, Grieve AP, Orgogozo JM, Ford GA; ASTIN Study Investigators. Acute Stroke Therapy by Inhibition of Neutrophils (ASTIN): an adaptive dose-response study of UK-279,276 in acute ischemic stroke. Stroke 2003; 34(11):2543–2548.

55. Lees KR, Diener H-C, Asplund K, Krams M, for the UK-279,276–301 Study Investigators. UK-279,276, a neutrophil inhibitory glycoprotein, in acute stroke: tolerability and pharmacokinetics. Stroke 2003; 34:1704–1709.

56. Dragalin V, Fedorov V. Adaptive model-based designs for dose-finding studies. J Stat Plan Infer 2005. In press.

57. Stallard N, Rosenberger WF. Exact group-sequential designs for clinical trials with randomized play-the-winner allocation. Stat Med 2002; 21(4):467–480.

58. Trnavský K, Fischer M, Vögtle-Junkert U, Schreyger F. Efficacy and safety of 5% ibuprofen cream treatment in knee osteoarthritis. Results of randomized, double-blind, placebo-controlled study. J Rheumatol 2004; 31:565–572.

59. Pope JE, Prashker M, Anderson J. The efficacy and cost-effectiveness of n of 1 studies with diclofenac compared to standard treatment with nonsteroidal antiinflammatory drugs in osteoarthritis. J Rheumatol 2004; 31:140–149.

60. Wegman ACM, van der Windt DAWM, de Haan M, Devillé WLJM, Fo CTCA, de Vries Th PGM. Switching from NSAIDs to paracetamol: a series of n of 1 trials for individual patients with osteoarthritis. Ann Rheum Dis 2003; 62:1156–1161.

61. Woodfield R, Goodyear-Smith F, Arroll B. N-of-1 trials of quinine efficacy in skeletal leg cramps of the leg. Br J Gen Pract 2005; 55:181–185.

62. Vozeh S, Steimer JL. Feedback control methods for drug dosage optimisation. Concepts, classification and clinical application. Clin Pharmacokinet 1985; 10(6):457–476.

63. Holford N, Kimko H, Monteleone J, Peck C. Simulation of clinical trials. Annu Rev Pharmacol Toxicol 2000; 40:209–234.

64. Hale M, Gillespie WR, Gupta SK, Tuk B, Holford NH. Clinical trial simulation—streamlining your drug development process. Appl Clin Trials 1996; 5:35–40.

65. Holford NH, Kimko HC, Monteleone JP, Peck CC. Simulation of clinical trials. Annu Rev Pharmacol Toxicol 2000; 40:209–234.

66. Chabaud S, Girard P, Nony P, Boissel JP. Clinical trial simulation using therapeutic effect modeling: application to ivabradine efficacy in patients with angina pectoris. J Pharmacokinet Pharmacodyn 2002; 29:339–363.

67. Gastonguay MR, Pentikis HS, Alexander MT, Lee L. Applying modeling and simulation to improve the design of a clinical efficacy trial. Clin Pharmacol Ther 1999; 65(2):181.

68. Wada DR, Engleman K, Ellis S, et al. Design of a Phase II efficacy trial for a GPIIB/IIIA antagonist using computer simulation. Clin Pharmacol Ther 1999; 65(2):182.

69. Pfister M, Martin NE, Haskell LP, Barrett JS. Optimizing dose selection with modeling and simulation: application to the vasopeptidase inhibitor M100240. J Clin Pharmacol 2004; 44(6):621–631.

70. Chan PL, Holford NH. Drug treatment effects on disease progression. Annu Rev Pharmacol Toxicol 2001; 41:625–659.

71. Holford NH, Peace K. The effect of tacrine and lecithin in Alzheimer's disease. A population pharmacodynamic analysis of five clinical trials. Eur J Clin Pharmacol 1994; 47:17–23.

72. Nutt JG, Holford NHG. The response to levodopa in Parkinson's disease: imposing pharmacological law and order. Ann Neurol 1996; 39:561–573.

73. Holford NH, Peace KE. Results and validation of a population pharmacodynamic model for cognitive effects in Alzheimer patients treated with tacrine. Proc Natl Acad Sci USA 1992; 89(23):11471–11475.

74. Frey N, Laveille C, Paraire M, Francillard M, Holford NH, Jochemsen R. Population PKPD modelling of the long-term hypoglycaemic effect of gliclazide given as a once-a-day modified release (MR) formulation. Br J Clin Pharmacol 2003; 55:147–157.

6

Biomarkers, Surrogate Endpoints, and Clinical Endpoints in the Development of Cardiovascular Drugs: A Regulatory Perspective[a]

Peter H. Hinderling and Patrick J. Marroum

Office of Clinical Pharmacology and Biopharmaceutics, Center for Drug Evaluation and Research, United States Food and Drug Administration, Silver Spring, Maryland, U.S.A.

The objectives of this chapter are to: (*i*) describe the current use of "proxy" endpoints during development and approval and after approval of cardiovascular and related drugs (CRD), (*ii*) identify issues that need to be addressed, and (*iii*) propose possible solutions.

THE CURRENT PARADIGM OF DRUG DEVELOPMENT

Medical interventions, whether diagnostic, prophylactic, or therapeutic, like any other intervention, are associated with benefits and risks. With drugs, biologics, and devices, the benefit, that is, efficacy, and the risk, toxicity, are determined in controlled clinical trials involving the population exhibiting the target disease. Efficacy of the intervention is usually assessed by measuring the impact on defined clinical endpoints. Only if the Food and Drug Administration (FDA) believes that there is net benefit does the Agency approve an application for marketing.

---

[a]The views expressed in this chapter do not reflect the official policy of the FDA. No official endorsement by the FDA is intended or should be inferred.

However, the development of a drug, biologic, or device usually does not start with investigations in the target population. The development of a new drug from discovery to market is a structured multi-phase process involving, usually, first in vitro and in vivo experiments in different animal species, followed by trials in human volunteers, and, finally, in patients with the target disease. Thus, during a good part of the development, a drug must be evaluated on the basis of "proxy" endpoints measured in "proxy" populations. The sequential process used in the development of a drug is dictated by concerns for the safety of the human volunteers and patients exposed to the drug. It is also mandated by alternating needs for "learning" from the information obtained and for "confirming" the results (1). The scientific, logistic, and strategic challenges to successful and efficient drug development are considerable. The development of a drug should be defined by a well-thought-out plan that specifies type and order of the individual studies required. The individual studies must be well-designed and informative. At each stage, the data obtained ought to be analyzed and the information should be used in designing future studies.

The traditional drug development paradigm assumes that information based on "proxy" effects of drugs measured in "proxy" populations is sufficiently predictive to separate effective and safe drugs from ineffective or hazardous drug candidates.

However, the large 50% attrition rate of drugs in Phase III (2) indicates that often a "learning" deficit exists as late as at the end of Phase II and, consequently, Phase III is not a pure "confirming" phase, as it ideally should be. To an important extent, the limited predictive power of the current paradigm is due to the often uncertain relationship between soft "proxy" endpoints and "hard" clinical outcomes.

DRUG RESPONSE MEASURES

There exist important distinctions between clinical endpoints, surrogate endpoints, and biomarkers. A biomarker is a characteristic that is objectively measured and evaluated as an indicator of normal biological processes, pathogenic processes, or pharmacological responses to a therapeutic intervention (3). A clinical endpoint has been defined as a direct measure of how a patient feels, functions, or survives. Among the clinical endpoints, intermediate clinical endpoints, such as, for example, symptoms and quality of life, have been differentiated from outcome endpoints, such as survival and irreversible morbidity. A surrogate endpoint, as defined in Subpart H of the Code of Federal Regulations (21 CFR 314, subpart H), is a biomarker intended to substitute for a clinical endpoint and reasonably likely to predict clinical benefit based on epidemiological, therapeutic, patho-physiologic, or other scientific evidence. Thus, a surrogate endpoint is a biomarker whose capability of forecasting a drug's effect on a clinical endpoint has been demonstrated. A drug's impact on a surrogate endpoint is not per se of any value to the patient, it is only its capability of predicting an outcome (4). Usually, establishment of a surrogate involves demonstration of the fact that the changes of the surrogate under different scenarios have the expected clinical consequences.

The expected clinical benefits have been realized with surrogate endpoints, such as viral load and CD4 count that predicted AIDS progression correctly (5); however, there are other examples where clinical benefits were not observed, such as with positive inotropic drugs in heart failure or PVC suppression with antiarrhythmic drugs (6,7). These examples indicate the criticality of choosing the right biomarker (BM), that is, a response marker that is more proximal but in the same disease pathway as the outcome, as shown in the following scheme:

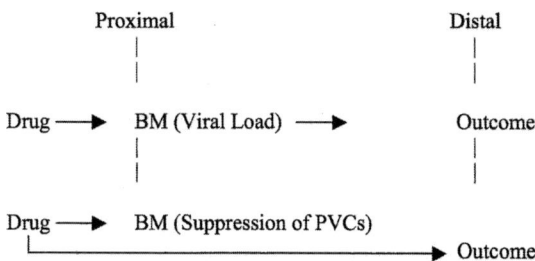

ACCEPTABLE SURROGATE ENDPOINTS AND BIOMARKERS FOR DEMONSTRATING EFFICACY OR ASSESSING THE TOXIC POTENTIAL OF DRUGS

Under Subpart H of the CFR, introduced in 1992 and signed into law in 1997, the FDA is entitled to approve drugs treating life-threatening or serious illnesses based on evidence obtained using surrogate endpoints, provided there is a commitment to study clinical benefit in Phase IV. With drugs indicated for non-life threatening diseases, demonstration of efficacy may also be based on surrogate endpoints, but confirmation of efficacy based on clinical endpoints is required prior to marketing approval. Unfortunately, the definition of a surrogate endpoint provided in Subpart H is vague. Thus, perhaps not surprisingly, to date, 13 years after introduction of Subpart H, a consensus has not been reached in the scientific community on a procedure and criteria for cross-validating biomarkers and clinical endpoints/outcomes. As a result, not many biomarkers have been elevated to surrogate endpoints since 1992. Surrogate endpoints presently accepted by the Agency to demonstrate efficacy of CRDs are listed in Table 1. It should be noted that most of these represent "grandfathered" surrogate endpoints, that is, biomarkers that have been used for a long time, but have not been correlated to outcomes with the statistical rigor proposed by some (8).

Table 1   Surrogate Endpoints for Cardiovascular and Related Drugs Acceptable to the FDA in the Past

Drug class efficacy	Indication	Surrogate endpoint	Endpoint
Antihypertensives	Hypertension	Blood pressure	Stroke
Hypotensives	Orthostatic hypotension	Blood pressure	Functioning in upright position
Lipid-lowering drugs	Hyperlipidemia	Lipid levels	Coronary artery disease
Antidiabetics	Hyperglycemia	Blood sugar, Hb1AC	Coronary artery disease
		Renal function	Renal failure
Miscellaneous	Acute renal failure	Renal function	Renal failure
Miscellaneous	Diabetic nephropathy with proteinuria	Renal function	Renal failure
Safety			
All	Safety	QTc interval	Torsades de pointes

"Proxy" endpoints to assess the safety of CRDs and other drugs are used routinely by sponsors and the Agency in assessing risk. Compared with the requirements for efficacy-related "proxy" endpoints, the expectations regarding the strength of the evidentiary linkage between safety-related surrogate and toxicity-related clinical endpoints are lower. The QTc interval is a case in point. QTc is an accepted surrogate endpoint believed to predict drug-induced pro-arrhythmic toxicity (Table 1). A draft ICH Guideline for Industry (9) recommends careful study of new drugs' effects on QTc to assess pro-arrhythmic potential. A drug is considered unequivocally safe if it causes a prolongation of the QTc interval that is below a critical cut-off, but it should be noted that drug-induced arrhythmias are quite rare and the true relationship between QTc and risk is poorly understood. Other safety-related biomarkers, such as, for example, liver function tests and forced expiratory volume, are acceptable to the Agency, but are outside of this review, which focuses on the cardiovascular system.

ACCEPTABLE BIOMARKERS WHEN EFFICACY AND SAFETY ARE ESTABLISHED BY OTHER DATA

Thus far, the discussion focused on the regulatory requirements for different drug response measures in the context of demonstrating efficacy and safety of new CRDs for which approval is sought. If efficacy of a drug is demonstrated by clinical endpoints or outcomes, biomarkers may be used to link different populations, ethnicities, formulations, routes of administrations, or regimens under certain conditions. This pertains to the pre- and the post-approval phases. In this context, not only response but also exposure biomarkers may be acceptable to the Agency. It is plausible that if the exposure measures, C_{max} and AUC, can be reproduced by a new formulation, route of administration or regimen, a drug's efficacy and safety profile in the target population does not change. Dose adjustments of drugs in adult subpopulations with renal or hepatic impairment are routinely based on a comparison of the exposure relative to subjects with normal renal or liver function (10,11). The underlying assumption is that the exposure–response relationship of a drug is not impacted by renal or hepatic disease, which may not always be true. In accordance with the pertinent FDA Guidance for Industry, linkage of co-medication and single-drug treatments may also be based on exposure, and, since these experiments are often conducted in healthy subjects, the same caveat is in order (12).

The linkage of pediatric and adult target populations has gained a lot of interest since the introduction of the Food and Drug Administration Modernization Act (FDAMA) in 1997. FDAMA addressed the need for improved information about efficacy and safety of drugs in the pediatric population by providing incentives to sponsors for conducting pediatric studies. A "decision tree" is used by the Agency to determine on a case-by-case basis type and the extent of information required for a linkage of the two populations (Fig. 1) (13). The decision tree exemplifies that the type of evidence required in the pediatric population varies, depending on the persuasiveness of existing information to link pediatric and adult patient populations. Depending on the persuasiveness of existing information, determination of exposure and/or response biomarkers, that is, surrogate endpoints or clinical endpoints/outcomes, may be required. The guiding principle is: the scarcer the pre-existing evidence, the

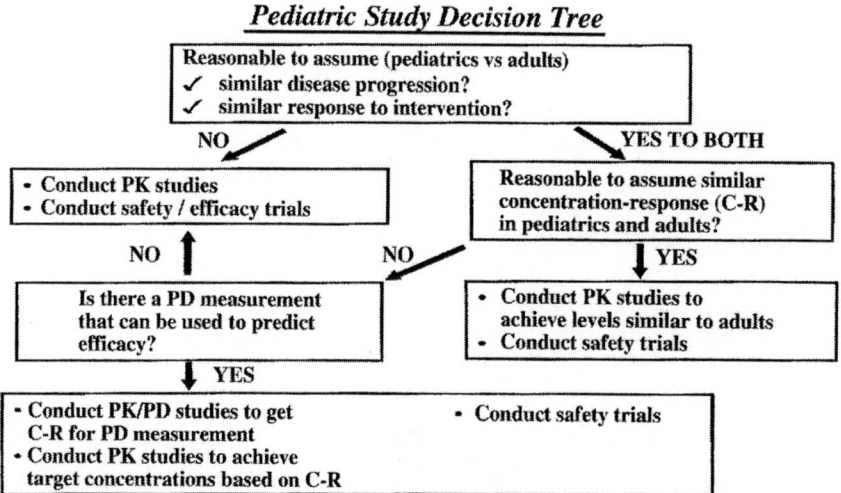

Figure 1   Pediatric decision tree. *Source*: Courtesy of the Food and Drug Administration.

Table 2 Drug Response and Exposure Biomarkers of Cardiovascular and Related Drugs that Were Acceptable in the Past for Linking of Populations, Ethnicities, Treatments, and Formulations

Drug/drug class	Response biomarker	Indication	Linkage From	Linkage To
Beta-blockers	Exercise induc. tachycardia	Hypertension	Ethnicity A	Ethnicity B
Digoxin	HR, LVET	AF, AFIB	Adults	Pediatrics
Sotalol	HR, QTc	AF, VT/VF	Adults	Pediatrics
Platelet agg. inhib.	Platelet agg. inhib.	MI, stroke	IR formul.	MR formul.
	Exposure biomarker			
All	AUC, C_{max}	All	Patients	Renal impairm. patients
All	AUC, C_{max}	All	Patients	Hepatic impairm. patients
All	AUC, C_{max}	All	Treatment	Treatment with interacting drug
All	AUC, C_{max}	All	IR formul.	New IR formul.
All	AUC, C_{max}	All	MR formul.	New MR formul.
All	AUC, C_{max}	All	Fasted	Fed

Abbreviations: HR, heart rate; LVET, left ventricular ejection time; AF, atrial flutter; AF, atrial fibrillation; VF, ventricular fibrillation; VT, ventricular tachycardia; MI, myocardial infarction; IRF, immediate release formulation; MRF, modified release formulation.

higher the requirements. The evidentiary requirements are lowest if pathophysiology and time course of the disease in pediatric and adult populations are similar. A concentration–response relationship based on biomarkers may be acceptable to connect different ethnicities, dependent on quality and strength of existing information (14,15). Examples of response and exposure biomarkers that may be acceptable to the Agency to link different ethnicities, populations, formulations, routes of administrations, and treatments are listed in Table 2. Three examples illustrating the use of biomarkers and surrogate endpoints to obtain regulatory approval can be found in the Appendix.

RELEVANCE OF AND CURRENT ISSUES WITH BIOMARKERS

Because of their promise to respond to therapeutic interventions earlier, to be easier, and more frequently measurable, less variable and more responsive than clinical endpoints to drug treatment, biomarkers and surrogate endpoints are of interest to drug developers and regulators alike. This interest is attested to by a number of excellent reviews on the use of biomarkers from academic, industrial, and regulatory viewpoints (5,16–19). Pharmaceutical companies with a portfolio of drugs competing for resources use biomarkers increasingly for internal decision-making at crucial junctures of the drug development process, that is, demonstration of proof of the principle in Phase I or IIa or in selecting doses for Phase II or III studies. Biomarkers may also be of use to define dose ranges and regimens of Phase III studies when the use of clinical endpoints in Phase II is not feasible or helpful. However, as discussed, reliance on biomarkers to predict efficacy is risky.

The number of surrogate endpoints acceptable to the Agency in the realm of CRDs and other drugs has not significantly increased since the introduction of Subpart H in 1992. Thus, an important opportunity to increase the efficiency of drug development remains largely unutilized. Identification of surrogate biomarkers should not be serendipitous and, thus, rare. Promising biomarkers in the cardiovascular arena have been identified some time ago (20). They include changes in coronary artery diameter as defined by angiography or intra-coronary ultrasound, late lumen loss, micro-albuminuria, left ventricular hypertrophy, brachial vaso-reactivity, and coronary vasomotor response to acetyl-choline and myocardial perfusion by radionuclide techniques or positron emission tomography. However, the concordance of these biomarkers with clinical endpoints has not been demonstrated to date.

Today, there is a clear need to improve the predictability and hence the efficiency of the "drug development by proxy" paradigm. The attrition rate of drugs in Phase III is too large (2) and the cost of development, particularly in the late phases of clinical development, has increased substantially (21). Unacceptable toxicity, lack of efficacy, or industrialization (the product cannot be manufactured at a commercial scale with consistently high quality) (22) are reportedly the major causes for the attrition of drugs during development. The Agency has responded with the Critical Path Initiative of 2003 (22) and is currently developing strategies to increase the efficiency of drug development without jeopardizing safety.

The predictability of the drug development by the "proxy" paradigm must be improved to increase safety and efficiency of the development of drugs. Systematic research and development of biomarkers, application of modeling and simulation techniques, and use of adaptive trials can increase the efficiency of the "learning" and "confirming" cycles and can provide tools with increased sensitivity and predictability to separate between "good" and "bad" drug candidates. Development and use of predictive biomarkers should become a routine part of the drug development process and start in the preclinical phase. The use of biomarkers should not stop after the proof of principle study in Phases I or II. Biomarkers should be assessed together with clinical endpoints or outcomes in the pivotal Phase III trials. It should be recognized that the development of predictive biomarkers is a process in its own right that will take time and cost money. The predominantly empirical approach used in the current drug development paradigm towards biomarkers must be replaced by a more mechanistic one that results in an improved understanding of the disease process, the patho-physiologic pathway, and the position of biomarkers in the chain of events causing diseases. Also, a better understanding of the sequence of events that take place before diseases become clinically manifest is necessary to increase the evidentiary level of biomarkers. To attain this more advanced stage of understanding, it may be necessary to measure panels of biomarkers and subsequently identify the relevant ones. An evaluation of drug effects on biomarkers and clinical endpoints across marketed compounds should be performed in epidemiological studies to find out about existing interrelationships. Also, the best use of already existing data should be made. Thus, there ought to be wider availability of collected data on disease factors and biomarkers. Systematic mining of data from submitted NDAs could provide important insights into process and time course of disease and impact on drug response measures. The ultimate goal of these initiatives is to create libraries of predictive biomarkers and important disease variables. As de facto repository of new and old information, the Agency should play a key role in this endeavor. In order to make explorations of such data practically feasible and efficient, a well-designed electronic database should be created with priority. A procedure should be identified that opens the database to regulatory and academic research, but protects proprietary information.

There should be incentives for organizations that are successful in demonstrating concordance of biomarkers and clinical endpoints/outcomes.

The Agency should also be the driving force in defining the process and criteria to be applied in elevating biomarkers to surrogate endpoints. Criteria may include a combination of quantitative measures of correlation with clinical endpoints and qualitative mechanistic elements in support of a common pathway. The correlation between biomarker and outcome must persist after adjusting for other potential prognostic factors. The effect of an intervention on biomarker and endpoint must be consistent and reproducibly demonstrated in clinical trials and the impact of the drug effect on the biomarker large and lasting (26). Parallel dose or exposure response curves of a biomarker and a clinical endpoint/outcome constitute a very persuasive finding.

The Agency should also take the lead in defining the standards for measuring response measures, particularly those for biomarkers. As with other exposure and response markers/endpoints, quality of measurement ought to be assured for promising biomarkers by demonstrating sensitivity, specificity, and reproducibility of the method used.

Recognition of the existence and magnitude of the outlined issues by all stakeholders, academia, pharmaceutical industry, and government, is required. A dialog among the stakeholders should be a first step towards a resolution.

APPENDIX

Example 1: Use of Biomarkers to Demonstrate Bioequivalence of a New Formulation

Biomarkers can play a vital role in the establishment of bioequivalence and interchangeability of formulations, especially if the concentration of the active moieties cannot be measured. A case in point is the novel platelet aggregation inhibitor, clopidogrel. Neither the parent compound nor the active intermediate metabolite is measurable in the biological fluids. The sponsor proposed to measure the inhibition of ADP-induced platelet aggregation by clopidogrel to assess whether two formulations containing different polymorphs of clopidogrel were bioequivalent. Because a 10% difference between test and standard formulations is considered not to be clinically relevant by the Agency (24), the sponsor was required to show that the 90% confidence intervals of the maximum achievable percent inhibition of aggregation (steady-state trough relative to baseline) was within the equivalence region of $\pm 10\%$. In addition, the 90% confidence intervals of C_{max} and AUC of the inactive metabolites of clopidogrel were to be within the 80–125% limits.

Example 2: Use of Biomarkers to Assess Drug–Drug Interactions

For an analog of clopidogrel with an established concentration–effect relationship, the drug's inhibition of platelet aggregation was used to assess the possible impact of another drug in a drug-interaction study. Absence of a drug interaction was to be declared if the difference in aggregation inhibition, as defined in Example 1, by the clopidogrel analog in the presence and absence of the second drug was <10%. Using this critical value and the known relationship between plasma concentration and inhibition of platelet aggregation, boundaries for AUC and C_{max} of the analog were calculated. It is entirely possible that the so defined upper and lower bounds for C_{max} and AUC exceed the traditional bioequivalence range of 80–125%. The criteria for the clinical significance of a drug interaction was defined in this example by a biomarker and not the target clinical endpoint (25).

Example 3: Use of a Surrogate Marker in the Approval of New Formulations

The approval of a new modified-release formulation for a drug that has an approved immediate-release formulation does not require the extensive clinical testing that is expected from new molecular entities. Moreover, provided the concentration–response relationship is well established and a surrogate endpoint is available, it is possible to get approval for modified release formulations by conducting PK/PD studies (26). A good illustration of this concept is the approval of the once-a-day formulation of metoprolol for angina (24). The basis for approval was: (*i*) the demonstration of effective beta blockade as evidenced by blunted exercise-induced tachycardia in healthy volunteers over the dose range and interval recommended for the modified release formulation (27), and (*ii*) demonstration of safety in four-week trials in patients.

ACKNOWLEDGMENTS

The authors would like to acknowledge the helpful comments of Douglas C. Throckmorton, MD, Deputy Director, CDER, FDA, and Norman Stockbridge MD, Ph.D., Director, Division of Cardio-Renal Products, CDER, FDA.

REFERENCES

1. Sheiner LB. Learning and confirming cycles in drug development. Clin Pharmacol Ther 1997; 61:275–291.
2. Lesko LJ, Woodcock J. Translation of pharmacogenetics and pharmacogenomics: a regulatory perspective. Nature Reviews 2000; 4:763–769.
3. Biomarkers Definitions Working Group. Biomarkers and surrogate endpoints: preferred definitions and conceptual framework. Clin Pharmacol Ther 2001; 69:89–95.
4. Temple R. Are surrogate markers adequate to assess cardiovascular disease drugs? J Am Med Assoc 1999; 28:790–795.
5. Colburn WA. Biomarkers in drug discovery and development: from target identification through drug marketing. J Clin Pharmacol 2003; 43:329–341.
6. Echt DS, Liebson PR, Mitchell B, CAST Investigators. Mortality and morbidity of patients receiving encainide, flecainide or placebo. The cardiac suppression trial. N Engl J Med 1991; 324:781–788.
7. The Cardiac Suppression Trial II Investigators. Effect of the antiarrhythmic agent moricizine on survival after myocardial infarction. N Engl J Med 1992; 327:227–233.
8. Prentice Rl. Surrogate endpoints in clinical trials: definition and operational criteria. Stat Med 1989; 8:431–440.
9. ICH Draft Consensus Guideline 2004. The Clinical Evaluation of QT/QTc Interval Prolongation and Pro-Arrhythmic Potential for Non-Arrhythmic Drugs, E14, released for consultation at Step 2 of the ICH process on June 10, 2004 by the ICH Steering Committee.
10. Food Drug Admin Cent Drug Eval Res, Cent Biol Eval Res 1998. Guidance for Industry. Pharmacokinetics in Patients with Impaired Renal Function—Study Design, Data Analysis, and Impact on Dosing and Labeling. http://.fda.gov/cber/guidelines.htm.
11. Food Drug Admin Cent Drug Eval Res, Cent Biol Eval Res 2003. Guidance for Industry. Pharmacokinetics in Patients with Impaired Hepatic Function: Study Design, Data Analysis, and Impact on Dosing and Labeling. http://www.fda.gov/cber/guidelines.htm.
12. Food Drug Admin Cent Drug Eval Res, Cent Biol Eval Res 1999. Guidance for Industry. In Vivo Drug Metabolism/Drug Interaction Studies—Study Design, Data Analysis, and Recommendations for Dosing and Labeling. http://www.fda.gov/cber/guidelines.htm.

13. Food Drug Admin Cent Drug Eval Res, Cent Biol Eval Res 1998. Draft Guidance for Industry. General Considerations for Pediatric Pharmacokinetic Studies for Drugs and Biologic Products. http://www.fda.gov/cber/guidelines.htm.

14. Food Drug Admin Cent Drug Eval Res, Cent Biol Eval Res 2003. Guidance for Industry. Exposure–Response Relationship—Study Design, Data Analysis, and Regulatory Application. http://www.fda.gov/cder/guidelines/htm.

15. Food Drug Admin Cent Drug Eval Res, Cent Biol Eval Res 2004. Guidance for Industry. E5-Ethnic Factors in the Acceptability of Foreign Clinical Data, Questions and Answers. http://www.fda.gov/cder/guidelines.htm.

16. Wagner JA. Overview of biomarkers and surrogate endpoints in drug development. Disease Markers 2002; 18:41–46.

17. Lesko LJ, Atkinson AJ Jr. Use of biomarkers and surrogate endpoints in drug development and regulatory decision making: criteria, validation, strategies. Annu Rev Pharmacol Toxicol 2000; 41:347–366.

18. Rolan P, Atkinson AJ Jr, Lesko LJ. Use of biomarkers from drug discovery through clinical practice: Report of the Ninth European Federation of Pharmaceutical Sciences Conference on Optimizing Drug Development. Clin Pharmacol Ther 2003; 73:284–291.

19. Jadhav PR, Mehta MU, Gobburu JVS. How biomarkers can improve clinical drug development. Am Pharmaceutical Review 2004; 7:62–64.

20. Lonn E. The use of surrogate endpoints in clinical trials: focus on clinical trials in cardiovascular disease. Pharmacoepidemiology and Drug Safety 2001; 10:497–508.

21. DiMasi JA, Hansen RW, Grabowski HG. The price of innovation: new estimates of drug development costs. J Health Economics 2003; 22:151–185.

22. Critical Path Initiative: Innovation or Stagnation. Food Drug Admin Cent Drug Eval Res, http://www.fda.gov/oc/initiatives/criticalpath/whitepaper.html.

23. Bucher HC, Guyatt GH, Cook DJ, Holbrook A, McAlister FA. User's Guide to the Medical Literature. XIX. Applying Clinical Trial Results A. How to Use an Article Measuring the Effect of an Intervention on Surrogate Endpoints. J Am Med Assoc 1999; 282:771–778.

24. Robbie G. Clinical Pharmacology and Biopharmaceutics Review. Food Drug Admin Cent Drug Eval Res, May 2000.

25. Uppoor R, Marroum PJ. Clinical Pharmacology and Biopharmaceutics Review. Food Drug Admin Cent Drug Eval Res, October 1997.

26. Guidance for providing clinical evidence of effectiveness for human drug and biological products Food Drug Admin Cent Drug Eval Res, May 1998. http://www.fda.gov/cder/guidelines.htm.

27. Lipicky RJ. Approvability Memorandum, Food Drug Admin Cent Drug Eval Res, July 1991.

7

PK and PD Variability—Estimation and Appraisal of Its Impact on Dose Optimization with an Example of Gender Differences

Vladimir Piotrovsky

Clinical Pharmacology and Experimental Medicine, Johnson & Johnson Pharmaceutical Research & Development, Beerse, Belgium

INTRODUCTION

As early as in the eighteenth century, it was mentioned that drug response (the duration of mydriasis observed following belladonna administration) depended on dose size (1), cited after Abdel-Rahman (2). Subsequent pharmacologic investigations have confirmed the presence of the dose–response relationship for the majority of drugs. However, drug response is subject to substantial inter-individual variability. Individuals receiving the same dose or dosage regimen may demonstrate responses that vary widely in onset, magnitude, and duration. Dose individualization is, therefore, the ultimate goal for those involved in drug development and evaluation: pharmaceutical industry, academia, and regulatory agencies. However, this does not seem to be an easy task, due to high between-individual variability (BIV) in pharmacokinetic (PK), pharmacodynamic (PD), physiological, and pathophysiological processes involved in clinical manifestation of drug effects. The goal of the late stage of drug development is thus the selection of a dose or doses to be recommended for therapeutic use, and the intention is to optimize the dosage and reduce the risk of under- or overdosing as much as possible.

If we construct a hypothetical distribution of optimal individual doses, loosely defined as those producing a maximal therapeutic outcome with an acceptable level of adverse effects (AE), we most probably will see a curve like that shown in Figure 1 (*continuous line*), which illustrates BIV of optimal doses in a target population. The peak corresponds to a population typical optimal dose, which is around 110 units. Individual doses vary considerably. The overall spread of individual optimal dose's distribution is determined by the variability in a number of PK, PD, and pathophysiological processes in the body, which lead to clinical outcomes. These processes depend to some extent on subject characteristics (e.g., gender, age, race, body size) that indirecty influence clinical responses and contribute to the variability in individual optimal doses. If we use the typical optimal dose to treat all patients, many of them will be under- or overdosed. To reduce the risk of inadequate dosing, we may perform a study (or studies) to identify one or more patients' characteristics that have a marked impact on the clinical outcome. Suppose it is the patients' gender. Properly designed and analyzed clinical studies can provide optimal doses separately for men and women; they will have narrower distribution (Fig. 1, *dotted lines*), and also typical optimal doses will differ (Fig. 1, *dotted vertical lines*). By administering the drug according to the patient's gender, we are able to reduce the risk of over- and underdosing.

This is a simplified scheme illustrating the dose optimization based on a single characteristic pertinent to a patient. Taking into account more than one

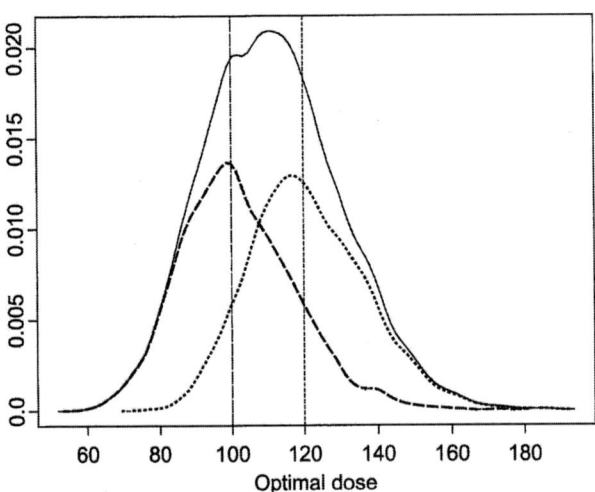

Figure 1   Hypothetical distribution of the optimal dose in the population (*see text for further explanation*).

characteristic may explain more of the variability, further reduce the spread of optimal doses, and diminish the risk of the inadequate therapy. Nevertheless, the random component of BIV of the optimal dose (i.e., not explained by patient characteristics and other known covariates) cannot be avoided, since individual PK, PD, and pathophysiological processes underlying clinical outcomes are subject to the uncontrollable variability. It is important to estimate parameters describing the random variability as it may help in individualizing the dosage regimen by means of therapeutic drug monitoring (3).

Estimation of BIV became possible with the development of the population PK and PK–PD methodology, which is now an established part of the drug development process (4). Population PK–PD modeling can provide a vital aid to the drug development process by generating reliable predictions of the individualized dose–exposure–response relationship, which is key to successful therapy (5). Understanding the variability associated with PK and PD of and clinical responses to treatment helps defining the therapeutic index, appropriate dosage regimen, and subpopulations at risk (6).

Drug development can be thought of as an information gathering process that consists of two successive "learning-confirming" cycles (5,7). The first cycle (clinical Phase I and Phase IIa) addresses the question of whether benefit over existing therapies in terms of efficacy and safety can be expected. It involves learning (Phase I) what is the largest short-term dose that may be safely administered, and then testing (Phase IIa) whether that dose induces some measurable short-term benefit in patients for whom the drug is intended to be prescribed. A positive answer at this first cycle justifies a more elaborate second cycle (traditionally, Phase IIb and Phase III). The aim of this second cycle is to first learn (Phase IIb) what is an optimal dosage regimen to achieve useful clinical outcome (i.e., an acceptable benefit–risk ratio), and then to perform one or more formal confirmatory trials (in Phase III) of that regimen versus a comparator (usually placebo). Implementation of PK–PD modeling in drug development seems to be quite natural. Among other benefits, it offers a scientifically valid tool to quantitatively evaluate the impact of patient characteristics on the response, to judge whether dose adjustment is needed, and to provide rules for that adjustment.

The aims of this chapter are:

1. To elucidate mechanisms behind BIV in PK and PD;
2. To summarize examples of clinical studies demonstrating effects of a subject characteristic, namely, gender, on PK and PD. The effect of gender is selected as it may have substantial clinical significance;
3. To give an overview of methods available in current PK, PK–PD, and PK-response modeling;
4. To outline the ways as to how dose optimization can be achieved at the stage of drug development.

MECHANISTIC CONSIDERATION

In this section, a high-level overview of a sequence of basic processes will be given, starting from drug administration and ending with a clinical effect manifestation. Figure 2 [adapted from Refs. (8) and (9)] summarizes the processes. This scheme will be used in the subsequent sections to help understanding BIV in plasma concentrations and in effects.

Physiochemical properties of a drug and biological properties of tissues at the site of drug administration determine the rate and extent to which the drug can enter the body. Biochemical properties and metabolic capacity of local

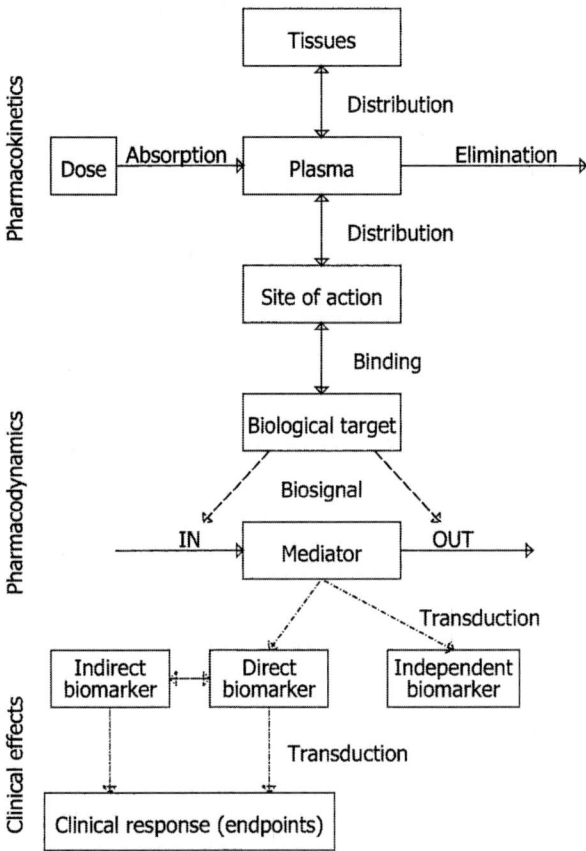

Figure 2 A simplified overview of processes involved in producing clinical effects of a drug. The *full arrows* indicate the mass transfer of the drug (unidirectional or bidirectional) and a mediator; *dashed arrows* depict single-step post-receptor events initiated by the drug–receptor interaction; *dashed-dotted arrows* show (multistage) complex processes triggered by a biosignal (transduction) leading to the observable response.

environments through which the drug traverses control the rate and degree to which it can reach the site of action. The genetic constitution of the host at the level of molecular targets influences the interaction between the drug and receptors. Finally, the pathophysiologic nature of the host may modulate post-receptor events initiated by the drug–receptor interaction, thereby influencing time course and intensity of the PD and clinical effect. Evidently, the system is extremely complicated, and rarely, if ever, can all processes involved in drug translocation, accumulation, subcellular localization, and receptor signaling be directly observed or quantitated (2). What we normally observe in clinical settings are plasma drug concentrations and some of the effects that the drug produces.

The processes under consideration can be grouped into three major categories (partly overlapping):

1. PK processes
2. PD processes
3. Processes involved in clinical effect generation

Here, only a superficial review of these basic processes will be provided. It is hardly feasible to give a more detailed general overview, since many of these processes, especially in what is related to PD and clinical effects, are drug-specific.

PK Processes

After being systemically absorbed, the drug distributes to the peripheral tissues and undergoes elimination out of the body via metabolism and/or excretion. These processes collectively define the shape of the plasma concentration–time profiles in individuals. Among other tissues, the drug may reach a site (or sites) of action (biophase), that is, the vicinity of molecular targets (usually receptors). The drug concentration at the site of action drives any further pharmacological events, including those of interest: clinical responses.

Only in rare cases can the anatomical location of the site of action be clearly identified. If receptors are distributed across the body, the site of action is the entire body. Moreover, sometimes the site of action cannot be kinetically distinguished from the plasma compartment. Simultaneous PK–PD modeling represents an adequate tool to evaluate the role of the site of action, which is represented by a hypothetical "effect" compartment (10). The equilibration rate constant between plasma and that compartment is the measure of the delay between changes in the plasma level and PD processes.

The drug metabolism leads to formation of compounds that may possess pharmacological properties either similar to those of the parent drug or different. The overall effect of the drug is, in this case, a result of combined effects of the parent compound and metabolites (the active moiety). Metabolites often have dissimilar PK properties, and their concentration–time profiles at the site of action may look completely different.

PD Processes

In order to produce any pharmacological response, the drug should bind to its biological targets. For short we will call them "receptors," keeping in mind that they are not necessarily membrane-bound proteins (classical receptors), which specifically bind drug molecules (11,12). The drug interaction with receptors produces a primary signal that triggers a series of pharmacological events, ultimately leading to clinical effects. This biosignal may consist in perturbing an intrinsic biochemical process (or processes) in the body. For example, formation or sequestration of certain mediators (hormones or proteins) may be accelerated or suppressed. Changes in the mediator level may, in their turn, initiate a cascade of events that we call "transduction," resulting in observable changes in body characteristics, or clinical effects.

Clinical effects are almost the only sources of information about the drug–receptor interaction and biosignals in man. Some new techniques such as proton emission tomography, that became recently available enable researchers to obtain direct information on the drug–receptor binding, and intensive researches are going on to find links between the receptor occupancy and clinical effects (13–15).

Clinical Effects

We will distinguish three categories of clinical drug effects that are observable due to changes in the following characteristics or variables (16,17):

1. A biomarker is a characteristic that is measured and evaluated as an indicator of normal biologic processes, pathogenic processes, or pharmacologic processes to a therapeutic intervention.
2. A surrogate endpoint is a biomarker that is intended to substitute for a clinical endpoint.
3. A clinical endpoint is a characteristic or variable that measures how a patient feels, functions, or survives.

One has to distinguish direct biomarkers that are in the causative pathway to clinical endpoints, and independent biomarkers, which are not. Indirect biomarkers depend on direct biomarkers, but still are in the causative pathway (9). There may be many combinations of these basic biomarkers and various clinical endpoints, depending on a specific drug or a therapeutic area. The linkage between a biomarker and the clinical outcome may sometimes be strongly based on the drug's mechanism of action, prior therapeutic experience, and well-understood pathophysiology. A properly selected biomarker may explain a large percentage of the ultimate clinical benefit and clinically relevant questions.

Biomarkers are either biochemical or clinical. For instance, in the case of asthma and chronic obstructive pulmonary disease, biochemical biomarkers are leukotrienes, chemokines, and cytokines; clinical biomarkers are pulmonary function tests. For diabetes mellitus, the biochemical biomarkers are glucose, fructosamine, glycosylated albumin, glycated haemoglobin, and cyto-kines; clinical biomarkers are retinal evaluations, nephropathy measures, and peripheral neuropathy assessments. In the case of hypertension, the biochemical biomarkers are angiotensin I, angiotensin II, plasma renin, aldo-sterone, and ACE activity; clinical biomarkers are blood pressure and heart rate measures.

Biomarkers do not necessarily confer any therapeutic benefit of a drug on a given disease process or provide any therapeutic benefit to a patient (18). As such, they are not considered as acceptable clinical endpoints of effectiveness or safety in assessing risk/benefit ratios prior to market authorization. On the other hand, biomarkers can usually be readily measured and are information-reachable in contrast to clinical endpoints. They often are more directly related to the time course of plasma drug or metabolite concentrations than clinical endpoints. Biomarkers can provide great value if they reflect the mechanism of action for the intervention, even if they cannot be used as surrogate endpoints. They are most suitable for PK–PD modeling and simulation, and can play a critical role in drug development.

A surrogate endpoint is a specific biomarker that may substitute for a clini-cal endpoint. Surrogates can predict the clinical effectiveness or safety when the pathophysiology of a disease and the mechanism of action of a therapy are very well understood (e.g., blood pressure, CD4 count, and viral load). Depending on the therapeutic area, the surrogate endpoint can also be a physiological response, a laboratory measurement, or a physical sign that is induced by the drug mecha-nism of action. The decision to use a biomarker as a surrogate endpoint is based on evidences demonstrating that changes in the biomarker correlate strongly with the desired clinical outcome. Typical examples of surrogate end-points are physiologic functions, such as pupil dilation in the case of narcotics, laboratory measurements, such as serum cholesterol in the case of HMG-CoA-reductase inhibitors, or biochemical markers, such as tumor marker (19). Before surrogate endpoints can be used to predict clinical outcomes, however, it is crucial to validate them in accordance with good clinical practice methods. This has to include the evidence of relevance (validity)—that is, changes in the marker are correlated to changes in disease state or clinical outcome—as well as measurement criteria (reliability) similar to those used in analytical method validation, such as repeatability, reproducibility, and sensitivity (20).

A clinical endpoint is a clinically defined, meaningful therapeutic outcome, such as survival, onset of serious morbidity, or symptomatic response that can be used as a primary response variable in a clinical trial of effectiveness or as a measure of safety. While the clinical outcome is the ultimate efficacy measure quantifying the direct benefit to a patient (e.g., cure or decreased morbidity), it is sometimes difficult to quantify and usually requires a large sample size since it is a categorical measurement (18).

BIV and Intraindividual Variability

Every process among those mentioned previously and depicted in Figure 2 may and does vary between individuals (21). Also, an intraindividual variability (e.g., with time) takes place.

PK processes vary since they depend on the individual body composition, enzymatic pattern, and the intensity of internal biochemical and physiological processes, and so on. This sort of BIV can at least partly be associated with and explained by subject-specific characteristics, among which the most important are gender, age, ethnicity, body size, and genotype. External factors like diseases, diet, physical activity, smoking, interaction with concomitant medication, and so on, may play a role as well.

The relationship of PD processes with subject characteristics is less obvious; nevertheless, one can anticipate that gender, age, race, etc. are important predictors. Since PK and PD processes determine clinical effects, the latter should depend on subject characteristics as well. However, the impact of these characteristics is often hidden by transduction processes, the nature of which is not always well-understood. Moreover, the intraindividual variability, particularly temporal variations, can mask the effects of subject characteristics.

As the goal of the late stage of drug development is the selection of an optimal dose to be recommended for therapeutic use, the developers are eager to reduce the negative impact of BIV in those processes on clinical outcomes. Taking subject characteristics into account is one of the obvious measures to diminish such an impact, and the modern PK–PD modeling and simulation technique is well suited for quantitating variabilities of various sorts and estimating optimal dosing regimens.

POPULATION MODELING: STATISTICAL FRAMEWORK

In this section, the notions of fixed and random effects will be introduced, and the statistical framework of population modeling based on mixed effects is briefly delineated. This framework is used when effects of subject characteristics on PK or PD are quantitatively evaluated.

PK data are longitudinal in nature, that is, several blood samples are collected from each individual in the course of a study. PD studies are also longitudinal, and most clinical efficacy/safety trials include multiple assessments, enabling the application of the statistical methodology, known as mixed-effects modeling (5,22,23).

Considering the PK data, theoretical plasma concentration–time profile in an ith individual, Cp_i, can be expressed as follows:

$$Cp_i = f_{pk}(\theta pk_i, D, \beta pk_i, t) \tag{1}$$

where f_{pk} denotes the functional form of the PK model (e.g., mono- or biexponential); θpk_i is a set of individual PK parameters, D is the dose (or dosing regimen in case of multiple or continuous dosing); βpk_i is a set of influential subject characteristics and other relevant covariates; and t is the time. In the cases of non-linear kinetics, f_{pk} may be not an analytical function, but a numerical solution of a system of partial differential equations defining the PK model.

Similarly, we can define a PD model for continuous direct effects (therapeutic or adverse). The drug concentration is the immediate driving force for changes of the effect variable, Eff_i, from the baseline value, $Eff_{0,i}$:

$$Eff_i = Eff_{0,i} + f_{pd}(\theta pd_i, Cp_i, \beta pd_i, t) \tag{2}$$

where f_{pd} is a PD function; θpd_i is a set of individual PD parameters; βpd_i is a set of influential patient characteristics and other relevant covariates (they may differ from those of the PK model). Note D is not in the list of PD model arguments, but Cp_i, which translates information on dosing into the PD model. This reflects the current paradigm that the dose may produce a response only through plasma concentration. On the contrary, the time is one of the arguments, since in some cases, for example, if tolerance develops, the effect may change with time even if Cp_i is constant. If the effect is indirect (the drug changes the effect variable through changes of rates of processes controlling the level of Eff_i), f_{pd} is not an analytical function anymore; it can be derived numerically by solving the system of partial differential equations representing the PD model.

Individual PK and PD parameters are distributed in a population, and the exact form of this distribution is usually unknown. In the framework of mixed-effects modeling, θpk_i and θpd_i are defined as deviations from population typical values, Θpk and Θpd:

$$\theta pk_i = \Theta pk + \eta pk_i \tag{3}$$
$$\theta pd_i = \Theta pd + \eta pd_i \tag{4}$$

where ηpk_i and ηpd_i are called random effects. The distribution of random effects ηpk_i and ηpk_i are usually assumed to be normal with zero mean and the standard deviations (SD) ω_{pk} and ω_{pd}. The additivity in Eqs. (3) and (4) allows individual parameters to take zero or negative values. Since all PK parameters and most of PD parameters must be positive, a convenient way to constrain them is as follows:

$$\theta pk_i = \Theta pk * \exp(\eta pk_i) \tag{5}$$
$$\theta pd_i = \Theta pd * \exp(\eta pd_i) \tag{6}$$

Population modeling offers a good way to summarize information; for each PK or PD model parameter, instead of long vectors of individual values, we have just two global parameters: a typical value, and SD of random effects. If model parameters are correlated in the population, a full variance–covariance matrix of random effects should be considered where diagonal elements represent BIV in parameters and off-diagonal elements correspond to covariance between parameters.

PK and PD model parameters are usually estimated by means of a maximum likelihood method [see statistical texts for technical details (24–26)], which also provides a useful tool to select the optimal model among several candidates: the likelihood ratio test, LRT. In particular, LRT is suitable for selecting influential subject covariates.

Fitting a population PK model to data gives estimates of Θpk and the corresponding random effects' SD that reflect the extent of random BIV. Influential covariates explain part of the random variability, and their effects on PK parameters are called fixed effects. The inclusion of fixed effects in the model should decrease the unexplained random BIV.

Suppose the drug clearance (CL) is different in men and women. We fit two rival models to the same data set, one without subject covariates (base model), and another one incorporating a fixed effect of gender on CL. From the point of view of implementation, this means that instead of one population typical CL, we consider two: CL in men and CL in women. Two resulting fits should differ in terms of SD representing the random part of BIV in CL: the model with gender effect on CL should have reduced SD. Besides this, the inclusion of influential covariate should significantly increase the likelihood of the data given the model.

Since population models include both fixed and random effects, they are called mixed-effects models. More detailed descriptions of mixed-effects modeling can be found in the previously cited texts.

BIV in PK and PD parameters translates into the variability in the optimal dose (dosing regimen). The following simple simulated example illustrates these relationships. Suppose the concentration–response relationship follows a sigmoidal E_{max} model (10,27,28), and the baseline effect is zero. Equation (2) becomes:

$$Eff_i = E_{max} \cdot Cp_i^h / (C_{50i}^h + Cp_i^h) \tag{7}$$

where E_{max} is a maximum response, C_{50i} is a concentration corresponding to the half-maximum response, and h is a sigmoidicity parameter. E_{max} and h have no subscript index i, thus the model assumes there is no BIV in these parameters. Only C_{50i} varies across individuals according to the statistical model represented by Eq. (6). Also, Cp_i is constant and may be regarded as that during constant rate steady-state intravenous (IV) infusion. Another assumption is that the same model works for both therapeutic and toxic effects. The only difference is in the typical C_{50} values: for the toxic effect it is higher (50 and 90 concentration units, respectively). This is thus an example of a low therapeutic window drug. E_{max} and h are 100 and 3, respectively. SD for BIV in C_{50i} was chosen to be 20%.

Two hundred pseudo-individuals were simulated, and Figure 3 (*panel A*) shows a small fraction of them, together with the typical profiles. Then the clinical benefit variable was created equal to the difference between efficacy and toxicity profiles, and plotted against Cp (*panel B*). Again, to improve the visibility, only a few profiles are plotted. The maximum clinical benefit identifies the optimal concentration, Cp_{OPTi}, which substantially varies between individuals (*panel C*). Finally, optimal concentrations were converted into optimal dosing regimens:

$$DR_i = Cp_{OPTi} \cdot CL_i \qquad (8)$$

where DR_i is the optimal dose rate in the ith individual, and CL varies between individuals according to Eq. (5). Typical CL was set to 10 and SD to 20%.

The resulting optimal dose rates are rounded for hundreds that are clinically meaningful and presented in *panel D* of Figure 3. BIV in CL and C_{50} thus translates into optimal dose rates that range between 300 and 1200 arbitrary units with the population typical value of 600. For more than 50% of the individuals, the optimal dosing range is within 500–700, and 600 can be considered as an appropriate dosing regimen for them. If the remaining individuals receive this dose rate, they may be under- or overdosed.

To illustrate the potential impact of subject characteristics, namely gender, another simulation was conducted using similar PD and PK models. The only difference was in the toxic effect model: two subpopulations were assumed to be differing in their typical values of C_{50}: 70 units for women and 100 for men. Also SD of random BIV was smaller (15% instead of 20% in the

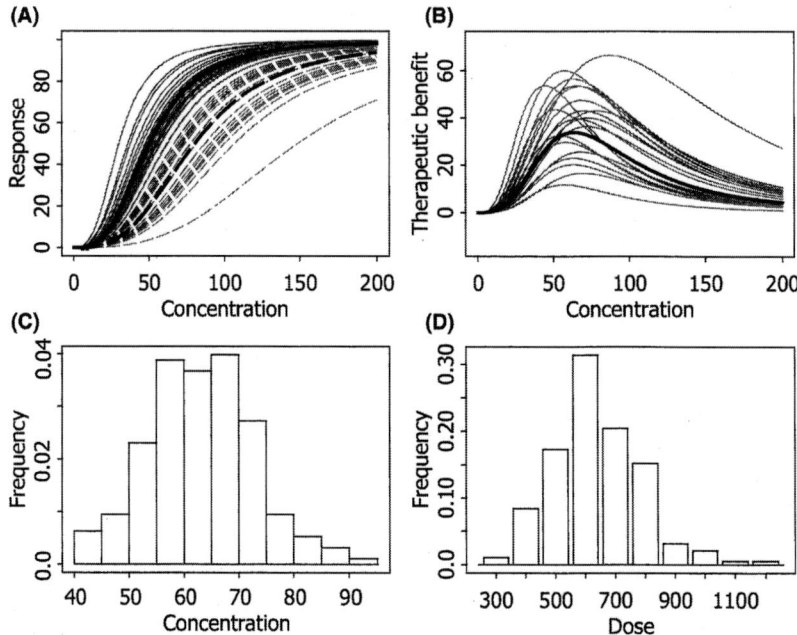

Figure 3 Simulation demonstrating how between-individual variability in PK and PD parameters is translated into optimal dose distribution (*see the text for more details*). *Abbreviations*: PK, pharmacokinetics; PD, pharmacodynamics.

previous example), mimicking a reduction of the random part of BIV after introducing the fixed effect of gender. The total number of simulated quasi-individuals was 200 (100 males and 100 females). Figure 4 shows the distribution of optimal doses separately for males and females. The overall spread is wider than that within one gender. Also, typical values differ: 600 and 700 units for females and males, respectively. The difference is not large and probably can be ignored in this case; however, there may be cases where the disparity is bigger and needs attention or even dose adjustment. In any event, this example visualizes the major point: by taking into account patient characteristics, one may reduce the random variability in optimal doses and thereby decrease the number of under- and overdosed patients.

Models represented by Equations 1 and 2 are not complete, as they represent an ideal case without measurement error. The complete PK and PD models include the residual error that usually associates with the measurement imprecision:

$$Cp_{ij} = f_{pk}(\theta pk_i, D, \beta pk_i, t_{ij}) \cdot \exp(\varepsilon pk_{ij}) \tag{9}$$

$$Eff_{ij} = Eff_{0,i} + f_{pd}(\theta pd_i, Cp_i, \beta pd_i, t_{ij}) + \varepsilon pd_{ij} \tag{10}$$

where εpk_{ij} and εpd_{ij} are random variables with zero mean and SD equal to σ_{pk} and σ_{pd}, respectively. The second subscript index j came into the picture as there are several observations in the ith individual at the times t_{ij}, and every

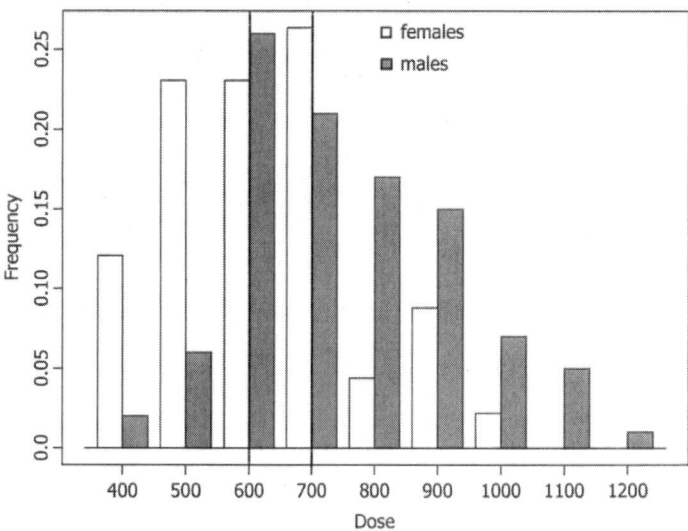

Figure 4   Distribution of simulated optimal doses in males and females (*see the text for more details*).

observation has its own error εpk_{ij} or εpd_{ij}. It is assumed, however, that SD of errors is common for all individuals. In the PK model [Eq. (9)], the residual errors follow the log-normal distribution, which is in line with the fact that concentrations are positive. On the contrary, the PD model [Eq. (10)] implies that the residual errors are normally distributed mimicking the fact that observations may be below the mean baseline level. There may be, of course, other residual model distributions, depending on the nature of the data.

One more source of random variability that is worse to mention is an intraindividual variability associated with repeated drug administrations at two or more occasions at different study days: between-occasion variability (BOV). In case of clinical studies, these are visits. To estimate BOV, more than one observation per visit (e.g., plasma samples) has to be made; otherwise, BOV becomes part of the residual variability. On the contrary, if an individual is tested only at one occasion, BOV cannot be separated from BIV.

When a PK or PK–PD model is fitted to the dense data of a single individual (many observations compared with the number of model parameters), and an appropriate statistical method is used [e.g., the extended least squares method (29)], the residual error can be estimated. If the structural model is adequate, σ_{pk} and σ_{pd} reflect the measurement imprecision. On the other hand, if one fits a model that has no random effects on parameters to data from more than one individual, estimated residual SD becomes higher than the measurement imprecision, as it now includes a contribution from BIV in model parameters. The inclusion of random effects on PK or PD parameters (ηpk_i and ηpd_i) will lead to a reduction of residual SD, and will result in precise estimates of σ_{pk} and σ_{pd} upon the condition that the number of individuals is sufficiently large. Besides this, a significant increase of the likelihood of the data given by the model will be observed. BIV in PK or PD parameters (ω_{pk} or ω_{pd}) is estimated together with the residual errors σ_{pk} and σ_{pd}. If one or more model parameters depend on subject charactistics, the model can be updated by corresponding fixed effects, and this should result in a decrease of certain elements of ω_{pk} or ω_{pd}, but not of σ_{pk} and σ_{pd}. This should be accompanied by a further significant increase of the likelihood.

This is the basic approach used in building population PK and PD models. Additional technical details on PK–PD modeling can be found elsewhere (30–33).

PK and PD modeling based on mixed-effects enables the estimation of population typical values and variabilities from sparse clinical data. Many researchers who are not familiar with this relatively new technique believe that population modeling is justified only in case of sparse data; if the data are dense, individual model fitting is the method of choice, and no population analysis is needed. This is a misunderstanding, since mixed-effects modeling in any case provides less biased estimates of typical population parameter values than straightforward averaging of individual values, and is undoubtedly preferable in estimating variance components.

Moreover, having in hand a population model with all parameters estimated, one can easily generate best individual estimates using a Bayesian forecasting technique, which is much more robust compared with individual model fitting (34,35). Particularly, Bayesian estimates are more stable with respect to outlying observations.

PK DIFFERENCES BETWEEN MALES AND FEMALES

Although the FDA mandated in 1998 that new drug applications must include data on safety and effectiveness by gender, a 2001 U.S. General Accounting Office investigation revealed that over one-third of the FDA-approved drugs in the preceding two years failed to provide such gender-specific information (36). Although women may be increasingly represented in clinical trials, failure to analyze gender-related differences in PK, side-effects, and efficacy limits the generalizability of such data to women. The importance of studying gender-based differences in PK, PD, and efficacy/safety is demonstrated by the increasing data on gender-related variation in basic processes involved in linking drug administration to clinical response. Gender-based differences in the major processes that contribute to interindividual PK variability (bioavailability, distribution, metabolism, and elimination) are theorized to stem from variations between men and women in factors such as body weight (BW), plasma volume, gastric emptying time, plasma protein levels, activity of drug-metabolizing enzymes, drug transporter function, and excretion activity (37–39). Gender-determined variations in PD have been more difficult to study due to the reasons mentioned in this section, but a number of recent studies have explored these differences (40–44).

In this section, differences in PK between the genders will be reviewed. First, the data collected in "classical" PK studies will be presented; they should, however, be regarded with caution. At the end, information obtained through thorough population PK modeling will be reviewed. Table 1 summarizes the various factors that contribute to each PK process and gender differences that have been identified or not, for these factors.

Absorption

Factors that influence drug absorption are gastric emptying time, gastric and intestinal pH, and the gastrointestinal blood flow (45), along with the effects of presystemic hepatic and gut metabolism and transport. Metabolism and active transport back into the lumen can also affect systemic bioavailability. Characteristics of stomach and proximal jejunal fluids, including pH, osmolality, electrolyte concentrations, and levels of bile acids and proteins, do not seem to vary significantly by gender (46–49), although it has been reported (50) that mean basal acid outputs were significantly higher for male patients than for female

Table 1 Gender Differences in PK Parameters

PK process	Components	Gender-based differences
Bioavailability	Gastrointestinal tract physiology	Gastric emptying time is slower in females than males, mainly secondary to the effects of estrogens
	Extrusion by drug transporters, such as intestinal Pgp	Intestinal Pgp levels do not seem to consistently vary by gender
	Gut enzymes, such as alcohol dehydrogenase and intestinal CYP3A4	Gastric levels of alcohol dehydrogenase are higher in males than females; intestinal CYP3A4 levels do not consistently vary with gender
Distribution	Body composition: body size, percent body fat, plasma volume, and organ blood flow	Women have lower body size than men; women have a higher proportion of body fat than men; plasma volume is greater in men than women, although volume varies throughout the menstrual cycle and during pregnancy; organ blood flow is greater in women than men
	Protein binding: extent of tissue and protein binding of the drug	Albumin concentrations do not seem to consistently vary with gender, but endogenous estrogens decrease the levels of AAG in the plasma, so women have lower concentrations of AAG than men. Exogenous estrogens increase levels of the serum-binding globulins (such as sex-hormone binding globulins, corticosteroid-binding globulin, and thyroxine-binding globulin)
Metabolism	Hepatic enzymes: Phase I metabolism reactions in the liver (oxidation, reduction, and hydrolysis mediated through the cytochrome P450 system)	Data on varying levels of CYP expression and activity using in vitro systems exist, but the majority of studies that examine CYP (mainly CYP3A4) substrates for differences in PK parameters in men and women are inconsistent; general trend toward higher rates of metabolism for CYP3A4 substrates in women versus men

(Continued)

Table 1   Gender Differences in PK Parameters (*Continued*)

PK process	Components	Gender-based differences
	Hepatic transporters: hepatic Pgp or MDR1	Men seem to have higher hepatic Pgp levels than women, with higher drug clearances in women versus men for drugs that are substrates of Pgp
Excretion	Renal clearance: renal excretion is dependent on filtration, secretion, and reabsorption	Renal clearance of drugs that are not actively secreted or reabsorbed is dependent on GFR, which is directly proportional to weight; gender differences for these drugs are attributable to weight differences. Drugs that are actively secreted by the kidney may show gender differences in excretion

Source: From Refs. 42, 171.
Abbreviations: PK, pharmacokinetics; AAG, α_1-acid glycoprotein.

patients with gastroesophageal reflux disease, gastric ulcer, and duodenal ulcer. Gastrointestinal motility is influenced by sex hormones (51,52), implying that gender-based disparity in motility may exist and that the transit time in women may vary throughout pregnancy and the menstrual cycle. Estrogen and its equivalents may inhibit gastric emptying (53,54), whereas the effects of progesterone depends on its concentration (55,56). Gastric transit time has been demonstrated by many researchers to be slower in females than males (57–61).

At least some drug-metabolizing enzymes located in the intestine also vary by gender (57,62,63). However, significant differences in gut expression of CYP3A isozymes in enterocytes between males and females have not been consistently observed (64,65). Potential gender differences in Pgp activity in the gut have been hypothesized based on the reports on differences in hepatic content (66). The data using oral fexofenadine as a probe of Pgp in humans, however, failed to find any gender differences in plasma concentration–time profiles of fexofenadine (67).

Several clinical PK studies reveal differences in bioavailability for certain drugs based on gender. A population PK analysis of mizolastine, an orally administered antihistamine, demonstrated a slower absorption of this drug in men versus women, contributing to variability in drug concentrations by gender (68). Two studies have demonstrated an increased absorption rate for some salicylate formulations in females compared with males (69,70), though other authors failed to show this difference (71).

In summary, while gastrointestinal motility and enzyme activity vary by gender, studies published thus far have not consistently shown a gender impact on drug bioavailability. Furthermore, studies that examine differences in bioavailability are few and confounded by variability in other PK processes, such as distribution, metabolism, and excretion. The present evidence, however, suggests that gender-based differences in bioavailability are not of great clinical significance.

Distribution

On average, women have a higher body fat percentage [the differences, however, decrease at older ages (72)], a smaller plasma volume, and a lower organ blood flow than men, with obvious implications for disparities in drug distribution. Moreover, the major protein groups responsible for binding in human plasma are influenced by sex hormone levels, so that plasma drug binding can clearly be influenced by gender. Note, however, that albumin is not greatly affected by gender (73). There were multiple reports of gender-related differences in α_1-acid glycoprotein (AAG) concentrations (74–79), gender-dependent stereospecific binding (80,81), and estrogen-mediated decreases in AAG production (82). Nevertheless, gender differences in unbound fractions of disopyramide are lacking despite differing AAG levels (75). Further investigations did not demonstrate gender-related differences in free fractions of highly bound drugs in patients or in subjects receiving hormone replacement therapy or oral contraceptive pills (83,84).

During pregnancy, the effects on binding proteins are complex. As pregnancy progresses, the concentration of albumin, along with other plasma proteins, decreases (85). The effect of pregnancy on the AAG level is under debate: two studies report an overall decrease in AAG concentration over the course of pregnancy (86,87); other studies report no change (88), or decreases in AAG levels throughout pregnancy (85). Unresolved questions still exist regarding drug protein-binding capacity in the setting of pregnancy. Some researchers report that there is a steady increase in the production of endogenous ligands, such as free fatty acids, during pregnancy that compete for drug-binding sites distinct from their own albumin (89,90). Furthermore, protein-binding capacity may be reduced secondary to intrinsic alterations in protein structure during pregnancy (91). In addition, exogenous estrogens increase levels of the serum-binding globulins, which include sex-hormone binding globulins, corticosteroid-binding globulin, and thyroxine-binding globulin (92).

The differences in body fat may account for the increased distribution volumes for lipophilic drugs, such as benzodiazepines (93,94). A larger volume of distribution of diazepam has been observed in females versus males (95,96), with differences in both body fat proportion and gender-dependent changes in protein binding being cited for this disparity. This may lead to prolonged duration of effect due to increased half-life. Increased fat stores and differences in organ blood flow in women versus men have been implicated in the faster onset of action and prolonged duration of neuromuscular blockade in females with lipophilic paralyzing agents, such as vecuronium (97–101) and rocuronium (102).

The water-soluble compound, metronidazole, demonstrates a smaller volume of distribution in women versus men, although increased CL of metronidazole in females versus males accounts for a lower AUC for this drug in females (103). A smaller volume of distribution for the water-soluble fluoroquinolones in women versus men was observed (104,105). Both the oral CL and the volume of distribution of prednisolone are significantly higher in men compared with women (106).

Metabolism

Although cardiac output and hepatic blood flow are lower in women than men, differences in hepatic enzymes seem to play the major role in determining PK variability by gender. Gender-based disparities in cytochrome P450-mediated drug metabolism have been examined through a variety of methods, including:

- The demonstration of gender differences in mRNA expression for various CYP enzymes in peripheral leukocytes (despite the uncertain clinical significance of those findings) and within hepatocytes.
- The direct examination of variability in CYP activity by gender.
- The demonstration of gender-based variability in PK parameters of drugs metabolized by these enzymes.

Multiple PK analyses reveal gender-based differences in drug concentrations that are attributed to gender disparities in hepatic enzyme expression. Gender-related PK differences in elimination are influenced by endogenous gender hormone production as well (107), and also hormonal changes associated with oral contraceptive use, pregnancy, and menopause. The following examples summarize some of the studies that attempt to demonstrate gender-based variability in drug metabolism.

Both expression and functional studies suggest that CYP1A2 activity, which is a prominent enzyme in the metabolism of antipsychotics (108), is higher in females than in males (109). Olanzapine is a CYP1A substrate (although glucuronidation also contributes to its metabolism). Combined analyses of studies of the PK of olanzapine in healthy volunteers, and also population studies of patients with schizophrenia, show CL of olanzapine (110) and clozapine (111) (another CYP1A substrate) to be higher in men compared with women.

Female livers had a significantly higher mean content of CYP3A4 (112), and in vitro liver microsome preparations exhibited a higher rate of the CYP3A4-mediated ifosfamide N-dechloroethylation reaction in females than in males (113). Erythromycin is metabolized through CYP3A-mediated N-demethylation, and an in vitro study used microsomes prepared from human livers to compare CYP3A4 activity in males versus females (114). It was 24% higher in women than men. However, Schmucker et al. (115) demonstrated that the mean amounts and activity of cytochrome P450-microsomal mono-oxygenases do not differ by gender. Another group used the liver microsome system to investigate a variety of CYP450 enzymes and found no clear gender-related differences in P450 levels or metabolizing activity, with the exception that CYP1A2 activity was higher in Caucasian women than men (109). A third study used the microsome system to evaluate the content of cytochrome P450 proteins in human livers and found that gender did not influence the expression of any of the CYP proteins (116). The results of these studies have to be interpreted with caution since the in vitro liver microsome assay lacks the systemic hormonal milieu of the male or female body, which may lead to disparate results from in vivo analyses.

Midazolam is a current "gold standard" metabolic probe for CYP3A. The majority of the studies evaluating gender differences in CYP3A4 activity using midazolam do not reveal any significant differences in IV or oral midazolam metabolism by gender (107,117–122), although others have shown greater clearance of the drug in women compared with men (123,124). Erythromycin is another well-studied substrate of CYP3A4 and its metabolism has been examined for gender differences. One group of investigators showed that erythromycin is cleared more rapidly after IV dosing in women versus men (125), which is thought to be a hepatic CYP3A4-mediated effect. In line with this, the erythromycin breath test has demonstrated greater CYP3A4 activity in women versus men (113,126).

The apparent CL of R-mephobarbital was much greater and the elimination half-life was much shorter in young men compared with women (127). This enantiomer also displayed an age-dependent gender effect and a gender-dependent age effect in its metabolism. The apparent CL of the S-enantiomer was much lower than that of the R-enantiomer in all subjects and did not differ between genders, although the elimination half-life was slightly but significantly shorter in young males. Alprazolam elimination half-life and oral CL were significantly different in men and women (128). Female subjects cleared ondansetron more slowly than males ($P < 0.05$), resulting in higher first-pass extraction and absolute bioavailability (129). Theophylline PK parameters were compared in healthy males and healthy premenopausal females who were matched for age and smoking status (130). Total body CL was significantly different in non-smoking females versus males, but did not reach statistical significance in smoking females versus males. Women (luteal phase) exhibited a greater methylprednisolone clearance (0.45 vs. 0.29 L/hr/kg) and shorter elimination half-life (1.7 vs. 2.6 hours) than men (131). Tirilazad CL was approximately 40% higher in young women than in young men (132). In patients with hypertension receiving oral nifedipine, a high-affinity CYP3A substrate, a similar higher CL in women compared with men has been reported (84). Gender differences in kinetics of triazolam, a CYP3A substrate benzodiazepine, were not apparent (133). However, among women, age had no significant effect on the drug CL in contrast to men, in which CL declined with age.

Oral CL of verapamil, another CYP3A substrate, is higher in men than women, and consequently absolute bioavailability is lower, which is thought to be a multifactorial phenomenon, including variations in hepatic metabolism. This was confirmed later using population modeling (134). Oral CL of sustained-release verapamil was 23.8 ± 2.3 mL/min per kilogram in women compared with 18.6 ± 3.4 mL/min per kilogram in men. Effects of age, formulation, and alcohol consumption were not detected. In a study by Gupta et al. (135), the mean plasma verapamil concentrations of each enantiomer after oral administration of the racemic drug were higher for women than for men at all time points, indicating lower CL.

In contrast, other studies have shown no differences in CL of oral verapamil between men and women (136,137), although these studies both had a total sample size of only 12 participants each. Overall, the weight of the evidence shows negligible gender differences in midazolam PK, whereas the data on verapamil kinetics more consistently reveals higher CL of the drug in women compared with men. A possible explanation of the inconsistency is based on the Pgp contribution (138): verapamil is a Pgp substrate. Drugs that encounter hepatocytes from the blood stream need to cross the cell membrane to become available for interaction with CYP3A4. Men may have higher hepatic Pgp levels than women (66), leading to higher intracellular drug concentrations in women with subsequent increases in CYP3A4 metabolism and CL of some drugs in this group. Midazolam is a substrate of CYP3A4, but not of Pgp, whereas verapamil is a substrate of both. The authors thus explain the gender-based disparity in verapamil versus midazolam PK as a consequence of the former drug's interaction with hepatic and/or intestinal Pgp (138). A literature survey to determine whether Pgp levels contribute to gender-related differences in the CL of CYP3A4 substrates reveals a general concordance between the predicted higher drug CL in women compared with men for drugs that are substrates of both Pgp and CYP3A4 (138). However, most of the studies that examined drugs that are substrates of CYP3A4, but not Pgp, demonstrated no significant gender-based PK differences.

Results from studies with sparteine (139) and debrisoquine (140,141), classical probes for CYP2D6-related phenotype, failed to find gender differences, whereas studies with dextromethorphan and metoprolol in subjects with the extensive metabolizer phenotype showed higher CL in men compared with women (142). Concentrations of sertraline, a CYP2D6 substrate, were reported to be higher in young men compared with young women volunteers (143), yet oral CL of desipramine has been reported to be higher in men compared with women (144). Mirtazepine is metabolized by CYP2D6 and CYP3A, and by CYP1A to a lesser extent. Higher CL and shorter elimination half-lives have been shown for mirtazepine in men compared with women (145). Gender differences in propranolol CL have been demonstrated in Caucasians (81,146) and in Chinese volunteers where propranolol CL was lower in women compared with men (147). Clomipramine and nortryptyline concentrations at steady-state have been reported to be higher in women compared with men (148,149). One study showed that tardive dyskinesia as a side-effect of various antipsychotic agents develops more frequently in female Chinese schizophrenic patients than in males secondary to the increased frequency of a defective CYP2D6 allele in Chinese women (150). However, these differences may have a PD rather than PK origin.

Data from studies of extensive CYP2C19 metabolizers who received mephenytoin (151) or (R)-mephobarbital (127) showed lower CL in women compared with men. However, for mephenytoin, the difference was attributed to oral contraceptive use (151) and a subsequent study has confirmed the inhibitory effects of oral contraceptives with respect to CYP2C19 activity (152).

There are limited data on gender differences in Phase II (conjugative) metabolism. Human liver biopsies have shown higher thiopurine methyltransferase (TPMT) levels in men compared with women (153,154), while erythrocyte TPMT activity can be higher in men (153). Glucuronidation of propranolol is faster in men compared with women (155). CL of labetalol (cleared by combined processes) was also higher in male hypertensive patients compared with female patients (156). Finally, higher doses of 6-mercaptopurine are needed for equivalent therapeutic efficacy in boys compared with girls with leukemia (157–159). However, the interpretation of this finding as a manifestation of PK differences is questionable.

Studies of glucuronosyltransferase activity using paracetamol and caffeine have demonstrated faster CL in men compared with women (139,160,161), whereas when caffeine was used as a probe of xanthine oxidase activity, it was equal or higher in women than in men (107,160). Gender differences are not universally found with substrates of the UDP glucuronosyltransferase superfamily of isozymes, such as clofibric acid or ibuprofen (162). The gender effect may vary with the isozyme, metabolic phenotype/genotype, study sample size, probe drug, or use of weight correction of parameters (107,163–165). Oral contraceptives have an important influence on the rate of glucuronidation in women and have been reported to increase it (165,166). There does appear to be differences in N-acetyltransferase activity, as assessed by isoniazid or caffeine (140,160) and in a small number of subjects studied with sulfamethazine (107).

Dihydrouracil dehydrogenase is an enzyme involved in the metabolism of an anticancer drug, fluorouracil. Its hepatic levels are higher in women than men (167). A series of clinical studies has shown that fluorouracil CL is dramatically lower in women than in men, and toxicity is higher (168,169). Fluorouracil CL in cancer patients $(L/hr/m^2)$ showed a wide dispersion for both men (median, 179; range, 29–739) and women (median, 155; range, 56–466). Values were lower significantly for women compared with men $(P = 0.0005)$ (170).

Gender differences in drug transporters are still much less studied than in metabolic enzymes. Some animal data suggest gender differences, however, evidence for humans are less apparent. Human multidrug-resistance gene (*MDR1*) product Pgp has been reported to be higher in livers of men compared with women (66), but phenotyping with fexofenadine did not demonstrate gender differences in CL. Gender-related hepatic Pgp differences may contribute to gender disparities in CL of CYP3A substrates that are also Pgp substrates (138,171).

Pgp and other drug transporters may play a significant role in determining clinical responses, where gender-related differences are potentially more pronounced (see Chap. 8).

Excretion

Renal clearance of drugs that are not actively secreted or reabsorbed is dependent on the glomerular filtration rate (GFR), which is directly proportional to weight (172), and, consequently, higher on average in men than women. Hence, gender differences in rates of renal excretion for most drugs are most likely attributable to weight differences (105,173). On the other hand, there are evidences of weight-independent gender differences in GFR (174). Many formulas used to calculate creatinine CL from serum creatinine, like the Cockcroft-Gault equation (175), include both weight and gender as predictors.

Drugs that are actively secreted by the kidney may show gender differences in excretion. One study in humans has shown increased renal CL of amantadine, an organic cation requiring secretion by the kidneys (176), in men compared with women.

Other examples of drugs in which elimination is primarily through renal excretion and is affected by gender are:

- Digoxin (177,178)
- Metildigoxin (179)
- Vancomycin (180)
- Cephalosporins (181,182)
- Fluoroquinolones (183)
- Methotrexate (184)

The renal clearance of these drugs in women was lower than in men.

All these data reinforce the need for gender-adjusted dosage selection for renally excreted drugs with low therapeutic to toxic ratios and/or adverse effects related to concentrations. Further study on gender-based differences in renal excretion in humans is required to clearly delineate the contribution of this factor.

Gender Effect on PK Through Population Modeling

The use of standard data analysis methods based on descriptive statistics and classical analysis of variance is not optimal in case of exploring effects of covariates on drugs' PK. Due to close association between gender and body size parameters, it is not a simple task to identify a primary effect unless an adequate statistical tool is carefully applied. Another serious problem of "classical" PK study designs is that they are underpowered. The number of subjects included is arbitrarily chosen, usually too low (e.g., 8 or 12 per group), and, therefore, the results of the studies are highly dependent on "outliers." Just one subject with a PK parameter (say, CL) accidentally deviating from others may lead to a wrong overall conclusion. Simulation based on a population PK model may help in properly designing studies.

Consequently, some, if not most, of the results of the studies cited previously should be considered with caution. The method of choice is population modeling that, among other advantages, enables researchers to take into account the intrinsic correlation between PK parameters (e.g., CL and volumes of distribution). Such a correlation may cause an illusive effect of a covariate on CL, whereas the true effect is on V.

Another serious problem of standard PK data analysis is that the results are inconclusive. Suppose the gender effect on CL is substantial and causes 50% difference. Should one adjust the dose for the clinical use accordingly? To answer this question, a detailed analysis, including PK, PD, and efficacy/toxicity data, is needed. The advantage of population modeling is that a PK model can be easily integrated in a PK–PD model, followed by drug efficacy/safety modeling. In this way, PK information is translated into clinical responses (endpoints) and the decision on the necessity of dose adjustment becomes well-founded.

In the remaining part of the subsection, an overview will be given of recent population analyses where gender effects on PK are addressed.

The first example presents a case where apparent gender differences in CL could be fully explained by the body size effect (185). Galantamine is a reversible, competitive inhibitor of acetylcholinesterase and an allosteric modulator of nicotinic acetylcholine receptors effective in Alzheimer's disease. It is cleared by renal and hepatic mechanisms, including metabolism by the CYP2D6 and CYP3A4 isoenzymes. Individual Bayesian estimates of CL show differences between male and female patients, though not very dramatic (Fig. 5). However, the final covariate model

$$CL(L/hr) = 9.4 - 0.033^*(AGE - 75) + 0.049^*(BW - 67) + 0.072^*CL_{CR}$$

did not include gender as a covariate. Thus, gender disparity was exclusively due to BW and CL_{CR} differences between males and females.

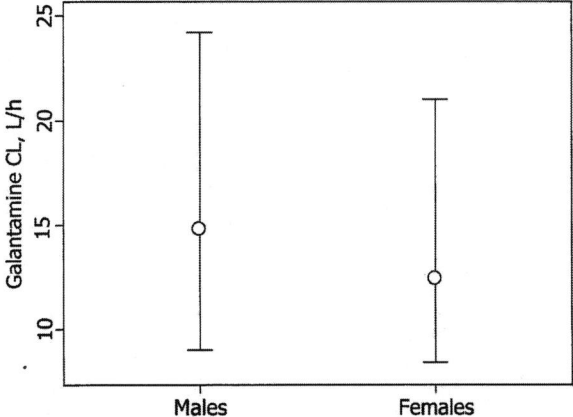

Figure 5 Galantamine oral clearance in Alzheimers' patients. The bars show 95% confidence intervals of the distributions of individual estimates.

Another example represents the case of significant and distinct BW and gender effects on steady-state volume of distribution (V_{ss}) of the anticancer drug vorozole (186). Figure 6 shows individual Bayesian estimates of V_{ss} plotted against weight (*left panel*). As can be seen, estimates for females (*F*) are systematically higher than for males (*M*). If the same values are plotted versus the difference between BW and the lean body mass (LBM) (this difference may represent the fat mass) two clouds of points overlap. This means that the gender disparity in V_{ss} could be caused by the higher fat content in females compared with males.

In a study in patients infected with HIV, population estimates of indinavir CL were 32.4 L/hr for females and 42.0 L/hr for males (187). CL was also moderately correlated with BW. Population PK of melphalan infused over a 24-hour period in patients with advanced malignancies demonstrated highly significant and pronounced gender effect on CL (188). The final model for a typical patient predicted 28% lower CL in females compared with males. Interestingly, no body size parameters, including body surface area (BSA), affected melphalan CL. Nevertheless, in the abstract, the authors reported BSA-normalized values: 14.3 ± 4.5 L/hr per m^2 in male versus 12.3 ± 4.5 L/hr per m^2 in female patients. Such a normalization of CL, which does not seem to be justified, reduced the gender differences from 28% to 14%.

In an extensive population PK analysis of darifenacin based on 18 clinical studies in healthy subjects and patients, Kerbusch et al. (189) found that CL was

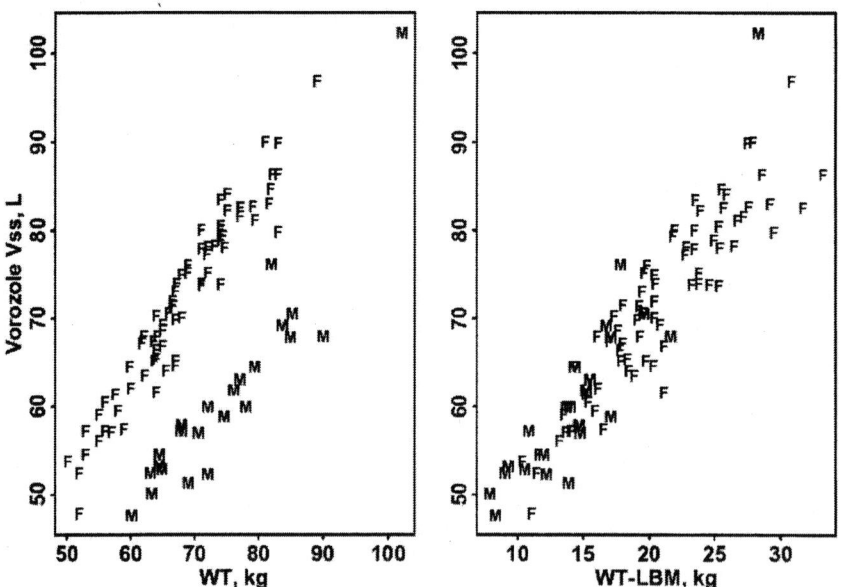

Figure 6 Individual Bayesian estimates of vorozole V_{ss} in healthy volunteers versus body weight (WT) (*left panel*); and body weight LBM difference (*right panel*).

31% lower in females compared with males. In the final model, the covariates race, gender, and circadian rhythm, accounted for approximately half of the variability in the estimated exposures to the drug. Population modeling of meloxicam concentration data collected in 586 rheumatoid arthritis patients showed slightly lower CL in females compared with males (0.347 vs. 0.377 L/hr, respectively) (190).

The metabolic pathways for capecitabine include 5′-deoxy-5-fluorocytidine (5′-DFCR) and 5′-deoxy-5-fluorouridine (5′-DFUR) formation, which are then converted to the pharmacologically active agent 5-fluorouracil (5-FU) (191). Systemic exposure to 5′-DFUR and alpha-fluoro-beta-alanine (FBAL), a catabolite of 5-FU, was predictive of dose-limiting toxicities. The authors developed a multi-response population PK model for the description of plasma concentrations of 5′-DFUR, 5-FU, and FBAL following oral administration of capecitabine. Statistically significant ($P < 0.001$) effects were found for the influence of gender, BSA, and total bilirubin on 5′-DFUR clearance and the influence of CL_{CR} on FBAL clearance. Gender differences were only marginal. PK and PD data of clinical trials of azimilide for prevention of supraventricular arrhythmia recurrence were analyzed using mixed-effects method (192). CL was found to depend on weight, gender and current tobacco use. The 17% increase for male patients compared with female patients were observed.

An anticancer drug pemetrexed disodium was administered as a 10-minute IV infusion, and concentration–time data were subject to population PK modeling (193). CL was dependent on CL_{CR}, weight, and, to a lesser extent, alanine transaminase and folate deficiency. Gender and weight were significant predictors of the central volume of distribution. 5-FU PK following IV infusion in patients with advanced colorectal cancer showed circadian changes of CL (194). The typical mean (through 24 hours) CL in the male subgroup was twice as large (125 L/hr) as that in the female subgroup (65 L/hr).

The population kinetic analyses of methotrexate in patients with rheumatoid arthritis after oral and intramuscular administration detected an effect of gender on renal clearance in the order of 17% even after adjustment for CL_{CR} and weight (184). In a study by Marino et al. (195), PK of pyridostigmine bromide was shown to be gender- and weight-dependent. The population PK study of amikacin in neonates revealed weight- and gender-dependent CL as 28% higher in girls than in boys (196). Theophylline PK was studied in the pediatric population (197), and gender, age, and weight were found to be the most important demographic fixed effects influencing CL. Race was not found to be important. Another study of theophylline in the same population (198) confirmed the significance of gender effect (CL for males was 25% higher than that for females); the race effect was found to be significant, too.

Population studies of riluzole in patients with amyotrophic lateral sclerosis showed 32% lower CL in women compared with men (199). The smoking status was the second main covariate to explain interpatient variability in CL. Only 5.7% lower valproic acid CL in females, compared with males, was identified in a population PK study (200). In another study by the same author, CL in females was about 11% less than in males (201). Other CL predictors were weight and the drug doses. A group of authors studied epirubicin PK in cancer patients (202). A significant proportion of the variability in CL could be attributed to gender, and also to age in women. For example, a 25-year-old man would display a mean CL of 95 L/hr, whereas a 70-year-old woman would exhibit a mean CL of 64 L/hr. Such differences might be important in the selection of dose regimens.

In conclusion, although gender disparity in PK has been identified for numerous drugs, differences are generally only subtle. For a few drugs, these differences have been shown to result in different PD responses, but their clinical relevance remains unproven.

GENDER DIFFERENCES IN PD AND CLINICAL ENDPOINTS

PD variability in humans is large, usually more pronounced than PK variability (203). PD disparities related to gender are one of the important causes of such variability; however, they have not been studied as extensively as PK differences. Gender effects on PD or clinical response can only be investigated by demonstrating that the same plasma concentration of a drug in the two genders does not yield the same pharmacologic outcome or, preferably, through extensive PK–PD modeling. These types of studies are still quite rare. Some studies that have examined PD differences between men and women are summarized in the following.

One study cited earlier showed that the oral clearance and the apparent volume of distribution of prednisolone were both higher in men than women, but these PK differences were not accompanied by PD differences (106). Specifically, the 50% inhibitory concentration (IC_{50}) values for effects of prednisolone on cortisol secretion and T-helper lymphocyte or neutrophil trafficking were not statistically different between men and women. However, another group found a significantly smaller IC_{50} value in women (0.1 vs. 1.7 ng/mL) for methylprednisolone suppression of cortisol secretion, indicating increased sensitivity (131). Gender-based differences in the pharmacodynamics of prednisolone may be mediated by endogenous estrogens; for instance, the IC_{50} values for effects of methylprednisolone on basophil trafficking are related to estradiol concentrations in a log-linear fashion in women, with increased sensitivity found at higher estradiol concentrations (131).

Earlier a study was cited that demonstrated increased bioavailability and decreased CL of oral verapamil in women compared with men (134,135); differences in pharmacologic effect secondary to these gender-based PK differences were observed, with greater reductions in blood pressure and heart rate observed in women compared with men taking oral verapamil (204,205). Unfortunately, PK–PD modeling was not attempted and that makes the findings of this extensive study inconclusive. Another study that examined gender-based PK differences for oral verapamil (both enantiomers) and norverapamil (both enantiomers) showed that the reduction in mean arterial blood pressure and PR-interval changes owing to the drug were closely correlated with its plasma concentration, and no impact of gender per se was observed (135).

Gender differences in response to various analgesics have been fairly well studied (206), mainly because men and women seem to respond differently to the syndrome of pain. The majority of the studies in humans point to greater analgesic effects with opioid agonists in females compared with males (207–209). Furthermore, women may have more side-effects than men when taking opioid agonists. For instance, women had a 60% higher risk of nausea and vomiting than men with the use of opiates, although efficacy did not differ between the two groups (210).

Gender differences in analgesic response have also been observed with nicotine and other cholinergic agents. Studies involving these agents have been rare in humans, but one group did investigate the analgesic effects of a nicotine patch in men and women (211). Ratings of electrocutaneous stimulation were obtained 2.5 hours after patch application from 30 male and 44 female smokers and non-smokers on either placebo or a nicotine patch (7–21 mg/24 hr transdermal). Nicotine increased the pain threshold and tolerance ratings of men, but had no effect on the pain ratings of women. Furthermore, there was no effect of smoking history on pain ratings among men, suggesting that the changes in pain perception reflect a direct inhibition of pain by nicotine, rather than relief from nicotine withdrawal symptoms.

Anesthetic agents have also been investigated for gender-based differences in PD and clinical responses (212). Females have 20–30% greater sensitivity to the muscle relaxant effects of vecuronium, pancuronium, and rocuronium (100,101) compared with men in terms of doses. The exact reason for the gender differences in the sensitivity is still unclear. The authors (107) incline to the PK differences (diverse distribution) as the likely explanation. Again, proper PK–PD modeling might help in indentifying the reason for gender diversities in this case.

PD differences seem to explain a 30–40% increase in sensitivity to the effects of propofol in males compared with females (213–216). Diazepam impairs psychomotor skills to a greater extent in women compared to men (217).

Many psychotropic medications also appear to exhibit gender-mediated differences in PD (43,218–220). Women show greater improvement in psychotic symptoms and more severe side-effects with typical antipsychotic agents than do men (221). For example, women appear to need much lower doses of fluspirilene than men to treat schizophrenia (222). The gender differences in the antipsychotic treatment responses may be at least partially a result of different hormone concentrations or hormonal effects on receptors (44,220). Detailed studies as to whether these differences are mediated through PK or PD mechanisms are needed (220,223). Females have higher risk of hyperprolactinemia as an adverse effect with risperidone and conventional antipsychotic agents (224).

A number of studies have also shown that men and women respond differently to antidepressants (220,225). For example, men may respond better to imipramine than do women (226). Another study showed that depressed men suffering from panic attacks are better treated by tricyclic antidepressant agents, whereas women with similar symptoms respond better to monoamine oxidase inhibitors (227). Women may also have a greater magnitude of response to serotonin (5-HT) agonists and serotonin reuptake inhibitors than do men (225). This difference may be related to differences in serotonin binding to serotonin uptake transporters. The binding of [3H]paroxetine to platelets, which may model serotonergic neurons was examined (228). Platelets of men had fewer binding sites and a lower affinity for paroxetine than did platelets of women. Consistent with these results, prolactin secretion in response to serotonin agonists is greater in women than in men (229).

The gender differences in nociception and response to ibuprofen were investigated in healthy subjects. Men had a significantly greater stimulus threshold, that is, lower nociception than women. However, only men exhibited a statistically significant analgesic response to ibuprofen. None of these results could be attributed to PK disparities, since the time courses of the plasma concentrations showed no gender differences (230). Women are more sensitive to insulin than men because of an enhanced insulin sensitivity in muscles (231).

There may also be gender differences in the response to cardiovascular drugs (232). Men and women may respond differently to antihypertensive agents (232,233) and antithrombotic therapy (232). A substantial amount of information was accumulated in the review by Makkar et al. on the incidence of the torsade de pointes (TdP) arrhythmias (234) associated with antiarrhythmic drugs, quinidine, procainamide, disopyramide, and amiodarone. Women made up 70% (95% confidence interval, 64% to 75%) of the 332 reported cases of cardiovascular-drug-related TdP, and a female prevalence exceeding 50% was observed in 20 (83%) of the 24 studies having at least four included cases. The authors suggest that TdP do not appear to be related to gender differences in drug levels, but rather to an intrinsic electrophysiological difference.

Tirilazad is an inhibitor of membrane lipid peroxidation. Its effectiveness for treatment of subarachnoid hemorrhage could only be shown in men, but was unproven for women (235). Gender differences in CL and the resulting differences in systemic exposure to tirilazad were discussed as a potential cause for the observed lack of efficacy in women (132). However, further investigations, including a population PK analysis of multiple studies, suggest that the effect of gender on tirilazad kinetics is only modest or even minimal during multiple-dose administration to a middle-aged population, the group most at risk for experiencing a subarachnoid hemorrhage (236). Thus, other factors, including PD differences, may have substantially contributed to the dramatic gender disparity in response to tirilazad.

Most of the studies reviewed before did not include any PK–PD modeling, and, in many cases, it is difficult to judge as to whether the observed differences in PD or efficacy/toxicity responses are "true," or caused by underlying PK differences, or both. Moreover, without detailed PD modeling, one cannot answer the question on the intrinsic target of gender effect: is it the drug potency that differs in men and women or the sensitivity? Another possibility is the difference in the drug transport to the site of action.

In a study by Parker and Hunter (237) of the neuromuscular blocking agent atracurium a detailed PK–PD modeling was performed. The model fitted to individual data included an "effect" compartment representing a delay between changes in the drug plasma concentration and PD effect. The response was described by a sigmoidal E_{max} model. The only gender effect identified was that on the transport rate constant to the "effect" compartment. No difference in the concentration corresponding to the half-maximum response between males and females was found (237).

The most common adverse event of all anticholinergic compounds used in patients with Alzheimer's disease is nausea. In population PK and PK–PD modeling of galantamine plasma concentrations, and adverse events data collected in several Phase III studies (185), a logistic regression model was fitted to nausea incidence with the peak plasma concentration (C_{max}) as predictor. C_{max} corresponding to 50% probability of nausea (CE_{50}) was estimated, and it turned out to be around 95 ng/mL in women, which was much lower than in men (>200 ng/mL, Fig. 7). This indicates that women are more susceptible to nausea, which is in concert with the findings by Cepeda et al. (210). In contrast, PK differences were small (185).

An interesting example of PK–PD modeling of the methylprednisolone suppressive effects on cortisol secretion and basophil and helper T-lymphocyte

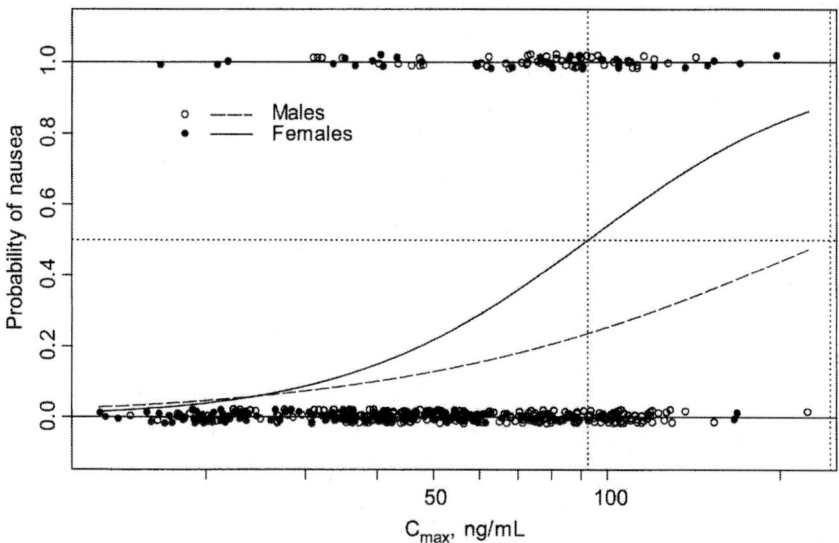

Figure 7 Probability of nausea in Alzheimer's patients as a function of the peak plasma concentration of galantamine (men and women shown separately). The *vertical dotted lines* show estimated CE_{50} values.

trafficking was published by Lew et al. (131). A dramatically smaller 50% inhibitory concentration (IC_{50}) value (0.1 vs. 1.7 ng/mL) was seen in women for suppression of cortisol secretion, indicating increased sensitivity. However, the areas under the effect-time curves were similar for both groups. The IC_{50} values for effects of methylprednisolone on basophil trafficking related to estradiol concentrations in a log-linear fashion in women, with increased sensitivity found at higher estradiol concentrations. Men displayed a greater 24-hour net suppression in blood basophil numbers, but no difference was observed in net cortisol and helper T-lymphocyte suppression between the genders. Thus, although women are more sensitive to methylprednisolone as measured by cortisol suppression, they eliminate the drug more quickly, generally producing a similar net response (131).

Plasma concentration and neuromuscular block data from 241 patients in eight prospectively designed Phase I–III trials were pooled and analyzed using population PK–PD modeling (238). The PD variable was percent block relative to a baseline control. The model included the "effect" compartment, and its PD part was the E_{max} model. Maximum effect parameter was fixed at 0% since at the concentration peak a complete block was observed. The only statistically significant gender effect was that on the "effect" compartment equilibration rate constant, which was 14% higher in females than in males.

In the article by Mougenot et al. (188) that was cited in the previous section, population modeling was applied to evaluate covariate effects on PK parameters of melphalan infused over a 24-hour period in patients with advanced malignancies. Highly significant and pronounced gender effect on CL was identified. In an attempt to establish an exposure–response relationship, the authors plotted the percentage decreases in red blood cells count, white blood cells count, and platelet count at the nadir during each chemotherapy course against AUC. As one could expect from such a simplistic analysis, no relationship was found. It seems the adequate mechanistic-based PK–PD analysis would use indirect-response models (239), in particular, models that take into account the cell turnover and cell life-span (240–244). The PK–PD modeling approach would enable researchers to explore the impact of patient covariates like gender on essential processes involved, including the drug effect.

The study by Gieschke et al. (245) of capecitabine PK included an attempt to find a relationship between the exposure (AUC and C_{max} of active metabolites) and the safety and efficacy parameters. Of 42 concentration–effect relationships investigated, only five achieved statistical significance. Thus, a positive association between the AUC of FBAL and grade 3–4 diarrhea ($P = 0.035$), a positive association between the AUC of 5-FU and grade 3–4 hyperbilirubinemia ($P = 0.025$), a negative association between the C_{max} of FBAL and grade 3–4 hyperbilirubinemia ($P = 0.014$), a negative association between the AUC of 5-FU (in plasma) and time to disease progression (hazard ratio = 1.626, $P = 0.0056$), and a positive association between the C_{max} of 5-DFUR and survival (hazard ratio = 0.938, $P = 0.0048$), were obtained. In general, there was a broad overlap in systemic exposures to capecitabine metabolites for all patients regardless of safety and efficacy outcomes. The overlap translates into absent or weak relationships between systemic exposure and safety/efficacy parameters. The basis of these findings may be that concentrations of 5-FU, 5-DFUR, and FBAL in plasma do not necessarily reflect concentrations in healthy tissues and tumors after capecitabine therapy. One should mention that the univariate logistic regression analysis and Cox proportional hazard regression using six predictors (AUC and C_{max} of each active metabolite) chosen by the authors (245) are inefficient due to the inherent multiple comparison. The reported *P*-values should therefore be regarded with caution.

In view of the potentially hazardous QTc prolongation caused by drugs, substantial efforts have been made to elucidate factors affecting processes involved in prolongation of QT intervals (246–250).

In a study of 91 healthy subjects, an effect of physical exercises on the QT interval was assessed (251). No drug was administered, and the aim of the work was, in fact, to explore the natural behavior of the QT interval without pharmacological intervention. QT was analyzed using the heart rate and subject gender and age as covariates. The gender differences were evident at the heart rate below 110 min. Unfortunately, only standard statistical methods were applied for the data analyses with no mixed-effects modeling, and the findings of this interesting study cannot be generalized.

An antiarrhythmic drug *d*-sotalol is known to prolong the QTc interval, and PK–PD modeling of data collected in 24 healthy subjects after i.v. infusion of the drug at three dose levels showed significant gender differences in baseline QTc: 0.40 versus 0.38 seconds in females and males, respectively (252). The drug effect was descibed by the sigmoidal E_{max} model, and no gender differences in E_{max}, EC_{50}, and Hill parameters were found. The authors used a standard two-step (STS) approach, namely, individual model-fitting followed by a statistical analysis, a procedure known to be less efficient compared with mixed-effects modeling. Particularly, STS usually overestimates BIV (253), which makes identification of covariate effects difficult. For example, the key parameter EC_{50} varied from 1.1 to 906 ng/mL (252).

The same STS method was applied in the study of 68 healthy subjects receiving an antiarrhythmics azimilide dihydrochloride through the i.v. route (254). The authors did not examine covariate effects, particularly the impact of gender was not studied since there were only seven women in the study group. A circadian rhythm in QTc was observed and estimated: peak circadian variation was equivalent to 14% E_{max} (254). A population analysis of azimilide PK–PD data was that of Phillips et al. (192). The circadian rhythm was not taken into account in this analysis, and also the between-day variability in baseline QTc. The linear, E_{max} and sigmoid E_{max} models were applied, and the second one was found to be optimal. The baseline QTc interval was dependent on gender: 392 and 400 ms in males and females, respectively. This is in fairly good agreement with the findings by Salazar et al. (252).

Shi et al. (255) carried out population PK and PD modeling of oral sotalol data in pediatric patients with supraventricular or ventricular tachyarrhythmia described in Chap. 12. A simple linear PD model relating QTc interval and plasma sotalol concentration was found to satisfactorily fit the data that were relatively sparse. The gender effect on the baseline QTc was significant, but weak, and was not included in the final model. The slope parameter did not depend on gender. Note that the study protocol did not foresee a placebo period, and circadian variation of baseline QTc was not considered in the analysis. Also, the between-day variability in the baseline was not incorporated as a separate variance term in the model.

All these PK–PD analyses of QT prolongation data had the common shortcoming: the QTc intervals were calculated from QT and RR intervals using the Bazett equation ($QTc = QT/RR^{0.5}$), known to be suboptimal (256, 257). The actual correction exponent is on average lower than 0.5 and substantially varies between individuals (258). The best way to model the QT prolongation caused by drugs is to incorporate the correction equation in the model in the form $QTc = QT/RR^W$ where the exponent W is a PD model parameter to be estimated together with other parameters. This approach was applied in an analysis of the results of the cardiovascular safety studies of two experimental compounds (A and B) discontinued from development (259). The PD model fitted to QT records was as follows:

$$QT = QTc_{bsl} \cdot (RR^W + CRC + E_{max} \cdot C^H/[C_{50}^H + C^H]) \tag{11}$$

where QTc_{bsl} is a corrected baseline value, and CRC represents a circadian rhythm submodel (the sum of two cosine functions). The E_{max} sigmoidal model was used as a drug effect submodel. The E_{max} parameter was expressed in terms of a fractional change from the baseline. All model parameters were subject to BIV, except the Hill parameter. For each individual, QTc_{bsl} varied between occasions (study days). Drug concentration C was predicted for each individual on the basis of a population PK model that was developed beforehand (Bayesian predictions). Placebo data and active treatment data (all doses) were combined in a single data set, and the population model was fitted to this set in one run (separately for each compound).

Table 2 summarizes the typical value estimates of the most important PD parameters. Baseline QTc intervals were higher in females than males in both studies. E_{max} expressed in terms of a fractional change from QTc_{bsl} did not show gender differences, but, as a result of differences in baseline values, the maximum QTc intervals ($QTc_{bsl} \cdot E_{max}$) were longer for females than males. The two compounds differed considerably with respect to their activity (E_{max}) and potency (C_{50}), and both showed a higher potency in females than in males. Figure 8 shows examples of the QTc data of compound A in two

Table 2 Estimates of the Typical Population Values of Parameters of the QT Prolongation Model

	Compound A	Compound B
QTc$_{bsl}$, ms		
Females	392	391
Males	380	382
E_{max} (fractional change from baseline)	0.076	0.006
Absolute QTc maximum, ms		
Females	422	393
Males	409	384
C_{50}, ng/mL		
Females	118	63
Males	154	84

individuals: a man and woman, expressed as changes from baseline, and the corresponding model fits (the drug effect part only). E_{max} estimates of the individuals slightly differ due to random BIV, while C_{50} for the man is higher than for the woman as the consequence of the gender effect.

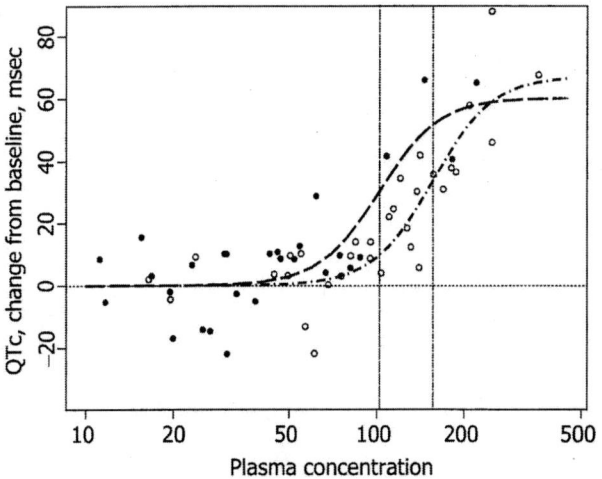

Figure 8 Examples of corrected QT intervals (changes from baseline) versus plasma concentration (the logarithmic scale) in a man and a woman, illustrating gender differences in compound A potency. *Closed circles* and *dashed lines* correspond to the woman; *open circles* and *dashed-dotted lines* to the man. *Vertical thin lines* show individual C_{50} values. *Bold lines* represent individual (Bayesian) fitted curves.

PITFALLS IN ESTIMATING AND INTERPRETING
EFFECTS OF SUBJECT DEMOGRAPHICS

Quantitative assessment of effects of subject demographics on PK and PD is a complicated problem, as many of those characteristics are mutually correlated. For example, all body size-related covariates (BW, HT, BSA, LBM, BW) are correlated, which makes selection of the best predictor difficult. Figure 9 shows plots of HT, BSA, LBM, ideal BW versus BW of 1361 unrelated adults (903 men and 458 women). BSA is especially tightly correlated. Taking into account that the impact of body size on the most important parameters like CL is usually not dramatic, it does not make a big difference which covariate to use as a predictor. The current practice in the oncology area to adjust doses per BSA does not have any reasonable background (260).

Not only oncologists, but also some pharmacokineticists, believe that expressing CL or dose per kilogram weight (or m^2 BSA) provides correction for the BW effect. This would be a right method if CL was proportional to BW; however, it is not typically the case. In fact, the effect of BW or other body size variables on CL is complex and depends on elimination mechanisms

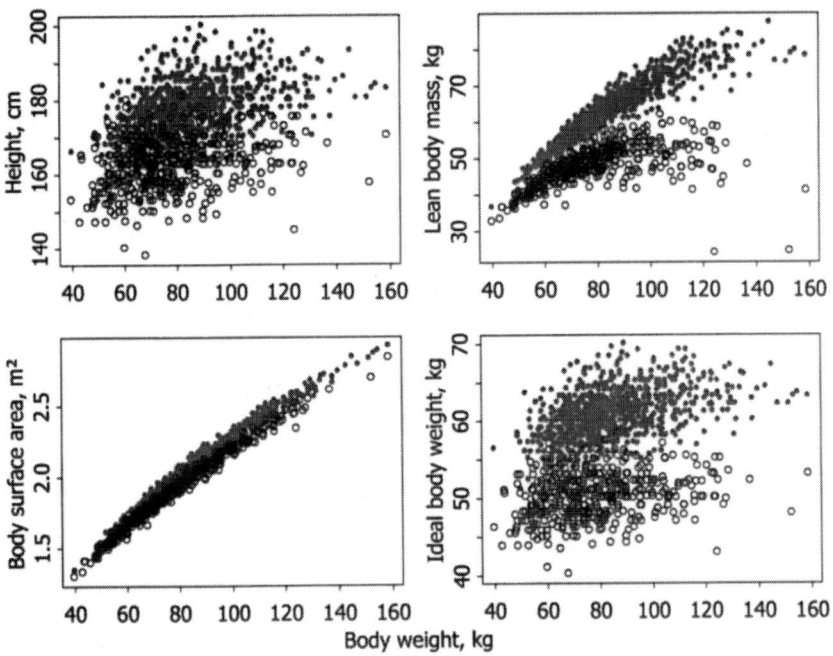

Figure 9 Body size parameters' correlation. *Closed* and *open circles* correspond to males and females, respectively.

involved. For example, in a study already cited (185), the following covariate model for galantamine CL has been developed (see p. 119).

CL_{CR} in this study was calculated using the Cockroft-Gault equation. For males:

$$CL_{CR}(mL/min) = BW \cdot SCR \, (140 - AGE)/72$$

where SCR is serum creatinine (mg/dL). For females, the coefficient 0.85 was applied. According to the model, for 75-year-old patients (note these were primarily Alzheimer's patients who were elderly) and SCR of 1 mg/dL, the typical profile of CL linearly depends on BW (Fig. 10, *panel A, solid line*). CL normalization to the median BW of 67 kg (dashed line) does not correct the parameter properly. Dose adjustment for body weight in this case may result, for example, in overdosing in lighter patients. On the other hand, if CL is proportional to body weight, normalization would work (*panel B*).

In the analysis by Gieschke et al. (191), it was found that a 10% increase in BSA resulted in a 12% increase in 5'-DFUR CL. This indicated a proportionality

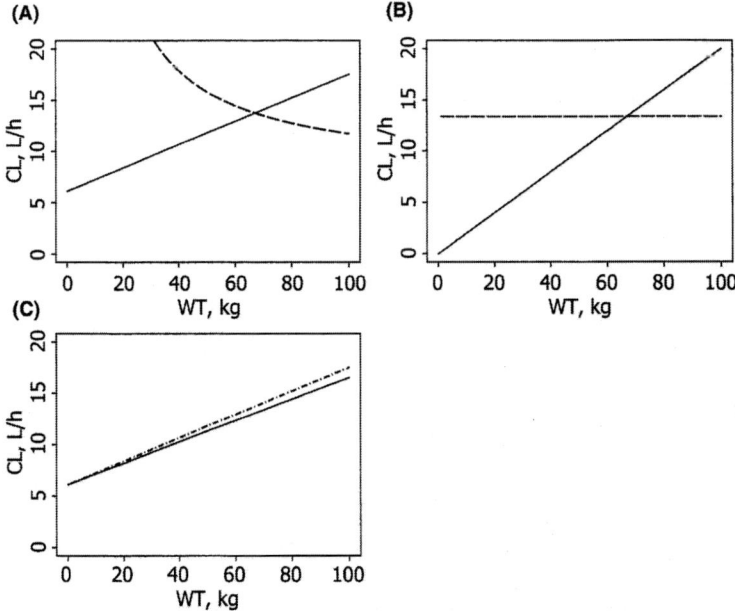

Figure 10 Normalization of galantamine clearance per kilogram body weight (*dashed lines*) assuming the actual linear (*panel A*) and the hypothetical proportional (*panel B*) models. *Panel C* compares clearance versus body weight relationships in males (*dotted line*) and females.

and justified dose abjustment. However, for most drugs, CL in the adult population is far from being proportional to the body size. According to some population PK analyses, it may even be independent of it [e.g., (261–265)]. Therefore, dose adjustment is strongly not recommended unless population PK analyses show proportionality. In pediatric patients, the situation is different: CL is often proportional to BW and dose adjustment is justified.

Panel C of Figure 10 illustrates the gender effect on the typical values of galantamine CL. The covariate model does not include gender effect on the metabolic part of CL (i.e., the part that does not depend on CL_{CR}). The observed differences in CL come from 15% lower CL_{CR} in females compared with males. These differences are small, and no dose adjustment is needed.

As can be seen from Figure 9, association between gender and BW is obvious: on average, men are larger than women. Due to this, the BW effect on any PK or PD parameter will automatically lead to apparent gender disparities. Hence, the observed gender differences can only be attributed to the "pure" gender effect if they remain significant after the body size effect is properly implemented in the model. To avoid the confusion, we will only consider differences between males and females as a true gender effect if they cannot be explained by just body size, but stem from variations in factors such as gastric emptying time, plasma protein levels, activity of drug-metabolizing enzymes, drug transporter function, excretion activity (PK factors), receptor density, intensity of transduction processes, and so on, translating into clinical effect differences (42). In view of this, the early studies where population modeling was not used have nowadays only a limited value.

The most serious problems are associated with evaluating effects of patient demographics on PD or clinical endpoints. The same patient characteristic, for example, gender, may affect either PK or PD of a drug, or both. Without rigorous PK modeling followed by detailed PK–PD modeling, one cannot conclude what specifically causes gender differences in a biomarker or clinical response. Due to this, many early reports of gender differences also have a limited value. From the point of view of therapeutic implications, the exact reason for gender-related disparities may be not critical; however, if the disparities require dose adjustment, one needs to know the actual source in order to estimate the right doses. The best way to do it is through simulation such as those performed in the previous sections. Additional examples will be given in the next section.

POPULATION MODELING AND SIMULATION AS A TOOL FOR DOSE OPTIMIZATION IN DRUG DEVELOPMENT

A final goal of Phase II is the identification of an optimal dosage regimen that provides a high probability of successful confirmation in Phase III that the compound is safe and efficacious (266). Frequently, however, dose-finding is being done in Phase III, and the goal of Phase II is being limited to identify a maximum safe dose. Dose optimization in Phase III is costly and inefficient; often it results in testing and even marketing of excessively high dosages that ultimately cause safety problems and may lead to a reduction in dosing after marketing and resultant reduction in sales, or the drug withdrawal from the market (267).

Population PK, PK–PD and PK-efficacy/safety modeling and simulation can help considerably in selecting optimal doses for further confirming in Phase III. However, this can only be achieved if sufficient information is collected in Phase II studies in target patients, including those with concomitant diseases that may alter drug PK or PD (hepatic, renal disfunction, and so on), and appropriate modeling is performed. All available information (including PK and safety data of Phase I) needs to be combined and a comprehensive model developed followed by extensive simulation. Simulation will not only enable the selection of optimal dosing regimen(s) to be run in Phase III. It is of high importance to ensure that the design is well suited to elucidate dose–response and will substantiate dose selection for Phase III based on the Phase II study outcome.

After the completion of Phase III studies (if the outcome is positive), one more M&S round is necessary after combining findings of the Phase III program. The goal is to generate final dosing recommendations. At this stage, the decision is to be taken whether dose adaptation for BW, gender, concomitant diseases, and so on, is needed. PK aspects have to be taken into account; however, the studies performed so far and reviewed earlier showed that gender disparities in PK did not play a significant role. The major emphasis should be on the efficacy and safety, and even substantial gender differences in CL can be ignored if they are not translated into efficacy/safety differences.

Simple examples of simulation were presented in the section on "Population Modeling." Simulation based on real data needs to include much more factors into account. Unfortunately, not so many examples can be found in the literature on using M&S to optimize dosing regimens. This reflects the past situation in the industry, where there was variable understanding of the value of this approach at the level of the development teams (268,269). The situation is now changing toward more extensive use of M&S in drug development (2,18,23,270–272). A few examples of dose selection using M&S will be reviewed here.

Probably the most successful application of PK and PK-efficacy/safety M&S in clinical development was that of docetaxel (Taxotere®) (273–275), an anticancer agent of the taxoid family. The population approach was implemented in Phase II studies to estimate and explain interpatient PK variability using pathophysiological covariates, generate individual estimates of patient PK parameters, and systemic exposure using Bayesian estimation, and investigate PK estimates as predictors of efficacy and safety endpoints through PK-efficacy/safety analysis. The population PK model was developed at the first course of treatment in 24 Phase II studies conducted in more than 50 centers in Europe and in three centers in the U.S. (266). Of the 18 covariates tested, five had a significant effect ($P < 0.005$) on docetaxel CL: BSA, α_1-acid glycoprotein and albumin plasma levels, age, and hepatic function.

PK-efficacy/safety analyses were conducted using logistic and Cox regression models on both efficacy and safety endpoints. Model development involved step-wise inclusion and deletion of covariates (274). Docetaxel CL was a strong predictor ($P < 0.0001$) of the odds of both Grade 4 neutropenia and febrile neutropenia at first treatment course, after adjustment for the effects of other covariates. According to the logistic regression model, a 50% decrease in CL is associated with a four- to fivefold increase of the odds of Grade 4 neutropenia and febrile neutropenia. Cumulative dose was the strongest predictor ($P < 0.0001$) for the time to onset of fluid retention, which is a cumulative side-effect. However, the exposure at the first course was also found to carry additional explanatory power ($P < 0.01$). As expected for a cumulative side-effect, the magnitude of CL influence was much less marked than that observed on first-course hematologic toxicity, with a 50% decrease in CL being associated with a 46% increase in the risk of experiencing fluid retention. With respect to efficacy, for breast cancer, no significant relationship was found between any estimate of docetaxel exposure (CL, peak plasma level, AUC, time above threshold concentrations) at the first course and either response rate or time to the first response. This may indicate the need of a more sophisticated PK-efficacy model. For non-small-cell lung cancer, docetaxel AUC at the first cycle was a significant ($P = 0.023$) independent prognostic factor for time to progression, with a decreased risk of progression in patients with higher exposure.

Thus, population PK and PK-safety M&S enabled the identification of a population of patients with elevated liver enzymes having decreased CL, which provided the rationale for making dosage recommendations (25% dose reduction) and allowed safety concerns with the drug to be addressed. M&S information obtained and its clinical relevance contributed to the accelerated approval of the drug based on Phase II data in metastatic breast cancer. This resulted in a significant shortening in registration time and time to market. Without these analyses, approval of docetaxel based on Phase II data alone would not have been obtained (270).

Another simulation example that received approval was that of titration schemes of galantamine in patients with Alzheimer's disease having moderate hepatic impairment (185). In patients without the concomitant disease, the recommended titration scheme was starting from 4 mg b.i.d. for one week with subsequent dose increase by 4 mg every week up to 16 mg b.i.d. The distributions of simulated concentration peaks at the end of each week of the titration period for patients with and without moderate hepatic impairment (850 patients in each group) are shown on Figure 11. The latter group has elevation of peak levels that is not desirable. The modification of the dosing regimen was recommended starting with 4 mg once daily for 1 week followed by weekly dose escalation: 4, 8 and 12 mg b.i.d. Figure 12 demonstrates that there are almost no differences between the two groups of patients any more. It is worthwhile to note that simulation was performed based on a population PK model developed using pooled data of Phase I–III studies, and there was only one Phase I study in

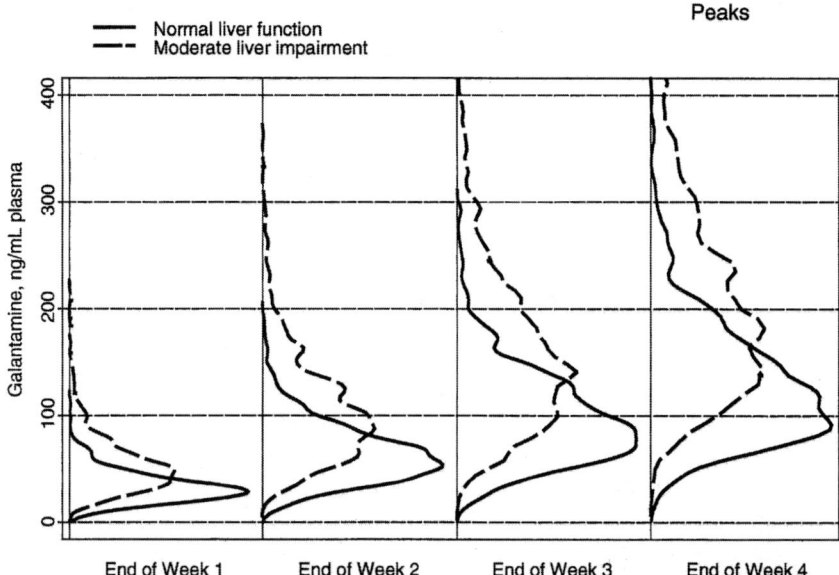

Figure 11 Distributions of simulated peak galantamine levels in patients with normal hepatic function and moderate hepatic impairment using standard titration scheme (4, 8, 12, 16 mg b.i.d.).

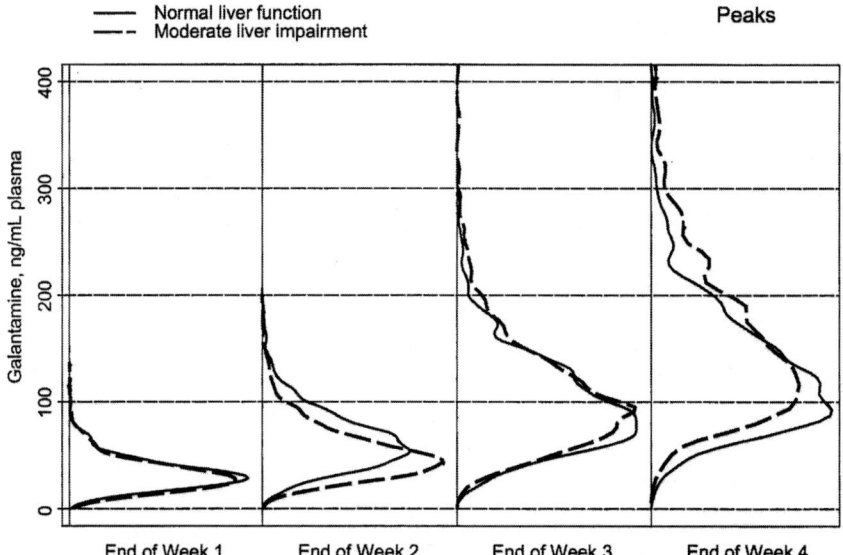

Figure 12 Distributions of simulated peak galantamine levels in patients with normal hepatic function (standard titration scheme: 4, 8, 12, 16 mg b.i.d.) and moderate hepatic impairment (modified titration scheme, 4 mg q.d., 4 mg b.i.d., 8 mg b.i.d., 12 mg b.i.d.).

non-Alzheimer patients with moderate hepatic impairment. Nevertheless, the regulatory authority agreed with the dose selection strategy based on simulation and approved the drug without additional study of the impact of moderate hepatic impairment in the target patient population.

In a paper by Lockwood et al. (276), a clinical trial simulation study is presented that evaluated how well two eight-week parallel group studies could identify doses that corresponded to a response of clinical interest for pregabalin, a drug for multiple indications, which includes pain relief in diabetic neuropathic patients. The response of interest was a one-point reduction in pain intensity on an 11-point numerical pain rating scale. The dose that produced this effect was defined as the minimum effective dose, as this change was considered the minimum clinically significant change. A PK model was based on that developed previously for gabapentine, a drug with similar PK properties and pain relief activity. It assumed the one-compartment disposition with zero-order input with the apparent volume of distribution proportional to weight and CL linearly related to CL_{CR}. The clinical efficacy model included a placebo effect developing with time, and a drug effect that depended on the average pregabalin plasma level according to the E_{max} equation:

$$E = \text{Base} \cdot \{1 + \text{PLM} \cdot (1 - \exp[-k_{pl} \cdot t]) + E_{max} \cdot C_{avg}^{n} / (C_{avg}^{n} + EC_{50}^{n})\} + \varepsilon$$

where E is an observed pain score (between 0 and 10); Base is a baseline score; PLM is the magnitude of the placebo effect; k_{pl} is the first-order rate constant describing the onset of the placebo effect (days^{-1}); t is the time since treatment initiation (days), E_{max} is the maximal drug effect; EC_{50} is the concentration at which the effect due to the drug is 50% of E_{max} ($\mu g/mL$); C_{avg} is the average gabapentine concentration based on dose, and estimated clearance ($\mu g/mL$); n is the Hill coefficient, and ε is the within-subject random effect. Between-subject random effects were associated with Base, PLM, and k_{pl}. No actual clinical efficacy data of pregabalin were available, and gabapentine historical data were used instead to estimate parameters of this model followed by scaling based on preclinical relative potency data.

The efficacy model suggested (276) by the authors does not seem to be optimal, as it assumes immediate development of a full drug effect as C_{avg} reaches the steady-state. Gabapentine half-life is relatively short: 5–7 hours in patients without renal impairment (277), and the steady-state is almost achieved already after one day of treatment. On the other hand, from the first figure of the article under consideration (276) it follows that the actual effect develops relatively slowly indicating a delay between the concentration change and the response change that can be related to transduction processes not taken into account by the PK-efficacy model. It is not surprising then that the model parameters could not be effectively estimated, the Hill coefficient in particular. Additional assumptions have been made, leading to excessive uncertainty.

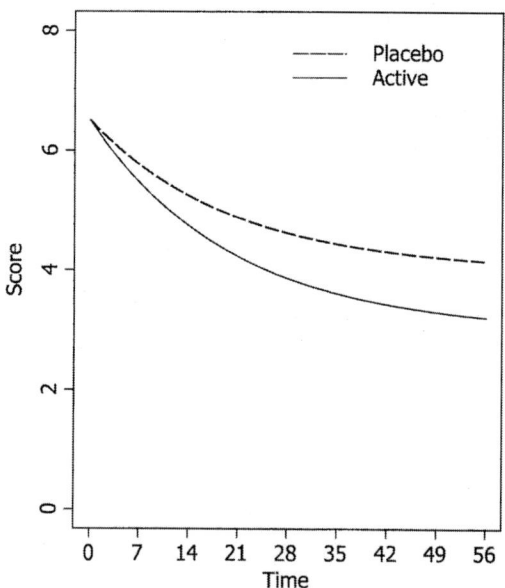

Figure 13 Profiles of a score versus time simulated with the PK-efficacy model that integrates the indirect response concept.

Nevertheless, the overall strategy was adequate, demonstrating the ability of M&S to explore rival study designs and to assess the likelihood of success given prior knowledge on PK and comparative efficacy. The major goal of the study was to compare two study designs with respect to their ability to estimate the dose that caused a one-point reduction in the pain score. The designs were as follows:

> *Study 1*: 2-wk titration; 4-wk stable treatment; daily doses 0,150,600 mg
> *Study 2*: 1-wk titration; 4-wk stable treatment; daily doses 0,75,300,600 mg

Analysis of the simulated data suggested that after accounting for the uncertainty, there was an 80% chance that the dose defining the clinical feature of interest was within 45% of the true value. The likelihood of the development program to estimate the dose with acceptable precision approximated 50% and ranged from 40% to 70%, depending on the key assumptions. The minimum dose that should be studied to have a reasonable chance of estimating the dose that caused a one-point change was 300 mg. This suggests that the identification of the selected dose–response feature with any real precision from the chosen design is borderline. Therefore, if the objective was to confirm the outcome in a future Phase III study, selecting a dose based on this single outcome might be "risky." To increase the likelihood, one might consider changing the number of treatments, the number of efficacy measurements, or the acceptance limits. Further options might be the gathering of additional information to reduce the uncertainty associated with key assumptions that influence how reliably a dose can be estimated. Investigating the impact of these options or combinations thereof may assist in identifying key failure points in a development program that, if remedied, may optimize decision-making and enable the selection of effective doses for confirmatory studies with a high level of confidence.

Another case study has been presented recently by Mandema and Wang (278). M&S was used to optimize the Phase II dose-finding strategy for a new 5-HT$_{1D}$ agonist indicated for the relief of moderate to severe migraine pain. A drug model was derived on the basis of literature, preclinical, and early clinical data of the drug, and other 5-HT$_{1D}$ agonists, such as sumatriptan, zolmitriptan, naratriptan, and rizatriptan. The model was used to explore the likely range of treatment outcomes for the new drug in comparison with the other 5-HT$_{1D}$ agonists and to design a dose-ranging study in terms of the number of treatment arms, spacing of active doses, and sample size, with the objective to confirm efficacy and to support dose selection with the appropriate profile for further development.

The severity of headache was measured on a four-point scale from $0 =$ none to $3 =$ severe pain. The primary clinical endpoint was the fraction of patients with the headache relief, and the relief was defined as none or mild pain. The following dose–response model relating the probability of pain relief to the drug dose was used:

$$\text{Pr(Pain Relief)} = g\{\beta + E_{\max} \cdot D_T{}^n/(D_T{}^n + \text{ED}_{50,T}{}^n) + \eta\}$$
$$g\{x\} = \exp(x)/[1 + \exp(x)]$$

where β corresponds to placebo response, $E_{\max}$ is the maximal drug effect, D_T is the dose of 5-HT$_{1D}$ agonist T, $\text{ED}_{50,T}$ is the dose giving 50% of the maximal effect, n is the Hill coefficient, and η is the random effect reflecting the between-study variability. This model was fitted to summary data of four known 5-HT$_{1D}$ agonist (triptans) obtained from seven trials, and parameters were estimated. It turned out that the only significant differences were in $\text{ED}_{50,T}$, but not in n and $E_{\max}$. The latter was 70% at a mean placebo response of 28%. This finding reflects the fact that all four drugs have the same mechanism of action and differ only in potency. Since the newly developed compound was of the same class of 5-HT$_{1D}$ agonists, the relative potency of 3 ± 0.5 (SD) was estimated from preclinical and Phase I studies compared with sumatriptan. The latter accounted for uncertainty in scaling from animal to man. From Phase I studies, it followed that 75 mg was the maximum tolerated dose. Through simulation it was found that the expected dose to achieve pain relief in 60% of the patients was 19 mg, with 80% probability that the dose is between 11 and 40 mg. Finally, two doses were recommended to include in a dose-finding study: 20 mg and 40 mg that had 54% and 88% chances, respectively, to exceed the minimum marketing target of migraine pain relief in 60% of the patients. Additional simulation was performed to identify the optimal study design and the sample size (278).

An M&S study briefly described in the review by Chaikin et al. (270) was aimed to optimize dosing regimens for the Phase II program in patients. A PK–PD model was used to simulate the dose of Klerval, a platelet GPIIb/IIIa receptor antagonist that would achieve the optimal inhibition of platelet aggregation. An E_{max} model that included contributions from Klerval and its active metabolite was fitted to pooled ex vivo data from normal volunteers and the parameters were estimated. The response variable was the percent inhibition of platelet aggregation induced by an agonist, such as collagen. The target platelet inhibition for simulation was between 50% and 80%. PK data from healthy volunteers were used to simulate the steady-state concentration of the parent compound and the metabolite after oral administration of 50, 100, 200, and 300 mg b.i.d. of Klerval, and the model was used to predict the steady-state effect. The 300 mg b.i.d. dose was judged as optimal in achieving the desired pharmacologic response. In actual Phase II studies conducted in patients with chronic stable coronary disease and patients with recent (< 14 days) and prior acute coronary syndrome (> 30 days), the observed response at each administered dose was close to that predicted by PK–PD simulations. The potency of the metabolite was twice that of the parent drug in normal healthy subjects and the patient populations studied (270).

An interesting example of M&S was published by Kimko et al. (279) although the goal of the analysis was not dose selection or design testing. An outcome of a Phase III trial of an antischizophrenic agent, quetiapine fumarate (seroquel), was predicted based on information collected in Phase I and II studies and compared with actual Phase III study results. The time course of quetiapine concentrations was described by the one-compartment linear PK model with first-order absorption. The clinical effect was assessed by a brief psychiatric rating scale (BPRS) and the corresponding model was as follows (the authors' notation is used):

$$BPRS = baseline\_BPRS + drft \times time - E_{max}C/(EC_{50} + C)$$

in which E_{max} is the maximum effect (shift in BPRS score from baseline) that can be attained as a result of exposure to drug concentrations C, EC_{50} is the drug concentration producing 50% of the maximum effect, and drift is the slope reflecting time course of disease progression and placebo response. Patient characteristics, like demographics, were shown not to be predictive covariates of both PK and PK-efficacy models. All parameters were subject to BIV, and the corresponding variances were estimated, although, due to the parallel group design of the Phase II study used to get parameter estimates of the PK-efficacy model, the variances were probably overestimated. Another shortcoming of the model was similar to that of the model by Lockwood et al.

(276): no delay was assumed between drug concentrations and the effect. As the half-life of quetiapine fumarate was short (according to the reported PK parameters, it was about three hours) the steady-state was reached soon after treatment initiation, resulting in a full development of the drug effect according to the E_{max} model. The authors did not present any goodness-of-fit plots to let the reader evaluate the model performance. Nevertheless, the simulation of the Phase III trial outcome was in good agreement with the actual trial, except that the placebo response showed deterioration of BPRS scores with time while simulation predicted an improvement.

The problem of delayed response is a common one for clinical endpoints based on scores. The score reflects the patient status (or disease status) and cannot change immediately after changing conditions (e.g., therapy). Without any treatment, the score versus time profile is defined by a spontaneous disease progression, and the indirect response model shown in the following is the way to express this paradigm:

$$dS/dt = v_d - v_a \tag{12}$$

where S is a score or any other clinically relevant variable reflecting the patient status, v_d and v_a are deterioration and amelioration rates, respectively. Equation 12 assumes that deterioration results in the increase of S.

An assumption important for the practical use of the model is v_a proportionality to the current value of S:

$$dS/dt = v_d - K_S \cdot S \tag{13}$$

where K_S is a rebalance rate constant, a core model parameter that determines how fast the system returns to equilibrium after perturbation. At time $t = 0$ when a patient is enrolled in the study $dS/dt = S_0'$, an unknown value, since we have no information about the disease progression before enrollment. Equation 13 becomes:

$$S_0' = v_d - K_s \cdot S_0 \tag{14}$$

where S_0 is a score at enrollment. We use equation 14 to exclude v_d in equation 13: $v_d = S_0' + K_S \cdot S_0$. Equation 13 now reads as follows:

$$dS/dt = S_0' + K_s \cdot S_0 - K_s \cdot S = S_0' + K_s \cdot (S_0 - S) \tag{15}$$

Usually the score S is constrained by definition. For example, in the case of pain score used in the analysis by Lockwood et al. (269), it is between 0 and 10. In the framework of the indirect response concept, we can consider an asymptotic value of the score due to disease progression, S_{max}, which corresponds to $t \to$ infinity. $dS/dt \to 0$ in this case. After taking the limit we get:

$$S_0' + K_S \cdot (S_0 - S_{max}) = 0 \tag{16}$$

From equation 16, S_0' can be expressed as $-K_S \cdot (S_0 - S_{max})$ and introduced into equation 15:

$$dS/dt = -K_S \cdot (S_0 - S_{max}) + K_S \cdot (S_0 - S) = K_S \cdot (S_{max} - S) \tag{17}$$

Note that despite the fact that S_0 vanished from the model equation, it remains a model parameter through the initial conditions defining the value of S at $t = 0$.

For patients treated with placebo, we assume that the effect is directed towards the deterioration rate, v_d, although the model allows an alternative target, too. The magnitude of the placebo effect is PL, a parameter that has the meaning of a fractional change. PL = 1 corresponds to no placebo effect; PL < 1 means some improvement. After repeating these rearrangements, we come up with the following equation:

$$dS/dt = K_S \cdot (PL \cdot S_{max} - S) \tag{18}$$

Most clinical studies do not include patients without treatment; a typical efficacy study design includes only placebo and active treatment groups, so estimation of the disease progression independently of the placebo effect is not feasible; that means PL and S_{max} in equation 18 are not estimable, but only their product, $PL \cdot S_{max}$, which we will denote as S_{PL}, an ultimate score on placebo.

$$dS/dt = K_S \cdot (S_{PL} - S) \tag{19}$$

Finally, the drug effect is also assumed to change the deterioration rate and is represented by a function of the plasma concentration, $E = 1 + f(Cp)$. Again, the effect on v_d is translated into the change of the ultimate score:

$$dS/dt = K_S \cdot (E \cdot S_{PL} - S) \tag{20}$$

$E = 1$ represents the case when the drug effect is lacking. There may be multiple ways to implement the concentration effect. The simplest variant is to assume a linear equation: $E = 1 + K \cdot Cp$, where K is a slope of the concentration–effect relationship. The advantage of the linear relationship is that the model equation has in this case a closed-form solution. If the drug half-life is short relative to the observed changes in S, like in the examples cited previously (i.e., it is much smaller than $\ln (2)/K_S$), Cp can be replaced by an average steady-state concentration. Figure 13 shows profiles simulated according to equations 19 and 20 with the following parameter values: $K_S = 0.05$; $S_0 = 6.5$; $S_{PL} = 4$; $K = -1$; $Cp = 0.25$. The profiles resemble mean pain score profiles observed in placebo- and gabapentin-treated groups presented in the first figure of the article by Lockwood et al. (276).

The function $f(\ )$ can be of an E_{max}-type, as those used in the articles by Lockwood et al. (276) and Kimko et al. (279). The model selection should be based on the goodness of fit criteria, as usual. If PK information is lacking, the model described can be used to explore dose–response relationships and help in dose-finding through M&S. In this case, E is a function of dose D, not concentration: $E = 1 + f(D)$. The impact of patient characteristics, including demographics, can be easily tested. If the PK component is included, one can evaluate the impact of patient covariates affecting PK on clinical response in terms of endpoints; this is the most suitable way to assess the actual role of those covariates. One important question to answer is: can the dose serve as a surrogate of concentration. In other words, does concentration as the predictor of the response have any advantages over just dose?

Currently, there are very few examples of use of this model (280,281); however, its generality, simplicity, and the fact that it is based on clearcut semi-mechanistic considerations will favor its wide application in the future.

Concluding the overview of M&S studies published in the literature, it should be stressed that this is probably only a small part of the studies performed, especially in the pharmaceutical industry. The majority of studies remains unpublished due to confidentiality issues. Therefore, the picture is rather fragmentary and biased. One can expect, however, more M&S studies published in the future in view of increasing interest from drug development teams in the companies and encouraging regulatory climate (282).

CONCLUSION

M&S is a general tool to evaluate complex systems that are hard to track analytically. This methodology can be incorporated in virtually every step of the drug development to improve efficiency and assist decision-making. For instance, it can be used to compare the information yield of competing trial strategies versus time, costs, and trial complexity. This enables the development team to balance the value versus cost of additional information derived from a study. The probabilistic study outcome models can be leveraged into a decision-making framework that can be further used to optimize the overall development strategy, also from a financial value perspective. This link is important because simulation can only determine the relationship between drug features, study features, and power or precision to make a certain decision. It cannot, however, determine what level of confidence one would like to achieve at a certain point in the development.

It is not surprising, therefore, that PK–PD and PK-efficacy/safety M&S are becoming more and more essential, especially in the later stages of clinical development, where there is a need to better understand the dosing regimen—concentration—efficacy/toxicity relationships in the target patient population. It is important to recognize that population M&S is one of the driving forces which can really help to overcome current problems in drug development that the U.S. FDA has called "stagnation" (282). The outcome of these kinds of analyses can have an impact on approval and final labeling decisions with respect to individualization of dosage for optimal therapeutic outcome and to properly balance benefit/risk.

REFERENCES

1. Daries PJA. De atropa belladonna. Dissertation, Leipzig. Ex Off. Langenhemia, 1776, pp. 1–40.
2. Abdel-Rahman SM, Kauffman RE. The integration of pharmacokinetics and pharmacodynamics: Understanding dose-response. Ann Rev Pharmacol Toxicol 2004; 44:111–136.
3. Jelliffe RW, Schumitzky A, Vanguilder M, et al. Individualizing drug dosage regimens—roles of population pharmacokinetic and dynamic models, Bayesian fitting, and adaptive control. Ther Drug Monit 1993; 15:380–393.
4. Graham G, Gupta S, Aarons L. Determination of an optimal dosage regimen using a Bayesian decision analysis of efficacy and adverse effect data. J Pharmacokinet Pharmacodyn 2002; 29:67–88.
5. Sheiner L, Wakefield J. Population modelling in drug development. Stat Meth Med Res 1999; 8:183–193.
6. Samara E, Granneman R. Role of population pharmacokinetics in drug development—a pharmaceutical industry perspective. Clin Pharmacokinet 1997; 32:294–312.
7. Sheiner LB. Learning versus confirming in clinical drug development. Clin Pharmacol Ther 1997; 61:275–279.
8. Jusko WJ, Ko HC, Ebling WF. Convergence of direct and indirect pharmacodynamic response models. J Pharmacokinet Biopharm 1995; 23:5–6.
9. Colburn WA, Lee JW. Biomarkers, validation and pharmacokinetic–pharmacodynamic modelling. Clin Pharmacokinet 2003; 42:997–1022.
10. Holford NH, Sheiner LB. Kinetics of pharmacologic response. Pharmacology & Therapeutics 1982; 16:143–166.
11. Kenakin T. A Pharmacology Primer. Theory, Application, and Methods. San Diego: Elsevier, 2004.
12. Kenakin TP. The study of drug-receptor interaction in in vivo systems. In: van Boxtel CJ, Holford NHG, Danhof M, eds. The In Vivo Study of Drug Action. Amsterdam: Elsevier; 1992:1–15.
13. Fischman AJ, Alpert NM, Rubin RH. Pharmacokinetic imaging—a noninvasive method for determining drug distribution and action. Clin Pharmacokinet 2002; 41:581–602.
14. Gupta N, Price PM, Aboagye EO. PET for in vivo pharmacokinetic and pharmacodynamic measurements. Eur J Cancer 2002; 38:2094–2107.
15. Paans AMJ, Vaalburg W. Positron emission tomography in drug development and drug evaluation. Curr Pharmaceut Design 2000; 6:1583–1591.
16. Biomarkers Definitions Working Group. Biomarkers and surrogate endpoints: preferred definitions and conceptual framework. Clin Pharmacol Ther 2001; 69:89–95.
17. Lathia CD. Biomarkers and surrogate endpoints: how and when might they impact drug development? Disease Markers 2002; 18:83–90.
18. Derendorf H, Lesko LJ, Chaikin P, et al. Pharmacokinetic/pharmacodynamic modeling in drug research and development. J Clin Pharmacol 2000; 40:1399–1418.
19. Colburn WA. Surrogate markers and clinical pharmacology. J Clin Pharmacol 1995; 35: 441–442.
20. Colburn WA. Selecting and validating biologic markers for drug development. J Clin Pharmacol 1997; 37:355–362.

21. Rowland M, Sheiner LB, Steimer JL, eds. Variability in Drug Therapy: Description, Estimation and Control. New York: Raven; 1985.
22. Piotrovsky VK. Population pharmacodynamic and pharmacokinetic modeling via mixed effects. Current Opinion in Drug Discovery and Development 2000; 3:314–330.
23. Sheiner LB, Steimer JL. Pharmacokinetic/pharmacodynamic modeling in drug development. Annu Rev Pharmacol Toxicol 2000; 40:67–95.
24. Vonesh EF, Chinchilli VM. Linear and nonlinear models for the analysis of repeated measurements. New York: Marcel Dekker, 1997.
25. Davidian M, Giltinan DM. Nonlinear models for repeated measurement data. London: Chapman & Hall, 1995.
26. Pinheiro J, Bates DM. Mixed Effects-Models in S and S-PLUS. New York: Springer, 2000.
27. Meibohm B, Derendorf H. Basic concepts of pharmacokinetic/pharmacodynamic (PK/PD) modelling. Int J Clin Pharmacol Ther 1997; 35:401–413.
28. Derendorf H, Meibohm B. Modeling of pharmacokinetic/pharmacodynamic (PK/PD) relationships: Concepts and perspectives. Pharm Res 1999; 16:176–185.
29. Peck CC, Beal SL, Sheiner LB, Nichols AI. Extended least squares nonlinear regression: a possible solution to the "choice of weights" problem in analysis of individual pharmacokinetic data. J Pharmacokinet Biopharm 1984; 12:545–558.
30. Aarons L. Population pharmacokinetics. Int J Clin Pharmacol Ther Toxicol. 1992; 30:520–522.
31. Sheiner LB, Ludden TM. Population pharmacokinetics/dynamics. Ann Rev Pharmacol Toxicol 1992; 32:185–209.
32. Mandema J, Verotta D, Sheiner LB. Building population pharmacokinetic-pharmacodynamic models. In: D'Argenio DZ, ed. Advanced Pharmacokinetic and Pharmacodynamic Systems Analysis. New York: Plenum Press; 1995; pp. 69–86.
33. Mandema JW, Verotta D, Sheiner LB. Building population pharmacokinetic-pharmacodynamic models. 1. Models for covariate effects. J Pharmacokinet Biopharm 1992; 20:511–528.
34. Sheiner LB, Beal SL. Bayesian individualization of pharmacokinetics: simple implementation and comparison with non-Bayesian methods. J Pharm Sci 1982; 71:1344–1348.
35. Thomson AH, Whiting B. Bayesian parameter estimation and population pharmacokinetics. Clin Pharmacokinet 1992; 22:447–467.
36. US Gen. Account. Office (GAO) 2001. Women Sufficiently Represented in New Drug Testing, but FDA Oversight Needs Improvement. (http://www.gao.gov/new.items/d01754.pdf).
37. Bonate PL. Gender-related differences in xenobiotic metabolism. J Clin Pharmacol 1991; 31:684–690.
38. Wilson K. Sex-related differences in drug disposition in man. Clin Pharmacokinet 1984; 9:189–202.
39. Schwartz JB. The influence of sex on pharmacokinetics. Clin Pharmacokinet 2003; 42:107–121.
40. Beierle I, Meibohm B, Derendorf H. Gender differences in pharmacokinetics and pharmacodynamics. Int J Clin Pharmacol Ther 1999; 37:529–547.
41. Tanaka E. Gender-related differences in pharmacokinetics and their clinical significance. J Clin Pharmacy Ther 1999; 24:339–346.

42. Gandhi M. Aweeka F. Greenblatt RM. Blaschke TF. 2004. Sex differences in pharmacokinetics and pharmacodynamics. Annu. Review Pharmacol. Toxicol. 44:499–523.

43. Harris R, Benet L, Schwartz J. Gender effects in pharmacokinetics and pharmacodynamics. Drugs 1995; 50:222–239.

44. Fletcher C, Acosta E, Strykowski J. Gender differences in human pharmacokinetics and pharmacodynamics. J Adolesc Health 1994; 15:619–629.

45. Martinez MN, Amidon GL. A mechanistic approach to understanding the factors affecting drug absorption: a review of fundamentals. J Clin Pharmacol 2002; 42:620–643.

46. Collen MJ, Sheridan MJ. Gastric ulcers differ from duodenal ulcers. Evaluation of basal acid output. Dig Dis Sci 1993; 38:2281–2286.

47. Dressman JB, Berardi RR, Derment-zoglou LC, et al. Upper gastrointestinal (GI) pH in young, healthy men and women. Pharm Res 1990; 7:756–761.

48. Lindahl A, Ungell AL, Knutson L, Lennernas H. Characterization of fluids from the stomach and proximal je-junum in men and women. Pharm Res 1997; 14:497–502.

49. Roland B, Grijalva CV. Gastric mucosal damage induced by lateral hypothalamic lesions in female rats: influence of age and ovariectomy. Behav Neural Biol 1991; 55:166–178.

50. Collen MJ, Abdulian JD, Chen YK. Age does not affect basal gastric acid secretion in normal subjects or in patients with acid-peptic disease. Am J Gastroenterol 1994; 89:712–716.

51. Hutson WR, Roehrkasse RL, Wald A. Influence of gender and menopause on gastric emptying and motility. Gastroenterology 1989; 96:11–17.

52. Singer AJ, Brandt LJ. Pathophysiology of the gastrointestinal tract during pregnancy. Am J Gastroenterol 1991; 86:1695–1712.

53. Coskun T, Sevinc A, Tevetoglu I, Alican I, Kurtel H, Yegen BC. Delayed gastric emptying in conscious male rats following chronic estrogen and progesterone treatment. Res Exp Med 1995; 195:49–54.

54. Wu CL, Hung CR, Chang FY, Pau KY, Wang JL, Wang PS. Involvement of cholecystokinin receptor in the inhibition of gastric emptying by oxytocin in male rats. Pflugers Arch 2002; 445:187–193.

55. Chen TS, Doong ML, Chang FY, Lee SD, Wang PS. Effects of sex steroid hormones on gastric emptying and gastrointestinal transit in rats. Am J Physiol Gastrointest Liver Physiol 1995; 268:G171–G176.

56. Liu CY, Chen LB, Liu PY, Xie DP, Wang PS. Effects of progesterone on gastric emptying and intestinal transit in male rats. World J Gastroenterol 2002; 8:338–341.

57. Baraona E, Abittan CS, Dohmen K, et al. Gender differences in pharmacokinetics of alcohol. Alcohol Clin Exp Res 2001; 25:502–507.

58. Bennink R, Peeters M, Van den Maegdenbergh V, et al. Evaluation of small-bowel transit for solid and liquid test meal in healthy men and women. Eur J Nucl Med 1999; 26:1560–1566.

59. Mearadji B, Penning C, Vu MK, et al. Influence of gender on proximal gastric motor and sensory function. Am J Gastroenterol 2001; 96:2066–2073.

60. Naslund E, Bogefors J, Gryback P, Jacobsson H, Hellstrom PM. Gastric emptying: comparison of scintigraphic, polyethylene glycol dilution, and paracetamol tracer assessment techniques. Scand J Gastroenterol 2000; 35:375–379.

61. Sadik R, Abrahamsson H, Stotzer PO. Gender differences in gut transit shown with a newly developed radiological procedure. Scand J Gastroenterol 2003; 38:36–42.
62. Frezza M, di Padova C, Pozzato G, Terpin M, Baraona E, Lieber CS. High blood alcohol levels in women. The role of decreased gastric alcohol dehydrogenase activity and first-pass metabolism. N Engl J Med 1990; 322:95–99.
63. Pastino GM, Flynn EJ, Sultatos LG. Genetic polymorphisms in ethanol metabolism: issues and goals for physiologically based pharmacokinetic modeling. Drug Chem Toxicol 2000; 23:179–201.
64. Johnson TN, Tanner MS, Tucker GT. A comparison of the ontogeny of enterocytic and hepatic cytochromes P450 3A in the rat. Biochem Pharmacol 2000; 60: 1601–1610.
65. Kolars JC, Schmiedlin-Ren P, Dobbins WO 3rd, Schuetz J, Wrighton SA, Watkins PB. Heterogeneity of cytochrome P450IIIA expression in rat gut epithelia. Gastroenterology 1992; 102:1186–1198.
66. Schuetz EG, Furuya KN, Schuetz JD. Interindividual variation in expression of P-glycoprotein in normal human liver and secondary hepatic neoplasms. J Pharmacol Exp Ther 1995; 275:1011–1018.
67. Kim R, Leake B, Choo E. Identification of functionally variant MDR1 alleles among European Americans and African Americans. Clin Pharmacol Ther 2001; 70:189–199.
68. Mesnil F, Mentre F, Dubruc C, Thenot JP, Mallet A, Thenot JP. Population pharmacokinetic analysis of mizolastine and validation from sparse data on patients using the nonparametric maximum likelihood method. J Pharmacokinet Biopharm 1998; 26:133–161.
69. Aarons L, Hopkins K, Rowland M, Brossel S, Thiercelin JF. Route of administration and sex differences in the pharmacokinetics of aspirin, administered as its lysine salt. Pharm Res 1989; 6:660–666.
70. Miaskiewicz SL, Shively CA, Vesell ES. Sex differences in absorption kinetics of sodium salicylate. Clin Pharmacol Ther 1982; 31:30–37.
71. Montgomery PR, Berger LG, Mitenko PA, Sitar DS. Salicylate metabolism: effects of age and sex in adults. Clin Pharmacol Ther 1986; 39:571–576.
72. Vahl N, Moller N, Lauritzen T. Metabolic effects and pharmacokinetics of a growth hormone pulse in healthy adults: relation to age, sex, and body composition. J Clin Endocrinol Metab 1998; 82:3612–3618.
73. Verbeeck R, Cardinal JA, Wallace S. Effect of age and sex on the plasma binding of acidic and basic drugs. Eur J Clin Pharmacol 1984; 27:91–97.
74. Piafsky K, Borga O. Plasma protein binding of basic drugs: importance of a1-acid glycoprotein for interindividual variation. Clin Pharmacol Ther 1977; 22:545–549.
75. Kishino S, Nomura A, Di Z. Alpha-1-acid glycoprotein concentration and the protein binding of disopyramide in healthy subjects. J Clin Pharmacol 1995; 35:510–514.
76. Brinkman-Van der Linden CM, Havenaar EC, Van Ommen CR, Van Kamp GJ, Gooren LJ. Oral estrogen treatment induces a decrease in expression of sialyl Lewis x on alpha 1-acid glycoprotein in females and male-to-female transsexuals. Glycobiology 1996; 6:407–412.
77. Succari M, Foglietti MJ, Percheron F. Microheterogeneity of alpha 1-acid glycoprotein: variation during the menstrual cycle in healthy women, and profile in women receiving estrogen-progestogen treatment. Clin Chim Acta 1990; 187:235–241.

78. Tuck CH, Holleran S, Berglund L. Hormonal regulation of lipoprotein(a) levels: effects of estrogen replacement therapy on lipoprotein(a) and acute phase reactants in postmenopausal women. Arterioscler. Thromb Vasc Biol 1997; 17:1822–1829.

79. Walle UK, Fagan TC, Topmiller MJ, Conradi EC, Walle T. The influence of gender and sex steroid hormones on the plasma binding of propranolol enantiomers. Br J Clin Pharmacol 1994; 37:21–25.

80. Walle U, Salle S, Bai S, Olanoff LS. Stereoselective binding of propranolol to human plasma alpha1-acid glycoprotein and albumin. Clin Pharmacol Ther 1983; 34:718–723.

81. Gilmore D, Gal J, Gerber J. Age and gender influence the stereoselective pharmacokinetics of propranolol. J Pharmacol Exp Ther 1992; 261:1181–1186.

82. Gleichmann W, Bachmann G, Dengler H. Effects of hormonal contraceptives and pregnancy on serum protein pattern. Eur J Clin Pharmacol 1973; 5:218–225.

83. Keefe D, Yee Y, Kates R. Verapamil protein binding in patients and in normal subjects. Clin Pharmacol Ther 1981; 29:21–26.

84. Krecic-Shepard ME, Park K, Barnas C, Slimko J, Kerwin DR, Schwartz JB. Race and sex influence clearance of nifedipine: results of a population study. Clin Pharmacol Ther 2000; 68:130–142.

85. Haram K, Augensen K, Elsayed S. Serum protein pattern in normal pregnancy with special reference to acute-phase reactants. Br J Obstet Gynaecol 1983; 90:139–145.

86. Aquirre C, Rodriguez-Sasiain JM, Navajas P, Calvo R. Plasma protein binding of penbutolol in pregnancy. Eur J Drug Metab Pharmacokinet 1988; 13:23–26.

87. Wood M, Wood AJ. Changes in plasma drug binding and alpha 1-acid glycoprotein in mother and newborn infant. Clin Pharmacol Ther 1981; 29:522–526.

88. Chu CY, Singla VP, Wang HP, Sweet B, Lai LT. Plasma alpha 1-acid glycoprotein levels in pregnancy. Clin Chim Acta 1981; 112:235–240.

89. Hill MD, Abramson FP. The significance of plasma protein binding on the fetal/maternal distribution of drugs at steady-state. Clin Pharmacokinet 1988; 14:156–170.

90. Notarianni LJ. Plasma protein binding of drugs in pregnancy and in neonates. Clin Pharmacokinet 1990; 18:20–36.

91. Perucca E, Crema A. Plasma protein binding of drugs in pregnancy. Clin Pharmacokinet 1982; 7:336–352.

92. Wiegratz I, Kutschera E, Lee JH, et al. Effect of four oral contraceptives on thyroid hormones, adrenal and blood pressure parameters. Contraception 2003; 67:361–366.

93. Greenblatt D, Wright C. Clinical pharmacokinetics of alprazolam: therapeutic implications. Clin Pharmacokinet 1993; 24:453–471.

94. Kirkwood C, Moore A, Hayes P. Influence of menstrual cycle and gender on alprazolam pharmacokinetics. Clin Pharmacol Ther 1991; 50:404–409.

95. Greenblatt DJ, Allen MD, Harmatz JS, Shader RI. Diazepam disposition determinants. Clin Pharmacol Ther 1980; 27:301–312.

96. Ochs HR, Greenblatt DJ, Divoll M, Abernethy DR, Feyerabend H, Dengler HJ. Diazepam kinetics in relation to age and sex. Pharmacology 1981; 23:24–30.

97. Houghton IT, Aun CS, Oh TE. Vecuronium: an anthropometric comparison. Anaesthesia 1992; 47:741–746.

98. Semple P, Hope DA, Clyburn P, Rodbert A. Relative potency of vecuronium in male and female patients in Britain and Australia. Br J Anaesth 1994; 72:190–194.

99. Takaya T, Takeyama K, Miura M, Takiguchi M. Influence of body fat on the onset of vecuronium induced neuromuscular blockade. Tokai J Exp Clin Med 2001; 26:107–111.

100. Xue FS, An G, Liao X, Zou Q, Luo LK. The pharmacokinetics of vecuronium in male and female patients. Anesth Analg 1998a; 86:1322–1327.

101. Xue FS, Liao X, Liu JH, et al. Dose-response curve and time-course of effect of vecuronium in male and female patients. Br J Anaesth 1998b; 80:720–724.

102. Xue FS, Tong SY, Liao X, Liu JH, An G, Luo LK. Dose-response and time course of effect of rocuronium in male and female anesthetized patients. Anesth Analg 1997; 85:667–671.

103. Carcas AJ, Guerra P, Frias J, et al. Gender differences in the disposition of metronidazole. Int J Clin Pharmacol Ther 2001; 39:213–218.

104. Bertino JS Jr, Nafziger AN. Pharmacokinetics of oral fleroxacin in male and premenopausal female volunteers. Antimicrob Agents Chemother 1996; 40:789–791.

105. Sowinski KM, Abel SR, Clark WR, Mueller BA. Effect of gender on the pharmacokinetics of ofloxacin. Pharmacotherapy 1999; 19:442–446.

106. Magee MH, Blum RA, Lates CD, Jusko WJ. Prednisolone pharmacokinetics and pharmacodynamics in relation to sex and race. J Clin Pharmacol 2001; 41:1180–1194.

107. Kashuba A, Nafziger A. Physiological changes during the menstrual cycle and their effects on the pharmacokinetic and pharmacodynamics of drugs. Clin Pharmacokinet 1998; 34:203–218.

108. Prior TI, Baker GB. Interactions between the cytochrome P450 system and the second-generation antipsychotics. J Psychiatry Neurosci 2003; 28:99–112.

109. Shimada T, Yamazaki H, Mimura M, Inui Y, Guengerich FP. Interindividual variations in human liver cytochrome P-450 enzymes involved in the oxidation of drugs, carcinogens and toxic chemicals: studies with liver microsomes of 30 Japanese and 30 Caucasians. J Pharmacol Exp Ther 1994; 270:414–423.

110. Callaghan J, Bergstrom R, Ptak L. Olanzapine: pharmacokinetic and pharmacodynamic profile. Clin Pharmacokinet 1999; 37:177–193.

111. Lane H-Y, Chang Y-C, Chang W-H. Effects of gender and age on plasma levels of clozapine and its metabolites: analyzed by critical statistics. J Clin Psychiatry 1999; 60:36–40.

112. Hunt CM, Westerkam WR, Stave GM. Effect of age and gender on the activity of human hepatic CYP3A. Biochem Pharmacol 1992; 44:275–283.

113. Schmidt R, Baumann F, Hanschmann H, Geissler F, Preiss R. Gender difference in ifosfamide metabolism by human liver microsomes. Eur J Drug Metab Pharmacokinet 2001; 26:193–200.

114. Hunt CM, Westerkam WR, Stave GM, Wilson JA. Hepatic cytochrome P-4503A (CYP3A) activity in the elderly. Mech Ageing Dev 1992; 64:189–199.

115. Schmucker DL, Woodhouse KW, Wang RK, Wynne H, James OF. Effects of age and gender on in vitro properties of human liver microsomal monooxygenases. Clin Pharmacol Ther 1990; 48:365–374.

116. George J, Byth K, Farrell GC. Age but not gender selectively affects expression of individual cytochrome P450 proteins in human liver. Biochem Pharmacol 1995; 50:727–730.

117. Greenblatt DJ, Abernethy DR, Locniskar A, Harmatz JS, Limjuco RA, Shader R. Effect of age, gender, and obesity on midazolam kinetics. Anesthesiology 1984; 61:27–35.

118. Holazo AA, Winkler MB, Patel IH. Effects of age, gender and oral contraceptives on intramuscular midazolam pharmacokinetics. J Clin Pharmacol 1988; 28:1040–1045.

119. Kinirons MT, O'Shea D, Kim RB, Groopman JD, Thummel KE. Failure of erythromycin breath test to correlate with midazolam clearance as a probe of cytochrome P4503A. Clin Pharmacol Ther 1999; 66:224–231.

120. Lown KS, Thummel KE, Benedict PE, et al. The erythromycin breath test predicts the clearance of midazolam. Clin Pharmacol Ther 1995; 57:16–24.

121. Nishiyama T, Matsukawa T, Hanaoka K. The effects of age and gender on the optimal premedication dose of intramuscular midazolam. Anesth Analg 1998; 86:1103–1108.

122. Kashuba AD, Bertino JS Jr, Rocci ML Jr, et al. Quantification of 3-month intraindividual variability and the influence of sex and menstrual cycle phase on CYP3A activity as measured by phenotyping with intravenous midazolam. Clin Pharmacol Ther 1998; 64:269–277.

123. Gorski JC, Jones DR, Haehner-Daniels BD, et al. The contribution of intestinal and hepatic CYP3A to the interaction between midazolam and clarithromycin. Clin Pharmacol Ther 1998; 64:133–143.

124. Greenblatt DJ, Locniskar A, Scavone JM, et al. Absence of interaction of cimetidine and ranitidine with intravenous and oral midazolam. Anesth Analg 1986; 65:176–180.

125. Austin KL, Mather LE, Philpot CR, McDonald PJ. Intersubject and dose-related variability after intravenous administration of erythromycin. Br J Clin Pharmacol 1980; 10:273–279.

126. Watkins PB, Turgeon DK, Saenger P, et al. Comparison of urinary 6-beta-cortisol and the erythromycin breath test as measures of hepatic P450IIIA (CYP3A) activity. Clin Pharmacol Ther 1992; 52:265–273.

127. Hooper WD, Qing MS. The influence of age and gender on the stereoselective metabolism and pharmacokinetics of mephobarbital in humans. Clin Pharmacol Ther 1990; 48:633–640.

128. Kristjansson F, Thorsteinsson SB. Disposition of alprazolam in human volunteers: differences between genders. Acta Pharm Nord 1991; 3:249–250.

129. Pritchard J, Bryson J, Kernodle A, Benedetti T, Powell J. Age and gender effects on ondansetron pharmacokinetics: evaluation of healthy aged volunteers. Clin Pharmacol Ther 1992; 51:51–55.

130. Nafziger A, Bertino J. Sex-related differences in theophylline pharmacokinetics. Eur J Clin Pharmacol 1989; 37:97–100.

131. Lew KH, Ludwig EA, Milad MA, et al. Gender-based effects on methylprednisolone pharmacokinetics and pharmacodynamics. Clin Pharmacol Ther 1993; 54:402–414.

132. Hulst L, Fleishaker J, Peters G, Harry J, Wright D, Ward P. Effect of age and gender on tirilazad pharmacokinetics in humans. Clin Pharmacol Ther 1994; 55:378–384.

133. Greenblatt DJ, Harmatz JS, von Moltke LL, Wright CE, Shader RL. Age and gender effects on the pharmacokinetics and pharmacodynamics of triazolam, a cytochrome P450 3A substrate. Clin Pharmacol Ther 2004; 76:467–479.

134. Kang D, Verotta D, Krecic-Shepard ME, Modi NB, Gupta SK, Schwartz JB. Population analyses of sustained-release verapamil in patients: effects of sex, race, and smoking. Clin Pharmacol Ther 2003; 73:31–40.

135. Gupta SK, Atkinson L, Tu T, Longstreth JA. Age and gender related changes in stereoselective pharmacokinetics and pharmacodynamics of verapamil and norverapamil. Br J Clin Pharmacol 1995; 40:325–331.
136. Sasaki M, Tateishi T, Ebihara A. The effects of age and gender on the stereoselective pharmacokinetics of verapamil. Clin Pharmacol Ther 1993; 54:278–285.
137. Sawicki W. Pharmacokinetics of verapamil and norverapamil from controlled release floating pellets in humans. Eur J Pharm Biopharm 2002; 53:29–35.
138. Cummins CL, Wu CY, Benet LZ. Sex-related differences in the clearance of cytochrome P450 3A4 substrates may be caused by P-glycoprotein. Clin Pharmacol Ther 2002; 72:474–489.
139. Bock K, Schrenk D, Forster A. et al. The influence of environmental and genetic factors on CYP2D6, CYP1A2 and UDP-glucuronosyltransferases in man using sparteine, caffeine, and paracetamol as probes. Pharmacogenetics 1994; 4:209–218.
140. May DG, Porter J, Wilkinson G, et al. Frequency distribution of dapsone N-hydroxylase, a putative probe for P4503A4 activity, in a white population. Clin Pharmacol Ther 1994; 55:492–500.
141. Pollock B, Altieri L, Kirshner M, et al. Debrisoquine hydroxylation phenotyping in geriatric psychopharmacology. Psychopharmacol Bull 1992; 28:163–168.
142. Labbe L, Sirois C, Pilote S, et al. Effect of gender, sex hormones, time variables, and physiological urinary pH on apparent CYP2D6 activity as assessed by metabolic ratios of marker substrates. Pharmacogenetics 2000; 10:425–438.
143. Ronfeld R, Tremaine L, Wilner K. Pharmacokinetics of sertraline and its N-demethyl metabolite in elderly and young male and female volunteers. Clin Pharmacokinet 1997; 32S:22–30.
144. Abernethy D, Greenblatt D, Shader R. Imipramine and desipramine disposition in the elderly. J Pharmacol Exp Ther 1985; 232:183–188.
145. Timmer CJ, Sitsen JM, Delbressine LP. Clinical pharmacokinetics of mirtazapine. Clin Pharmacokinet 2000; 38:461–474.
146. Walle T, Byington R, Furberg C, et al. Biologic determinants of propranolol disposition: results from 1308 patients in the beta-blocker heart attack trial. Clin Pharmacol Ther 1985; 38:509–518.
147. Hong-Guang X, Xiu C. Sex differences in pharmacokinetics of oral propranolol in healthy Chinese volunteers. Acta Pharmacol Sin 1995; 16:468–470.
148. Gex-Fabry M, Balant-Gorgia A, Balant L, et al. Clomipramine metabolism: model-based analysis of variability factors from drug monitoring data. Clin Pharmacokinet 1990; 19:241–255.
149. Dahl M, Bertilsson L, Nordin C. Steady-state plasma levels of nortriptyline and its 10-hydroxy metabolite: relationship to the CYP2D6 genotype. Psychopharmacology (Berlin) 1996; 123:315–319.
150. Lam LCW, Garcia-Barcelo MM, Ungvari GS, et al. Cytochrome P450 2D6 genotyping and association with tardive dyskinesia in Chinese schizophrenic patients. Pharmacopsychiatry 2001; 34:238–241.
151. Tamminga A, Wemer J, Oosterhuis B, et al. CYP2D6 and CYP2C19 activity in a large population of Dutch healthy volunteers: indications for oral contraceptive-related gender differences. Eur J Clin Pharmacol 1999; 55:177–184.

152. Laine K, Tybring G, Bertilsson L. No sex-related differences but significant inhibition by oral contraceptives of CYP2C19 activity as measured by the probe drugs mephenytoin and omeprazole in healthy Swedish white subjects. Clin Pharmacol Ther 2000; 68:151–159.

153. Szumlanski C, Honchel R, Scott M, et al. Human liver thiopurine methyltransferase pharmacogenetics: biochemical properties, liver—erythrocyte correlation and presence of isozymes. Pharmacogenetics 1992; 2:148–159.

154. Klemetsdal B, Tollefsen E, Loennechen T, et al. Interethnic differences in thiopurine methyltransferase activity. Clin Pharmacol Ther 1992; 51:24–31.

155. Walle T, Walle U, Cowart T, et al. Pathway-selective sex differences in the metabolic clearance of propranolol in human subjects. Clin Pharmacol Ther 1989; 46:257–263.

156. Johnson J, Akers W, Herring V, et al. Gender differences in labetalol kinetics: importance of determining stereoisomer kinetics for racemic drugs. Pharmacotherapy 2000; 20:622–628.

157. Lennard L, Lilleyman J, Van Loon J, et al. Genetic variation in response to 6-mercaptopurine for childhood acute lymphoblastic leukaemia. Lancet 1990; 336: 225–229.

158. Chessells J, Richards S, Bailey C, et al. Gender and treatment outcome in childhood lymphoblastic leukaemia: report from the MRC UKALL trials. Br J Haematol 1995; 89:364–372.

159. Lennard L, Welch J, Lilleyman J. Thiopurine drugs in the treatment of childhood leukaemia: the influence of inherited thiopurine methyltransferase activity on drug metabolism and cytotoxicity. Br J Clin Pharmacol 1997; 44:455–461.

160. Relling M, Lin J, Ayers G, et al. Racial and gender differences in N-acetyltransferase, xanthine oxidase, and CYP1A2 activities. Clin Pharmacol Ther 1992; 52:643–658.

161. Miners J, Robson R, Birkett D. Gender and oral contraceptive steroids as determinants of drug glucuronidation: effects on clofibric acid elimination. Br J Clin Pharmacol 1984; 18:240–243.

162. Greenblatt D, Abernethy D, Matlis R, et al. Absorption and disposition of ibuprofen in the elderly. Arthritis Rheum 1984; 27:1066–1069.

163. Divoll M, Abernethy D, Ameer B, et al. Acetaminophen kinetics in the elderly. Clin Pharmacol Ther 1982; 31:151–156.

164. Abernethy D, Divoll M, Greenblatt D. Obesity, sex, and acetaminophen disposition. Clin Pharmacol Ther 1982; 31:151–156.

165. Macdonald J, Herman R, Verbeeck R. Sex-difference and the effects of smoking and oral contraceptive steroids on the kinetics of diflunisal. Eur J Clin Pharmacol 1990; 38:175–179.

166. Miners J, Attwood J, Birkett D. Influence of sex and oral contraceptive steroids on paracetamol metabolism. Br J Clin Pharmacol 1983; 16:503–509.

167. Lu Z, Zhankg R, Diasio R. Population characteristics of hepatic dihydropyrimidine dehydrogenase activity, a key metabolic enzyme in 5-fluorouracil chemotherapy. Clin Pharmacol Ther 1995; 58:512–522.

168. Port R, Daniel B, Ding R, et al. Relative importance of dose, body surface area, sex, and age for 5-fluorouracil clearance. Oncology 1991; 48:277–281.

169. Zalcberg J, Kerr D, Seymour L, et al. Haematological and non-haematological toxicity after 5-fluorouracil and leucovorin in patients with advanced colorectal cancer is significantly associated with gender, increasing age and cycle number. Eur J Cancer 1998; 34:1871–1875.

170. Milano G, Cassuto-Viguier E, Thyss A, et al. Influence of sex and age on fluorouracil clearance. J Clin Oncol 1992; 10:1171–1175.

171. Meibohm B, Beierle I, Derendorf H. How important are gender differences in pharmacokinetics? Clin Pharmacokinet 2002; 41:329–342.

172. Rowland M, Tozer T. Clinical Pharmacokinetics: Concepts and Applications. 3rd ed. Philadelphia, PA: Williams and Wilkins, 1995.

173. Hermann R, Ferron GM, Erb K, et al. Effects of age and sex on the disposition of retigabine. Clin Pharmacol Ther 2003; 73:61–70.

174. Gross J, Friedman R, Azevedo M. Effects of age and sex on glomerular filtration rate measured by 51Cr-EDTA. Braz J Med Biol Res 1992; 25:129–134.

175. Cockcroft DW, Gault MH. Prediction of creatinine clearance from serum creatinine. Nephron 1976; 16:31–41.

176. Gaudry SE, Sitar DS, Smyth DD, McKenzie JK, Aoki FY. Gender and age as factors in the inhibition of renal clearance of amantadine by quinine and quinidine. Clin Pharmacol Ther 1993; 54:23–27.

177. Yukawa E, Mine H, Higuchi S, et al. Digoxin population pharmacokinetics from routine clinical data: role of patient characteristics for estimating dosing regimens. J Pharm Pharmacol 1992; 44:761–765.

178. Yukawa E, Honda T, Ohdo S, Higuchi S, Aoyama T. Population-based investigation of relative clearance of digoxin in Japanese patients by multiple trough screen analysis: an update. J Clin Pharmacol 1997; 37:92–100.

179. Yukawa E. New and simple method for estimating metildigoxin dosing regimens by multiple trough screen analysis. Int J Clin Pharmacol Ther 1995; 33:605–611.

180. Ducharme M, Slaughter R, Edwards D. Vancomycin pharmacokinetics in a patient population: effect of age, gender, and body weight. Ther Drug Monit 1994; 16:513–518.

181. Barbhaiya R, Knupp C, Pittman K. Effects of age and gender on pharmacokinetics of cefepime. Antimicrob Agents Chemother 1992; 36:1181–1185.

182. Frame B, Facca B, Nicolau D, Triesenberg SN. Population pharmacokinetics of continuous infusion ceftazidime. Clin Pharmacokinet 1999; 37:343–350.

183. Reigner BG, Welker H. Factors influencing elimination and distribution of fleroxacin: metaanalysis of individual data from 10 pharmacokinetic studies. Antimicrob Agents Chemother 1996; 40:575–580.

184. Godfrey C, Sweeney K, Miller K, Hamilton R, Kremer J. The population pharmacokinetics of long-term methotrexate in rheumatoid arthritis. Br J Clin Pharmacol 1998; 46:369–376.

185. Piotrovsky V, Van Peer A, Van Osselaer N, Armstrong M, Aerssens J. Galantamine population pharmacokinetics in patients with Alzheimer's disease: modeling and simulations. J Clin Pharmacol 2003; 43:514–523.

186. Piotrovsky VK, Huang M-L, Van Peer A, Langenaeken C. Effect of demographic variables on vorozole pharmacokinetics in healthy volunteers and in breast cancer patients. Cancer Chemother Pharmacol 1998; 42:221–228.

187. Csajka C, Marzolini C, Fattinger K, et al. Population pharmacokinetics of indinavir in patients infected with human immunodeficiency virus. Antimicrob Agents Chemother 2004; 48:3226–3232.

188. Mougenot P, Pinguet F, Fabbro M, et al. Population pharmacokinetics of melphalan, infused over a 24-hour period, in patients with advanced malignancies. Cancer Chemother Pharmacol 2004; 53:503–512.

189. Kerbusch T, Wahlby U, Milligan PA, Karlsson MO. Population pharmacokinetic modelling of darifenacin and its hydroxylated metabolite using pooled data, incorporating saturable first-pass metabolism, CYP2D6 genotype and formulation-dependent bioavailability. Br J Clin Pharmacol 2003; 56:639–652.

190. Meineke I, Turck D. Population pharmacokinetic analysis of meloxicam in rheumatoid arthritis patients. Br J Clin Pharmacol 2003; 55:32–38.

191. Gieschke R, Reigner B, Blesch KS, Steimer JL. Population pharmacokinetic analysis of the major metabolites of capecitabine. J Pharmacokinet Pharmacodyn 2002; 29:25–47.

192. Phillips L, Grasela TH, Agnew JR, Ludwig EA, Thompson GA. A population pharmacokinetic-pharmacodynamic analysis and model validation of azimilide. Clin Pharmacol Ther 2001; 70:370–383.

193. Ouellet D, Periclou AP, Johnson RD, Woodworth JR, Lalonde RL. Population pharmacokinetics of pemetrexed disodium (ALIMTA) in patients with cancer. Cancer Chemother Pharmacol 2000; 46:227–334.

194. Bressolle F, Joulia JM, Pinguet F, et al. Circadian rhythm of 5-fluorouracil population pharmacokinetics in patients with metastatic colorectal cancer. Cancer Chemother Pharmacol 1999; 44:295–302.

195. Marino MT, Schuster BG, Brueckner RP, Lin E, Kaminskis A, Lasseter KC. Population pharmacokinetics and pharmacodynamics of pyridostigmine bromide for prophylaxis against nerve agents in humans. J Clin Pharmacol 1998; 38:227–235.

196. Botha JH, du Preez MJ, Miller R, Adhikari M. Determination of population pharmacokinetic parameters for amikacin in neonates using mixed-effect models. Eur J Clin Pharmacol 1998; 53:337–341.

197. Botha JH, Tyrannes I, Miller R, Wesley A. Determination of theophylline clearance in South African children. Eur J Clin Pharmacol 1993; 44:369–375.

198. Driscoll MS, Ludden TM, Casto DT, Littlefield LC. Evaluation of theophylline pharmacokinetics in a pediatric population using mixed effects models. J Pharmacokinet Biopharm 1989; 17:141–168.

199. Bruno R, Vivier N, Montay G, et al. Population pharmacokinetics of riluzole in patients with amyotrophic lateral sclerosis. Clin Pharmacol Ther 1997; 62:518–526.

200. Yukawa E, Honda T, Ohdo S, Higuchi S, Aoyama T. Detection of carbamazepine-induced changes in valproic acid relative clearance in man by simple pharmacokinetic screening. J Pharm Pharmacol 1997; 49:751–756.

201. Yukawa E. A feasibility study of the multiple-peak approach for pharmacokinetic screening: population-based investigation of valproic acid relative clearance using routine clinical pharmacokinetic data. J Pharm Pharmacol 1995; 47:1048–1052.

202. Wade JR, Kelman AW, Kerr DJ, Robert J, Whiting B. Variability in the pharmacokinetics of epirubicin: a population analysis. Cancer Chemother Pharmacol 1992; 29:391–395.

203. Levy G. Predicting effective drug concentrations for individual patients—determinants of pharmacodynamic variability. Clin Pharmacokinet 1998; 34:323–333.
204. Krecic-Shepard ME, Barnas CE, Slimko J, Jones M, Schwartz JB. Gender-specific effects on verapamil pharmacokinetics and pharmacodynamics in humans. J Clin Pharmacol 2000; 40:219–230.
205. Krecic-Shepard ME, Barnas CR, Slimko J, Schwartz JB. Faster clearance of sustained release verapamil in men versus women: continuing observations on sex-specific differences after oral administration of verapamil. Clin Pharmacol Ther 2000; 68:286–292.
206. Craft RM. Sex differences in drug-and non-drug-induced analgesia. Life Sci 2003; 72:2675–2688.
207. Craft RM, Bernal SA. Sex differences in opioid antinociception: kappa and mixed action agonists. Drug Alcohol Depend 2001; 63:215–228.
208. Gordon NC, Gear RW, Heller PH, Paul S, Miaskowski C, Levine JD. Enhancement of morphine analgesia by the GABA-B agonist baclofen. Neuroscience 1995; 69:345–349.
209. Sarton E, Olofsen E, Romberg R, et al. Sex differences in morphine analgesia: an experimental study in healthy volunteers. Anesthesiology 2000; 93:1245–1254.
210. Cepeda MS, Farrar JT, Baumgarten M, et al. Side effects of opioids during short-term administration: effect of age, gender, and race. Clin Pharmacol Ther 2003; 74:102–112.
211. Jamner LD, Girdler SS, Shapiro D, Jarvik ME. Pain inhibition, nicotine, and gender. Exp Clin Psychopharmacol 1998; 6:96–106.
212. Pleym H, Spigset O, Kharasch ED, Dale O. Gender differences in drug effects: implications for anesthesiologists. Acta Anaesthesiol Scand 2003; 47:241–259.
213. Schuttler J, Ihmsen H. Population pharmacokinetics of propofol: a multi-center study. Anesthesiology 2000; 92:727–738.
214. Apfelbaum JL, Grasela TH, Hug CC Jr, et al. The initial clinical experience of 1819 physicians in maintaining anesthesia with propofol: characteristics associated with prolonged time to awakening. Anesth Analg 1993; 77:S10–S14.
215. Gan TJ, Glass PS, Sigl J, et al. Women emerge from general anesthesia with propofol/alfentanil/nitrous oxide faster than men. Anesthesiology 1999; 90:1283–1287.
216. Vuyk J, Oostwouder CJ, Vletter AA, Burm AG, Bovill JG. Gender differences in the pharmacokinetics of propofol in elderly patients during and after continuous infusion. Br J Anaesth 2001; 86:183–188.
217. Palva ES. Gender-related differences in diazepam effects on performance. Med Biol 1985; 63:92–95.
218. Yonkers KA, Kando JC, Cole JO, Blumenthal S. Gender differences in pharmacokinetics and pharmacodynamics of psychotropic medication. Am J Psychiatry 1992; 149:587–595.
219. Yonkers KA, Harrison W. The inclusion of women in psychopharmacologic trials. J Clin Psychopharmacol 1993; 13:380–382.
220. Yonkers KA, Brawman-Mintzer O. The pharmacologic treatment of depression: is gender a critical factor? J Clin Psychiatry 2002; 63:610–615.
221. Chouinard G, Annable L. Pimozide in the treatment of newly admitted schizophrenic patients. Psychopharmacology 1982; 76:13–19.

222. Chouinard G, Annable L, Steinberg S. A controlled clinical trial of fluspirilene, a long-acting injectable neuroleptic, in schizophrenic patients with acute exacerbation. J Clin Psychopharmacol 1986; 6:21–26.

223. Frackiewicz EJ, Sramek JJ, Cutler NR. Gender differences in depression and antidepressant pharmacokinetics and adverse events. Ann Pharmacother 2000; 34:80–88.

224. Kinon BJ, Gilmore JA, Liu H, Halbreich UM. Hyperprolactinemia in response to antipsychotic drugs: characterization across comparative clinical trials. Psychoneuroendocrinology 2003; 28:S69-S82.

225. Dawkins K, Potter WZ. Gender differences in pharmacokinetics and pharmacodynamics of psychotropics: focus on women. Psychopharmacol Bull 1991; 27:417–426.

226. Risch SC, Huey LY, Janowsky DS. Plasma levels of tricyclic antidepressants and clinical efficacy. J Clin Psychiatry 1979; 40:58–69.

227. Davidson J, Pelton S. Forms of atypical depression and their response to antidepressant drugs. Psychiatry Res 1986; 17:87–95.

228. Klompenhouwer JL, Fekkes D, van Hulst AM, Moleman P, Pepplinkhuizen L, Mulder PG. Seasonal variations in binding of 3H-paroxetine to blood platelets in healthy volunteers: indications for a gender difference. Biol Psychiatry 1990; 28:509–517.

229. Mueller EA, Murphy DL, Sunderland T. Neuroendocrine effects of M-chlorophenylpiperazine, a serotonin agonist, in humans. J Clin Endocrinol Metab 1985; 61: 1179–1184.

230. Walker JS, Carmody JJ. Experimental pain in healthy human subjects—gender differences in nociception and in response to ibuprofen. Anesth Analg 1998; 86:1257–1262.

231. Nuutila P, Knuuti MJ, Maki M, et al. Gender and insulin sensitivity in the heart and in skeletal muscles. Studies using positron emission tomography. Diabetes 1995; 44:31–36.

232. Kitler ME. Coronary disease: are there gender differences? Eur Heart J 1994; 15:409–417.

233. Anastos K, Charney P, Charon RA, et al. Hypertension in women: what is really known? Ann Intern Med 1991; 115:287–293.

234. Makkar RR, Fromm BS, Steinman RT, Meissner MD, Lehmann MH. Female gender as a risk factor for torsades de pointes associated with cardiovascular drugs. JAMA 1993; 270:2590–2597.

235. Kassell NF, Haley EC Jr, Apperson-Hansen C, et al. Randomized, double-blind, vehicle-controlled trial of tirilazad mesylate in patients with aneurysmal subarachnoid hemorrhage: a cooperative study in Europe, Australia, and New Zealand. J Neurosurg 1996; 84:221–228.

236. Fleishaker JC, Fiedler-Kelly J, Grasela TH. Population pharmacokinetics of tirilazad: effects of weight, gender, concomitant phenytoin, and subarachnoid hemorrhage. Pharm Res 1999; 16:575–583.

237. Parker CJ, Hunter JM. Pharmacokinetic/pharmacodynamic modelling of atracurium. Br J Anaesth 1993; 70:111–112.

238. Schmith VD, Fiedler-Kelly J, Phillips L, Grasela TH Jr. Prospective use of population pharmacokinetics/pharmacodynamics in the development of cisatracurium. Pharm Res 1997; 14:91–97.

239. Mager DE, Wyska E, Jusko WJ. Diversity of mechanism-based pharmacodynamic models. Drug Metab Dis 2003; 31:510–518.
240. Friberg LE, Brindley CJ, Karlsson MO, Devlin AJ. Models of schedule dependent haematological toxicity of 2′-deoxy-2′-methylidenecytidine (DMDC). Eur J Clin Pharmacol 2000; 56:567–774.
241. Friberg LE, Henningsson A, Maas H, Nguyen L, Karlsson MO. Model of chemotherapy-induced myelosuppression with parameter consistency across drugs. J Clin Oncol 2002; 20:4713–4721.
242. Krzyzanski W, Ramakrishnan R, Jusko WJ. Basic models for agents that alter production of natural cells. J Pharmacokinet Biopharm 1999; 27:467–489.
243. Krzyzanski W, Jusko WJ. Multiple-pool cell lifespan model of hamatologic effects of anticancer agents. J Phamacokinet Pharmacodyn 2002; 29:311–337.
244. Perez-Ruixo JJ, Kimko HC, Chow AT, Piotrovsky V, Krzyzanski W, Jusko WJ. Population cell life span models for effects of drugs following indirect mechanisms of action. J Pharmacokinet Pharmacodyn 2005; 32:767–793.
245. Gieschke R, Burger HU, Reigner B, Blesch KS, Steimer JL. Population pharmacokinetics and concentration-effect relationships of capecitabine metabolites in colorectal cancer patients. Br J Clin Pharmacol 2003; 55:252–263.
246. Roden DM. Drug-induced prolongation of the QT interval. New Eng J Med 2004; 350:1013–1022.
247. De Ponti F, Poluzzi E, Montanaro N. QT-interval prolongation by non-cardiac drugs: lessons to be learned from recent experience. Eur J Clin Pharmacol 2000; 56:1–18.
248. Haddad PM, Anderson IM. Antipsychotic-related QTc prolongation, Torsade de Pointes and sudden death. Drugs 2002; 62:1649–1671.
249. Owens RC. QT prolongation with antimicrobial agents—understanding the significance. Drugs 2004; 64:1091–1124.
250. Sheridan DJ. Drug-induced proarrhythmic effects: assessment of changes in QT interval. Br J Clin Pharmacol 2000; 50:297–302.
251. Mayuga KA, Parker M, Sukthanker ND, Perlowski A, Schwartz JB, Kadish AH. Effects of age and gender on the QT response to exercise. Am J Cardiol 2001; 87:163–167.
252. Salazar DE, Much DR, Nichola PS, Seibold JR, Shindler D, Slugg PH. A pharmacokinetic-pharmacodynamic model of d-sotalol QTc prolongation during intravenous administration to healthy subjects. J Clin Pharmacol 1997; 37:799–809.
253. Steimer J-L, Vozeh S, Racine-Poon A, Holford N, O'Neill R. The population approach: rationale, methods and applications in clinical pharmacology and drug development. In: Welling PG, Balant LP, eds. Pharmacokinetics of Drugs. Berlin: Springer-Verlag, 1994:405–450.
254. Corey A, Agnew J, Brum J, Parekh N, Valentine S, Williams M. Pharmacokinetics and pharmacodynamics following intravenous doses of azimilide dihydrochloride. J Clin Pharmacol 1999; 39:1263–1271.
255. Shi J, Ludden TM, Melikian AP, Gastonguay MR, Hinderling PH. Population pharmacokinetics and pharmacodynamics of sotalol in pediatric patients with supraventricular or ventricular tachyarrhythmia. J Pharmacokinet Pharmacodyn 2001; 28:555–575.

256. Malik M, Camm AJ. Evaluation of drug-induced QT interval prolongation—Implications for drug approval and labelling. Drug Safety 2001; 24:323–351.
257. Malik M. If Dr. Bazett had had a computer ... Pacing Clin Electrophysiol 1996; 19:1635–1639.
258. Batchvarov VN, Ghuran A, Smetana P, et al. QT-RR relationship in healthy subjects exhibits substantial intersubject variability and high intrasubject stability. Am J Physiol—Heart Circ Physiol 2002; 282:H2356-H2363.
259. Piotrovsky V. Pharmacokinetic-pharmacodynamic modeling in the data anlysis and interpretation of drug-induced QT/QTc prolongation. AAPS J. 2005; 7:Article 63. http://www.aapsj.org/view.asp?art=aapsj070363.
260. Reilly JJ, Workman P. Normalisation of anti-cancer drug dosage using body weight and surface area: is it worthwhile? A review of theoretical and practical considerations. Cancer Chemother Phrmacol 1993; 32:411–418.
261. Deleu D. Aarons L. Ahmed IA. Population pharmacokinetics of free carbamazepine in adult Omani epileptic patient. Eur J Clin Pharmacol 2001; 57:243–248.
262. Gobburu JVS, Tammara V, Lesko L, et al. Pharmacokinetic-pharmacodynamic modeling of rivastigmine, a cholinesterase inhibitor, in patients with Alzheimer's disease. J Clin Pharmacol 2001; 41: 1082–1090.
263. Huitema ADR, Mathot RAA, Tibben MM, Schellens JHM, Rodenhuis S, Beijnen JH. Population pharmacokinetics of thioTEPA and its active metabolite TEPA in patients undergoing high-dose chemotherapy. Br J Clin Pharmacol 2001; 51:61–70.
264. Jackson KA, Rosenbaum SE, Kerr BM, Pithavala YK, Yuen G, Dudley MN. A population pharmacokinetic analysis of nelfinavir mesylate in human immunodeficiency virus-infected patients enrolled in a Phase III clinical trial. Antimicrob Agents Chemother 2000; 44:1832–1837.
265. Jorga K, Fotteler B, Banken L, Snell P, Steimer JL. Population pharmacokinetics of tolcapone in parkinsonian patients in dose finding studies. Br J Clin Pharmacol 2000; 49:39–48.
266. Lesko LJ, Rowland M, Peck CC, Blaschke TF. Optimizing the science of drug development: Opportunities for better candidate selection and accelerated evaluation in humans. Pharmaceut Res 2000; 17:1335–1344.
267. Heerdink ER, Urquhart J, Leufkens HG. Changes in prescribed drug doses after market introduction. Pharmaceoepidemiol Drug Safety 2002; 1:447–453.
268. Reigner BG, Williams PEO, Patel JH, Steimer JL, Peck C, Vanbrummelen P. An evaluation of the integration of pharmacokinetic and pharmacodynamic principles in clinical drug development—experience within Hoffmann-La-Roche. Clin Pharmacokinet 1997; 33:142–152.
269. Olson SC, Bockbrader H, Boyd RA, et al. Impact of population pharmacokinetic-pharmacodynamic analyses on the drug development process—experience at Parke-Davis. Clin Pharmacokinet 2000; 38:449–459.
270. Chaikin P, Rhodes GR, Bruno R, Rohatagi S, Natarajan C. Pharmacokinetics/pharmacodynamics in drug development: An industrial perspective. J Clin Pharmacol 2000; 40(12 Part 2):1428–1438.
271. Meibohm B, Derendorf H. Pharmacokinetic/pharmacodynamic studies in drug product development. J Pharm Sci 2002; 91:18–31.

272. Bonate PL. Clinical trial simulation in drug development. Pharmaceut Res 2000; 17:252–256.

273. Bruno R, Vivier N, Vergniol JC, De Phillips SL, Montay G, Sheiner LB. A population pharmacokinetic model for docetaxel (Taxotere): model building and validation. J Pharmacokinet Biopharm 1996; 24:153–172.

274. Bruno R, Hille D, Riva A, et al. Population pharmacokinetics/pharmacodynamics of docetaxel in phase II studies in patients with cancer. J Clin Oncol 1998; 16:187–196.

275. Veyrat-Follet C, Bruno R, Olivares R, Rhodes GR, Chaikin P. Clinical trial simulation of docetaxel in patients with cancer as a tool for dosage optimization. Clin Pharmacol Ther 2000; 68:677–687.

276. Lockwood PA, Cook JA, Ewy WE, Mandema JW. The use of clinical trial simulation to support dose selection: Application to development of a new treatment for chronic neuropathic pain. Pharmaceut Res 2003; 20:1752–1759.

277. McLean MJ. Clinical pharmacokinetics of gabapentin. Neurology 1994; 44(6 Suppl. 5):17–22.

278. Mandema J, Wang W. Use of modeling and simulation to optimize dose-finding strategies. In: Kimko HC, Duffull SB, eds. Simulation for Designing Clinical Trials. A Pharmacokinetic-Pharmacodynamic Modeling Perspective. New York: Marcel Dekker, 2003:289–312.

279. Kimko HC, Reele SSB, Holford NHG, Peck CC. Prediction of the outcome of a phase 3 clinical trial of an antischizophrenic agent (quetiapine fumarate) by simulation with a population pharmacokinetic and pharmacodynamic model. Clin Pharmacol Therapeut 2000; 68:568–577.

280. Piotrovsky V. Drug efficacy analysis as an exercise in dynamic (indirect-response) population PK–PD modeling. Abstracts of the Annual Meeting of the Population Approach Group in Europe, Paris 2002, Abstr 305. ISSN 1871-6032. http://www.page-meeting.org/?abstract=305.

281. Piotrovsky V. Indirect-response model for the analysis of concentration-effect relationships in clinical trials where response variables are scores. Abstracts of the Annual Meeting of the Population Approach Group in Europe, Pamplona, 2005. Abstr 773. ISSN 1871-6032. http//www.page-meeting.org/?abstract=773.

282. Innovation or Stagnation: Challenge and Opportunity on the Critical Path to New Medical Products. The US FDA, 2006. http//www.fda.gov/oc/initiatives/criticalpath/whitepaper.html

8

Pharmacogenetics (PGx) and Dose Response: Dose Individualization

Wolfgang M. Schmidt and Markus Müller
Department of Clinical Pharmacology, Medical University of Vienna, Vienna, Austria

SUMMARY

Recent achievements in molecular genetics have led to a substantial accumulation of knowledge about the mechanisms of interindividual variability in drug response. According to a recent report of the British Department of Health, the greatest impact of novel genetic tools and technologies will be realized in the field of pharmacogenomics (1). Pharmacogenomics is set to provide a relevant contribution to our understanding of adverse drug reactions and non-responsiveness to drug therapy. The most intriguing application of pharmacogenomics in drug treatment will likely change the way in which we apply drugs to routine care. It is widely proposed that genetic information of individuals could be used to avoid "trial-and-error" scenarios during medication. Based on genotype-based dose recommendations, medicine is expected to evolve from the commonly used "one dose fits all" strategy to a patient-tailored drug selection and dose optimization. So far, however, most promises related to the vision of individualized therapies have remained unfulfilled. The greatest challenges for the field of pharmacogenomics relate to the issues of genotype–phenotype and genotype–environment interactions, optimal selection of study designs, predictivity and ethical aspects. Besides other factors, such as drug interactions or poor compliance, pharmacogenetic variability constitutes a potentially relevant factor for drug response variability. Although its current impact on the routine of medicine is minimal, pharmacogenomics might, thus, provide useful contributions to the future practice of drug therapy.

INTRODUCTION

A Primer to the *"Omics"* Sciences

Ambitious genome sequencing projects, powered by significant technological advances, resulted in the successful deciphering of the genetic information of the human and many other organisms during the past decade (2,3). The genetic information of an organism in its entirety can now be described by an exact order of base pairs within the DNA sequence. The human genome contains ~3.2 billions of base pairs, organized into 23 chromosomes, each holding between 47 million and 246 million base pairs and containing ~30,000 genes. While the genome of any living organism harbors the complete genetic information in terms of both structural and functional blueprints of life, each cell, carrying out specific roles, makes use of RNA, which serves as "working copy" during protein synthesis. During the process of gene expression, a gene is transcribed into an RNA copy, which is then processed to a mature, active messenger RNA (mRNA) copy that contains the exact plan needed for the synthesis of the protein encoded by the gene. The total mRNA content of a human cell, the transcriptome, is estimated to consist of ~100,000 different gene transcripts. Compared with the total gene count, the higher number of transcripts is a result of alternations and shuffling introduced during mRNA maturation, for example, by alternative splicing. The total protein content in a given cell, tissue or organism, the proteome, is even an additional order of magnitude higher: the human proteome is estimated to contain up to 1 million different protein species.

Initiated by *"genomics"* research, the life science scene has seen the creation of several other *"omics"* research fields. While genomics usually includes both, the genome-wide analysis of gene function and the global analysis of gene activity (*"transcriptomics"*), *"proteomics"* research includes the assessment of protein content, activity, modification, localization, and interaction. Proteomics is a rapidly growing discipline, enabled by highly sophisticated technology, such as protein chips (4), and holds significant promise to refine our understanding of cellular processes in health and disease. Genomics- and proteomics-based approaches will benefit clinical research by driving both the discovery of new drug targets and the development of new diagnostic markers (5,6).

The *"omics"* confusion did not stop in front of the world of small molecules. Recently, the terms *"metabonomics"* and *"metabolomics"* have been coined. Metabonomics comprises techniques (usually based on NMR technology) for examining dynamic changes in the metabolome, the small molecular inventory of the cell, and targets metabolites or important cellular compounds, such as nucleotides, vitamins, or catecholamines. Thus, metabonomics and metabolomics constitute an interface between genomics, proteomics, and chemical biology and will also play an important role in the future development of drugs (7,8).

PGx and Pharmacogenomics: A Definition and Short History

Although the terms pharmacogenetics (PGx) and pharmacogenomics are often used interchangeably, they do not exactly match. While genetics looks at single genes, genomics is trying to look at all genes globally and to determine how they interact and influence biological pathways. PGx can best be defined as the discipline based on the identification of genetic variations (polymorphisms) that affect the inherited response to drugs, aiming at providing molecular genetics-based diagnostic tests that can be used to personalize drug treatment (9,10). Pharmacogenetic research is usually focusing on genetic polymorphisms in genes encoding drug-metabolizing enzymes, drug targets, receptors, and transporters. Pharmacogenomics aims at an even more ambitious goal, that is, analyzing a multitude of genes in parallel to assess the transcriptome. Pharmacogenomics-based research would, for instance, include the application of genome-wide expression profiling approaches, such as the GeneChip technology, which can be deployed to simultaneously assess the activity of thousands of genes at the RNA level (11). This allows for study of the total gene expression output of cells in order to discern functions and interplay of genes, for example, in response to different drugs and/or doses. Thus, pharmacogenomics usually refers to the field of novel drug discovery and development. Genomics-based approaches, however, will also help to tailor drug therapies based on a patient's individual genetic trait.

Historically, it has long been recognized that patients show substantial variability in their response to drugs and that unusual drug responses may be clustered in families. These observations have led to the notion that at least some part of the variability in response to therapeutic interventions may be inherited. This view was also supported by Karl Landsteiner's discovery of blood groups in 1901. Concepts about genetically determined reagibility to exogenous compounds in a narrower sense were first formulated by Archibald Garrod in the thirties, and pursued by phenotype studies by Vogel and Motulsky in the fifties, and by twin studies by Vesell and Page in the sixties (12,13). The first routine aspect of PGx, albeit rather on a proteomic level, was screening for a genetic deficiency in glucose-6-phosphate dehydrogenase (14). Other notable milestones were the recognition of a close relationship between inherited deficiencies in serum cholinesterase and susceptibility to muscle relaxants by Kalow and Genest in 1957 and the description of "slow" and "rapid" metabolizers in 1960. The era of molecular PGx started with the cloning and characterization of the gene encoding the drug-metabolizing enzyme, debrisoquine hydroxylase, which is identical with cytochrome P (CYP) 450 2D6 (15). This event triggered the discovery of many other genetic variants of metabolizing enzymes and drug targets, fueling the emerging science of PGx.

With the increased understanding of molecular biology and the completion of the sequence of the entire human genome (2,3), the concept of studying the whole genome to predict drug action became feasible and was termed *pharmacogenomics* (16). Today, pharmacogenomics pursues two main goals (17–21): first, the pharmaceutical industry devotes intense efforts into pharmacogenomics for drug target characterization in drug development (19). Present drug therapy targets only about 500 molecules, but genomic target validation may help to exploit a theoretical number of ~30,000 protein targets for drug therapy. The second line of research aims at elucidating the genetic basis for predicting drug responses in routine care. Conceptually, this process follows two different approaches. The traditional approach in detecting a pharmacogenetic trait was based on the observation of a relevant phenotype, that is, an unusual drug response in a patient or an unusual metabolic phenotype, for example, by measuring metabolite ratios in plasma or urine. Consecutively, individual patients or families were studied to elucidate inheritance patterns and to identify a responsible gene. This could be achieved by candidate gene approaches or by screening techniques, such as differential display or positional cloning strategies. In contrast, strategies in the *"post-genomic"* era capitalize on databases generated from the human genome project, comprising ~30,000 genes, to identify polymorphisms or mutations that are associated with drug response phenotypes (20,21). The mechanisms involved in potential genotype–phenotype associations need not necessarily be known a priori. This approach allows for the localization of genetic traits by statistical association to specific regions in the genome and enables identification of allelic variants that have only subtle clinical consequences. These are most often characterized by point mutations, which cannot be visualized cytogenetically. Therefore, the identification and analysis of such genetic variation is pivotal to post-genomic approaches.

Genetic Variation in the Human Genome: The Basis of PGx

To date, it is estimated that the human genome harbors approximately 20,000–25,000 genes, a surprisingly low number, meaning that only a small percentage of the genome (~3%) consists of (known) functional roles. Embedded into large stretches of non-coding DNA and many thousands of interspersed repeats (often called "junk DNA"), approximately every 60–100 kbps, there are stretches of DNA encoding a functional product, namely genes. Genes can exist in alternative forms, the so-called alleles. Because each individual inherits two different alleles, one from each parent's chromosomes, the genetic constitution is built up from either homozygous (two identical, either normal or variant alleles) or heterozygous (the normal and the variant allele) genotypes. Except for monozygotic twins, humans differ on average in every 100th to 1000th of the total 3.2×10^9 base pairs per haploid genome. Different alleles arise from mutations, caused either de novo by spontaneous changes in the DNA sequence or by DNA damage. Among those mutations, three major types can be distinguished, namely: (*i*) insertions/deletions, (*ii*) repeat length variations in repetitive DNA (called mini- and microsatellites), and (*iii*) point mutations. Depending on the exact nature, a mutation might cause the synthesis of an altered or inactive protein. Genetic sequence variations occurring with higher frequency among individuals or populations are called polymorphisms. The human genome is scattered with millions of such polymorphisms (22), most of them are bi-allelic and affect a single nucleotide, the so-called single-nucleotide polymorphisms (SNPs). It is estimated that the human genome between any two individuals is identical by only 99.9%; SNPs account for the majority of the genetic variation within human populations and constitute the molecular basis for interindividual variation of inherited traits. SNPs significantly contribute to the dynamics of genomes and can be regarded as the driving force of evolution (23,24). The relationship between SNPs and possibly associated changes in gene function is illustrated (Fig. 1).

By definition, genes are considered genetically *"polymorphic"* if at one given locus more than one allelic variant occurs with a frequency of >1% in a certain population. Because only a minor fraction of the genome contains coding sequence, many of these polymorphisms, of which more than 10 million can be expected to exist in the human genome, can be considered *"silent"* without any functional effect. However, SNPs serve as genetic markers because they are inherited together if they reside in close physical proximity on a chromosome (linkage disequilibrium, LD). SNPs in LD build haplotypes, between few and several tens of thousands base pair-long genetic blocks that can be used in genotype prediction in order to assess long stretches of DNA sequence instead of measuring every single SNP (25).

There is a continually growing list of polymorphisms found in genes encoding drug-metabolizing enzymes, drug transporters and drug targets, and also disease-modifying genes that have been linked to drug effects in humans. Of the pharmacogenetically important polymorphisms, most rare alleles are associated with reduced activity of an encoded protein, but there are also examples of allelic variants, for example, gene duplications, which lead to enhanced activity.

PGx, DRUG DOSE, AND SAFETY

Genotype-Guided Dose Optimization

The current understanding about how PGx will influence drug dose selection in future clinical routine is most advanced with respect to allelic variants affecting genes that encode drug-metabolizing enzymes, such as the *CYP2D6* and the *CYP2C9* genes. While *CYP2D6* metabolizes ~20–25% of clinically important drugs (26) and affects the pharmacokinetics (PK) of ~50% of the drugs in clinical use (27), *CYP2C9* metabolizes 10–20% of the commonly prescribed drugs (28). A plethora of allelic variants in *CYP2D6* result in either poor, intermediate,

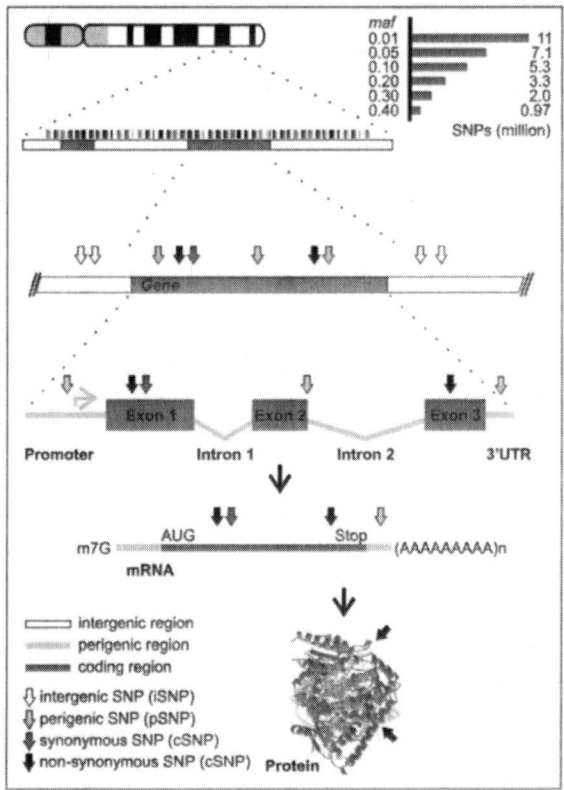

Figure 1   Relationship between SNPs and changes in gene function. To date ∼10 million human SNPs have been identified, ∼4 million of which have been validated as double-hit by the international HapMap consortium (164). It is estimated that ∼5 million SNPs occur with a minor allele frequency (*maf*) of 10%, which equals a prevalence of one every 600 bp. The bar graph schematically plots the estimated number of SNPs in the human genome, occurring with frequencies between 1% and 40% (24). Shown is a typical sub-chromosomal region with scattered, random SNPs (indicated as *vertical lines*). The majority of SNPs are located in intergenic regions (iSNPs, *white arrows*). Perigenic SNPs (pSNPS, *light gray arrows*) are located either inside, or in the flanking regions of genes and affect the promoter, intron, or downstream untranslated (3′-UTR) regions. These SNPs can affect, for example, the transcriptional activity, stability, or correct splicing of the mRNA copy. Coding-region SNPs (cSNPs) affect exon sequences and lead—as "non-synonymous" changes—to an altered amino acid pattern of the gene product (ns-SNPs, *black arrows*). This might ultimately cause, for example, higher, lower or absent enzyme activity (in case of a non-conservative amino acid exchange). It is estimated that every exon within a human gene harbors at least two cSNPs. Non-conservative cSNPs are found at a lower rate and with lower allele frequencies than silent substitutions, likely due to selection during human evolution (165). Note that synonymous codon changes do not change the gene product but can be used—if in linkage disequilibrium due to physical vicinity to functional ns-SNPs—as genetic markers (*dark gray arrows*).

efficient or ultrarapid metabolizer phenotypes and the six common *CYP2C9* genotypes can be correlated either to normal, reduced, or very low enzyme activity. Both genes have been studied extensively and are often cited as well established, classic examples of how predictive genotyping could be applied to dose selection and adjustment during pharmacotherapy. Figure 2 illustrates how the *CYP2C9* genotype, for instance, might be used to predict warfarin dosing requirements in anticoagulant therapy. The *S*-isomer of warfarin, a commonly used vitamin K antagonist, is primarily metabolized by *CYP2C9* through a typical Phase I hydroxylation reaction. The low activity-conferring *CYP2C9* alleles therefore cause a reduction in warfarin metabolism and may explain an increased warfarin drug response in the carriers of these alleles. Clinical studies demonstrated increased plasma levels of *S*-warfarin, decreased clearance, increased frequency of bleeding, and prolongation of hospitalization in patients carrying variant *CYP2C9* genotypes (29). Pharmacogenetic screening may therefore be a perfect means of identifying patients who require lower initiation and maintenance doses of warfarin, and who are at risk for warfarin-associated bleeding and certain drug interactions (28,30–32).

Genetic testing for variants of the *CYP2D6* genotype could be used to identify subjects carrying multiple gene copies. They will metabolize drugs more rapidly; therapeutic drug plasma levels will not be achieved with commonly prescribed drug doses. On the other side, subjects lacking functional *CYP2D6* alleles will metabolize drugs more slowly, indicating lower drug dose requirements and smaller therapeutic effect of pro-drugs activated by *CYP2D6* (33). The genotype–phenotype relationship for the *CYP2D6* gene is shown schematically (Fig. 3). The power of *CYP2D6* genotyping has been shown, for instance, for predicting plasma clearance of antidepressants and neuroleptics, as the dosage of nearly half of the currently used antipsychotics is dependent on the *CYP2D6* genotype (34). A few years ago, first dosing recommendations considering pharmacogenetic differences in drug metabolic capacity were published for a set of antidepressants: for tricyclic antidepressants, for example, the authors recommended dose reductions around 50% for poor metabolizers (35).

Adverse Drug Reactions

Case Study

The issue of inherited differences in response to drugs has recently gained broader attention due to a report in *Fortune Magazine* (36) on the death of a nine-year-old boy. Michael Adams-Conroy, afflicted with the brain damage of fetal alcohol syndrome and attention-deficit hyperactivity disorder, died in 1995 due to a prolonged grand mal seizure. An autopsy showed a massive overdose of fluoxetine, which he was taking to control his emotional outbursts. This finding prompted a murder charge against his parents and led juvenile authorities to take away their other children pending the outcome of a homicide investigation.

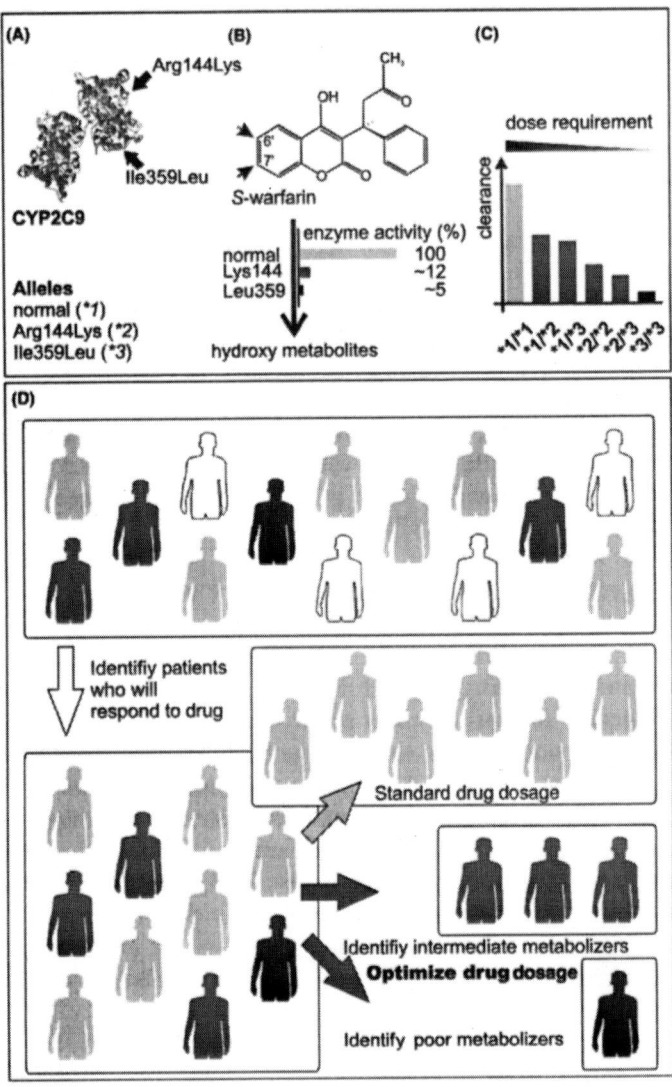

Figure 2 CYP2C9 and warfarin dosing. (**A**) Main *CYP2C9* variants. Two SNPs within the *CYP2C9* gene, called *CYP2C9*2* and *CYP2C9*3*, occur with a frequency of 10–15% and 5–10% of white populations, respectively. Both SNPs are non-synonymous cSNPs (*black arrows*), causing altered gene products (cysteine exchanged for arginine at amino-acid position 144, and leucine for isoleucine at position 359). (**B**) Reduced enzyme activity of CYP2C9 variants. CYP2C9 catalyzes the conversion of *S*-warfarin to 6- and 7-hydroxy metabolites (indicated by *arrows*). The enzyme variants encoded by the variant alleles display markedly reduced activity and impaired hydroxylation (*graph*). The Leu359 variant has a lower affinity and a lower intrinsic clearance for *S*-warfarin 7-hydroxylation (166), while the lower activity of the Cys144 variant probably (*Continued*)

Eventually, it turned out that Michael harbored an unsuspected deficiency in the *CYP2D6* gene that led to drug levels exceeding any previous reports in cases of fluoxetine overdose.

PGx has repeatedly been proposed as diagnostic and predictive tool for preventing adverse drug reactions (ADR) (13,37,38). Approved drugs frequently require a warning statement on the product label because of foreseeable ADRs. Although such warnings are necessary for around 15% of the registered drugs, ADRs still account for 7–13% of all hospital admissions in Europe (39). In the United States, it has been estimated that the overall incidence of serious ADRs is around 6% of the hospitalized patients with ∼100,000 deaths per year, making these reactions a leading cause of death (40,41). Besides their importance in routine drug therapy, ADRs are perhaps the most important reason for attrition in the costly drug development process. These frequent unpredictable reactions to medications seem strongly influenced by genetic factors (13). Some genetic causes of ADRs have been identified, including mutations responsible for anesthetic-induced malignant hyperthermia and for prolonged apnea after succinylcholine administration.

Table 1 lists commonly observed ADRs with relevance to PGx. An important example of a genetic determination of a Phase II reaction is the intolerance to 6-mercaptopurine, a standard anti-ALL (acute lymphoblastic leukemia) drug, due to the deficiency of thiopurine methyltransferase (TPMT) (42). The *TPMT* genotype is associated with risk of relapse in ALL and extreme intolerance has been shown among patients with deficiencies in TPMT activity leading to severe and even fatal cases of bone marrow aplasia. Reducing the dose of 6-mercaptopurine in *TPMT* heterozygotes and use of a full treatment protocol with other types of chemotherapy in deficient patients allows us to maintain high thioguanine nucleotide concentrations.

A recent example of a successful elucidation of a "type-B" reaction based on SNP-mapping is the case of abacavir hypersensitivity (43,44). Hypersensitivity to abacavir, an anti-HIV reverse-transcriptase inhibitor, is a potentially

---

Figure 2 *(Continued)* results from altered interaction of the cytochrome P450 with the NADPH:cytochrome P450 oxidoreductase (167). (**C**) *CYP2C9* genotypes and *S*-warfarin clearance. Together with the reference "wild-type" *CYP2C9* allele, the two variant alleles build six common *CYP2C9* genotypes, which can be correlated either to normal, reduced, or very low enzyme activity (168). The genotype therefore can be correlated to different, individual warfarin dose requirements (28). (**D**) Concept of genotype-guided dose optimization. In a first step, patients who will respond to warfarin are selected, taking into consideration possible drug interactions (169) or specific molecular factors modulating anticoagulant therapy such as, for example, coagulation factor IX (170,171) or factors II and VII (172). In the next step, the *CYP2C9* genotype could be used to stratify patients into poor, intermediate, and normal metabolizers and to predict the likely optimal (starting) dose for therapy.

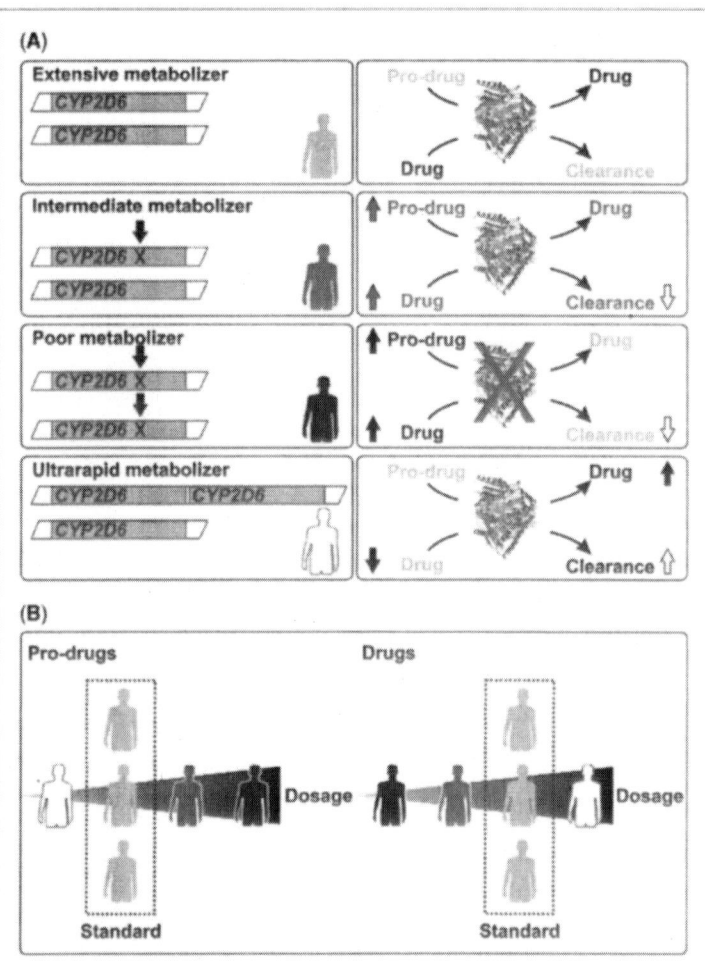

Figure 3 Implications of *CYP2D6* Genotypes for Dose Optimization. (**A**) Simplified relationship between common *CYP2D6* genotypes and metabolizer phenotypes. SNPs within the *CYP2D6* gene (*gray*) conferring low-enzyme activity are indicated as *black vertical arrows* and *x-marks*. While the heterozygous genotype is associated with an intermediate metabolizer phenotype, carriers of the homozygous variant genotype are poor metabolizers. Carriers of multiple gene copies, for example, through gene duplication, present excessive enzyme activity and are ultrarapid metabolizers. Drug clearance is moderately reduced in intermediate and markedly reduced in poor metabolizers, potentially increasing the risk of adverse drug effects. On the other hand, efficacious drug levels may not be achieved in ultrarapid metabolizers due to rapid clearance. In contrast, in the case of pro-drugs, poor metabolizers will likely be non-responders, whereas ultrarapid metabolizers will be at higher risk of adverse drug effects due to excess drug activation at standard drug doses. (**B**) Dose adjustments from standard dosing depending on *CYP2D6* metabolizer status and the type of drug.

Table 1 Examples of Adverse Drug Effects with Relevance to Pharmacogenetics

Gene name	Symbol	Drug (class)	Adverse drug reaction	Reference(s)
Cytochrome P450 2D6	CYP2D6	Antipsychotics Codeine	Extrapyramidal symptoms Intoxication	(84–87) (47)
Cytochrome P450 2C9	CYP2C9	Warfarin Phenytoin Tolbutamide Diphenylhydantoin	Hemorrhage Increased toxicity Hypoglycemia Cutaneous ADR	(29) (88–91) (92,93) (94)
Bradykinin receptor B2	BDKRB2	ACE inhibitors	Therapy-related cough	(95,96)
Dihydropyrimidine dehydrogenase	DPYD	5-Fluorouracil	Severe toxicity	(97–99)
Dopamine receptor D3	DRD3	Antipsychotics	Tardive dyskinesia	(100)
Fc fragment of IgG, low affinity IIa, receptor (CD32)	FCGR2A	Heparin	Heparin-induced thrombocytopenia	(101)
Major histocompatibility complex, class I, B	HLA-B	Abacavir	Toxicity syndromes, hypersensitivity	(43,44); reviewed in (102,103)
"Long QT loci"	KCNQ1, HERG, SCN5A, KCNE1, KCNE2	Antiarrythmics, terfenadine, others	Long QT syndrome, sudden cardiac death	(104,105)
N-acetyltransferase 2	NAT2	Isoniazid, rifampicin	Hepatotoxicity	(106,107)
Thiopurine S-methyltransferase	TPMT	6-Mercaptopurine, thioguanine, azathiopurine	Myelotoxicity	Reviewed in (108–111)
Thymidylate synthase	TYMS	5-Fluorouracil	Toxicity	(112)
UDP glycosyltransferase 1A1	UGT1A1	Irinotecan	Severe toxicity, neutropenia	Reviewed in (113)

life-threatening idiosyncratic ADR affecting ~4% of the patients treated. Abacavir was selected for a proof-of-concept experiment for whole-genome SNP-mapping because the ADR has a typical clinical phenotype and occurs frequently enough to allow identification of sufficient numbers of affected patients and matched controls. The goal of the experiment was to identify a genetic pattern defined by SNPs that are associated with the ADR in patients. Using this approach, polymorphisms in three HLA candidate genes were found to be highly associated with abacavir hypersensitivity. Subsequent clinical studies confirmed the relevance of these loci in that withholding abacavir in individuals with *HLA-B*5701*, *HLA-DR7*, and *HLA-DQ3* reduced the prevalence of hypersensitivity from 9% to 2.5% without withholding abacavir from a patient who would benefit from the drug.

PK AND DRUG METABOLISM

Genetic Variants Affecting PK

Inherited differences in molecules determining PK frequently follow monogenic traits, and in many cases, mutations are inactivating in character. For molecules that apparently do not have critical endogenous substrates, the molecular mechanisms of inactivation include "loss of function" mutations, such as splice mutations resulting in exon skipping, point mutations resulting in early stop codons, or complete gene deletions. Missense mutations causing amino acid substitutions that alter protein stability or catalytic activity and microsatellite nucleotide repeats have also been described. Usually these inactivating mutations affect single proteins and lead to extreme phenotypes with excessively higher plasma concentrations. This is particularly relevant for drugs with a narrow therapeutic index, for example, cancer drugs like mercaptopurine. Although most mutations are inactivating in character, gene duplications may also occur, rendering the resulting phenotype hyperfunctional. This is the case for *CYP2D6* where gene duplications due to unequal cross-over lead to 10 times higher dosing requirements for nortryptiline compared with the wild-type. Table 2 lists examples for genetic variants in genes with functional roles in drug metabolism and PK.

Drug distribution may be affected by membrane transporters, for example, P-glycoprotein (P-gp), the product of the *ABCB1* (formerly called *MDR-1*) gene, which was first identified by its overexpression in various tumors. Later, P-gp was also shown to be expressed in various human tissues involved in gastrointestinal absorption and excretion into the bile. Disruption of one or both *MDR-1* genes in mice was associated with increased bioavailability and reduced urinary clearance and similar results were obtained in humans when P-gp inhibitors were administered. Recently, it was shown that an *MDR-1* gene polymorphism in exon 26 affects absorption of digoxin also in humans (21) and response to antiepileptics (45).

Table 2 Examples of Genetic Variants Affecting Pharmacokinetics

Gene name	Symbol	Variant	Molecular/clinical phenotype	Drug (class)	Reference(s)
ATP-binding cassette, sub-family B (MDR/TAP), member 1	*ABCB1*	C>T Pos. 3435 Exon 26 (Ile1144Ile)	Duodenal expression of *P*-glycoprotein (MDR-1), increased plasma levels	Digoxin, fexofenadine, ciclosporin, talinolol	(21,114,115)
ATP-binding cassette, sub-family C (CFTR/MRP), member 8 (sulfonylurea receptor)	*ABCC8*	Many	Decreased insulin response	Tolbutamide	(116)
Cytochrome P450 11B2	*CYP11B2*	T>C Pos. −344 Promoter	Variations in aldosterone and 11-deoxycortisol production, positive response to candesartan treatment	Candesartan	(117)
Cytochrome P450 2A6	*CYP2A6*	Gross deletions	Poor metabolizer, impaired nicotine metabolism	Tegafur	(118)
Cytochrome P450 2C19	*CYP2C19*	Twenty alleles (nine common variants)	Enzyme deficiency, poor metabolizer	Antidepressants, antipsychotics, proton pump inhibitors	Reviewed in (28,32,119,120)
Cytochrome P450 2C9	*CYP2C9*	Twenty alleles (two common variants)	Intermediate, poor metabolizer, warfarin hypersensitivity	*S*-warfarin, tolbutamide, glipizide, celecoxib, fluvastatin	(28,34)

(Continued)

Table 2 Examples of Genetic Variants Affecting Pharmacokinetics (*Continued*)

Gene name	Symbol	Variant	Molecular/clinical phenotype	Drug (class)	Reference(s)
Cytochrome P450 2D6	*CYP2D6*	Ninety-one alleles	Poor, intermediate, extensive, ultrarapid metabolizers	Many, for example, beta-blockers, analgesics, antiarrythmics, antidepressants, antipsychotics	(27,34,121)
Dihydropyrimidine dehydrogenase	*DPYD*	Many	Enzyme deficiency, 5-fluorouracil toxicity	5-Fluorouracil	(122,123)
N-acetyltransferase 2	*NAT2*	Eight alleles (three common variants)	Slow, intermediate, rapid acetylation	antiarrythmics, procainamide, isoniazid	(124)
Sulfotransferase 1A1	*SULT1A1*	Arg213His	Reduced enzyme activity	Minoxidil	(121)
Thiopurine S-methyltransferase	*TPMT*	Many	Deficiency, toxicity	6-Mercaptopurine, thioguanine, azathiopurine	Reviewed in (108,109)

Most human drug-metabolizing enzymes responsible for modification of functional groups (Phase I reactions) or conjugation with endogenous substituents (Phase II reactions) exhibit common genetic polymorphisms that are clinically relevant. These genetic variants are most likely the result of dietary adaptation to various food challenges by alkaloids or plant toxins (27,39). One reason for the relatively high frequency may be that some enzymes are redundant and thus dispensable for life. The frequency of almost all known polymorphisms differs between the ethnic groups—a finding that proved decisive in the discovery of acetylator subtypes. The most important class of metabolizing enzymes is the cytochrome P450 (CYP) family, in which 58 different CYPs are known. Most CYPs are polymorphic and there are a relatively large number of pseudogenes—that is, archaically conserved genes without function. Only two CYPs, CYP1A1 and CYP2E1, are well conserved—indicating that they have a function in the metabolism of endogenous substrates (39). Interestingly, no mutation causing complete inactivation has been described so far for the main enzyme involved in drug metabolism, namely CYP3A4. In contrast, to date, more than 90 alleles of the *CYP2D6* gene are known for and an important inactivating mutation in the *CYP2D6* gene affects the metabolism of many commonly prescribed drugs in about 6% of the Europeans. Another example of a clinically relevant polymorphism affects the *CYP2C19* gene and occurs predominantly in Asians. This mutation renders omeprazole therapy and eradication of *Helicobacter pylori* much more effective in Japanese as compared with Caucasians (41). Apart from their role in metabolism, drug-metabolizing enzymes may also act as activators of pro-drugs. This is the case for a number of opioids, for example, codeine is activated by the polymorphic enzyme CYP2D6 and carriers of non-functional *CYP2D6* alleles may exhibit varying degrees of codeine resistance (46). In contrast, *CYP2D6* gene duplications lead to enhanced conversion of codeine to morphine and corresponding side-effects (47). Enzymes responsible for Phase I reactions can make substrates more reactive through insertion of oxygen in the molecule. When Phase II reactions are reduced, the phenotype is particularly characterized by a predisposition for ADRs. In addition, some cancers have been linked to polymorphisms in drug-metabolizing enzymes and an impaired ability to inactivate exogenous or endogenous mutagenic molecules (48). Other examples of clinically relevant variants are aldehyde dehydrogenase *ALDH2* mutations causing antabus side-effects following ethanol consumption and long-term cancer risk or dihydropyrimidine-dehydrogenase (*DPYD*) variants leading to increased myelo- and neurotoxicity of 5-fluorouracil.

In contrast to the current knowledge on the genetic determinants in metabolism, our knowledge about inherited aspects of elimination is still limited. In the last decade, a large number of renal transporter proteins have been cloned and their role in the handling of a wide variety of drugs have been established. Expression of the cloned transporters in cell culture systems allows for the examination of the pharmacological efficacy of individual transporter gene products.

It is likely that a similar situation as described for CYP polymorphisms also exists for organic anion transporters (OATs). Indeed, three different polymorphisms have been identified in the human *SLC22A5* gene (formerly called *OCTN2*). Given that as many as half-a-dozen OAT family members may be expressed in the kidney, it is likely that SNPs in these will give rise to different drug elimination phenotypes.

PD AND DRUG EFFICACY

Genetic Variants Affecting PD and Responsiveness

About 30–60% of the patients treated with various drugs do not respond to treatment (39). So far, the reasons for non-responsiveness have largely remained unknown. The presence of non-responsiveness is usually detected clinically and the reasons for the lack of drug effects often remain "idiopathic." PGx studies are expected to bring about a change in this situation. Several publications on PGx of drug targets underline the importance of inherited determinants of drug response and have helped to elucidate the mechanisms responsible.

Pharmacodynamics (PD) focuses on target molecules, that is, receptors or enzymes that determine cellular reactions to drugs and can best be described by the term "events indicating what the drug does to the body." In contrast to PK, the genetic basis of PD is far less well established and results have had a much smaller impact on the practice of drug therapy so far. Information has been mostly obtained by postgenomic genotype-to-phenotype approaches. Inherited differences in molecules determining PD frequently follow polygenic traits. The underlying genetic mutations, such as SNPs in promoters, rarely inactivate a gene but are affecting gene regulation. The effect is mostly subtle, affects multiple proteins, and thus leads to more subtle phenotypes. Presently, there is no established routine application but several proof-of-concept studies have already been published.

A number of functionally polymorphic drug targets that influence pharmacotherapy have been described. Examples of clinically relevant polymorphisms in drug targets comprise the angiotensin-converting enzyme (ACE), the sulfonylurea-, and 5-hydroxtryptamine receptor, apolipoprotein E, and the cholesteryl ester transfer protein. Finally, the risk of ADRs has been linked to genetic polymorphisms that predispose to toxicity, such as dopamine D3 receptor polymorphism and the risk of drug-induced tardive dyskinesia. Other associations have been found for a β2-adrenergic receptor gene polymorphism and drug–response in asthma, drug–response and *CYP2C9* in epilepsia, *P2RY12* mutations and clopidogrel response, and mutations in potassium channel genes and their association with drug-induced QT-prolongation syndromes. Table 3 summarizes important examples of gene variants study with respect to PD and responsiveness to therapy. A genetic variant in α-adducin, for example, a transporter responsible for renal sodium reabsorption, was associated with a lower risk of combined myocardial infarction and stroke during diuretic therapy as compared with the other antihypertensive therapies (17). Another notable example relates to responsiveness to albuterol and a β2-receptor polymorphism (18,49).

Genetic Variants Influencing Dose Selection

With regard to patient-tailored therapies, SNPs within genes encoding either drug targets or key components of pathways are of greatest interest. In recent studies, several such SNPs have been suggested to be predictive of drug selection, which is illustrated by the two following examples. During antihypertensive therapy in patients with left ventricular hypertrophy, for instance, SNPs in the angiotensinogen gene (*AGT*) and the apolipoprotein B (*APOB*) predicted the change in left ventricular mass in response to irbesartan, while a SNP in the α2A-adrenoreceptor gene (*ADRA2A*) was associated with response to the β1-adrenoreceptor blocker atenolol (50). Another SNP within the *APOB* gene was also associated with the blood pressure response to irbesartan but not to atenolol (51). The predictive power of these SNPs could therefore be potentially deployed for the genoytpe-guided selection of either an angiotensin-II type 1 receptor antagonist or beta-blockade-based strategy in antihypertensive therapy. Another important example for genotype-based prediction of response to a specific pharmacotherapy was published recently with regard to total cholesterol reduction in pravastatin therapy. The gene encoding HMG-CoA reductase, the target of pravastatin therapy, was reported to harbor two common SNPs in linkage disequilibrium, which were significantly associated with smaller reductions in cholesterol in heterozygous carriers and, thus, reduced efficacy of pravastatin therapy (52). Genotyping of the *HMGCR* gene could help in selecting patients suitable for additional or alternative therapeutic strategies in cholesterol reduction.

PHARMACOGENOMICS, EXPRESSION SIGNATURES, AND PREDICTIVE BIOMARKERS

Pharmacogenomic identification of non-responders may change the way the pharmaceutical industry is developing and marketing drugs. Over the next few years, pharmaceutical companies are likely to abandon the "chemical blockbuster model" and adopt the "biological individualized" model of drug development. Table 4 lists important examples of recent approaches deploying predictive biomarkers for stratification of patients in order to achieve safer and/or more efficacious therapy. On a similar path, regulators like the FDA are more likely to grant provisional approval on the basis of a surrogate/biomarker measure clinical benefit in a single uncontrolled trial. This will also force industry to define subpopulations of patients who are likely responders. Recent examples include the use of a diagnostic test that detects overexpression of the HER-2 antigen to identify breast cancer patients likely to benefit from herceptin. Although the HER-2

Table 3 Examples of Genetic Variants Affecting Pharmacodynamics

Gene name	Symbol	Variant	Molecular phenotype	Drug (class)	Clinical phenotype	Reference(s)
Angiotensin-1 converting enzyme 1	*ACE*	Ins > Del 286 bp Intron 16	Higher plasma and tissue angiotensin-II	ACE inhibitors, beta-blockers, fosinopril, imidapril, irbesartan, enalapril	Response to antihypertensive therapy	Reviewed in (125,126)
Adducin 1 (alpha)	*ADD1*	Gly460Trp	Renal sodium retaining effect	Thiazide diuretics	Response to salt-sensitive hypertension therapy and salt restriction	(127)
Adrenergic receptor alpha-2A	*ADRA2A*	A1817G		Atenolol	Change in left ventricular mass in response to atenolol	(50)
Adrenergic receptor, beta-1	*ADRB1*	Ser49Gly Gly389Arg	Enhanced down-regulation, enhanced receptor function	Metroprolol, carvedilol, timolol, propanolol	Response to beta-blockade, predisposition and survival in heart failure	(128–131), reviewed in (121,132)

Adrenergic receptor, beta-2	ADRB2	Arg16Gly Gln27Glu Thr164Ile	Enhanced down-regulation, decreased responsiveness	Atenolol, bisoprolol, albuterol	Bronchodilator response to albuterol, response to beta-blockers, higher resting heart rate	(18,133) (49,134–135), reviewed in (126,136)
Angiotensinogen	AGT	Met235Thr	Plasma level of angiotensinogen	ACE inhibitors, irbesatan	Response to ACE inhibitor (mono)therapy, change in left ventricular mass in response to irbesatan	(50,137,138)
Angiotensin-II receptor, type 1	AGTR1	A>C Pos. 1166 3'UTR		ACE inhibitors, losartan	Humoral and renal hemodynamic responses to losartan	(139,140)
Aldehyde dehydrogenase 2	ALDH2	Glu487Lys	Decreased ability to clear acetaldehyde	Antabus (disulfiram)	Ethanol toxicity, long-term cancer risk	(141)
Apolipoprotein B	APOB	C>T Pos. 711 G>A Pos. 10108	Increased cholesterol	Irbesatan	Change in left ventricular mass in response to irbesatan, response to antihypertensive therapy	(50,51)

(Continued)

Table 3 Examples of Genetic Variants Affecting Pharmacodynamics (*Continued*)

Gene name	Symbol	Variant	Molecular phenotype	Drug (class)	Clinical phenotype	Reference(s)
Apolipoprotein E	*APOE*	Cys112Arg (*E4*) Arg158Cys (*E2*)	Increased cholesterol, decreased cholesterol	Tacrine, simvastatin	Interaction with cholesterol in Alzheimer's disease, response to simvastatin therapy	(142,143)
Cholesteryl ester transfer protein, plasma	*CETP*	C>A Pos. −629 Promoter Arg451Gln ("Taq1B1/ B2")	CETP serum level and mass	Statins	Response to statin therapy	(144–146)
Guanine nucleotide-binding protein (G-protein), beta polypeptide 3	*GNB3*	C>T Pos. −92 Exon 10	Increased signal transduction	Endogenous hormones, thiazide, sildenafil, sibutramine	Antihypertensive therapy with diuretics and endothelin blockade, weight loss	Reviewed in (147)

Gene	Symbol	Variant	Effect	Drug	Response	Ref
3-Hydroxy-3-methylglutaryl-Coenzyme A reductase	HMGCR	Chr. 5 Pos. 74726928 (A>T) & 74739571 (T>G)	Unknown	Pravastatin	Response to lipid-lowering therapy	(52)
5-Hydroxytryptamine (serotonin) receptor 2A	HTR2A	Ile197Val	Reduced antagonist sensitivity	Clozapine	Associated with higher dose to inhibit serotonin stimulation	(148)
Integrin, beta-3 (platelet glycoprotein IIIa antigen, CD61)	ITGB3	Leu33Pro	Increased platelet activation	Antiplatelet agents	Sensitivity to aspirin, clopidogrel loading dose in patients with coronary stent	(149,150)
Low-density lipoprotein receptor	LDLR	C>T Pos. 16730		Atenolol	Response antihypertensive therapy	(51)
Matrix metalloproteinase 3 (stromelysin 1)	MMP3	5A>6A Pos. −1171 Promoter	Enhanced activity	5-Fluorouracil, cisplatin	Chemosensitivity in head and neck cancer patients	(151)
Purinergic receptor P2Y 12	P2RY12	Small deletion in codon 238	Platelet ADP receptor defect	Clopidogrel	Bleeding disorder	(152)

Table 4 Examples of Predictive Biomarkers

Predictive test	Biomarker	Drug (therapy)	Reference(s)
Protein-based tests			
Predict clinical benefit from herceptin therapy in breast cancer (approved by the FDA)	*ERBB2* (HER-2)	Trastuzumab (herceptin)	(153)
Screening for all stages of ovarian cancer in high-risk and general populations	Proteomic serum patterns generated by SELDI-TOF-MS	Early detection of neoplastic cells	(154)
Testing for specific gene activity			
Testing for *bcl-2* expression in bladder cancer	*Bcl2*-mRNA expression	Blc2-antisense therapy	(155–157)
Testing for somatic mutations ("oncogenomics")			
Selection for adenoviral gene therapy in patients with head and neck cancers	*TP53* (mutations)	Oncolytic adenovirus	(158–160)
Clinical response of lung-cancer patients to gefitinib	*EGFR* (mutations)	Gefitinib (Iressa)	(19,161)
Clinical response to imatinib in patients with advanced gastrointestinal stromal tumors	*c-KIT/PDGFRA* (mutations)	Imatinib (Gleevec)	(162,163)
Gene expression profiling			
Prediction of outcome in breast cancer, selection of patients who will benefit from adjuvant therapy	72-gene expression signature	Adjuvant therapy in breast cancer	(53,54)
Prediction of therapeutic response to docetaxel in breast cancer	92-gene expression signature	Docetaxel	(55)
Prediction of chemotherapy response in estrogen-receptor positive breast cancer	44-gene expression signature	Tamoxifen	(56)
Prediction of drug resistance in pediatric acute lymphoblastic leukemia	124-gene expression signature	Prednisolone, vincristine, asparaginase, daunorubicin	(57)

test is a "proteomic," rather than a genetic test, it provides a good example of where development is going to be in a few years from now. Recently, it was reported that somatic mutations in the tyrosine kinase genes in patients with non-small cell lung cancer may predict sensitivity to gefitinib (19).

Great potential for genomic testing lies in therapy-specific diagnostics ("theranostics") of the chemotherapy of cancer, where predictive biomarkers can be applied to select patients who will benefit from specific drug treatments. Brilliant examples for such approaches in the therapy of breast cancer have been published during recent years. Nearly 80% of the breast cancer patients undergo adjuvant therapies, designed to destroy remaining cancer cells and prevent metastatic spread. According to two studies, patterns of gene activity within breast cancer cells significantly predicted the aggressiveness of the cancer and the clinical outcome. This gene expression signature outperformed all currently used standard diagnostic criteria in predicting metastasis and overall survival and could therefore be used to predict the need of adjuvant chemotherapy after surgical intervention in breast cancer (53,54). Likewise, other transcriptomics-based tests have been recently published and predict the therapeutic response to docetaxel (55) or response to tamoxifen in estrogen-receptor positive breast cancer (56). Another important example has shown that gene expression values of four different sets of genes predict resistance to drugs commonly used to fight ALL in children (57).

Overall, pharmacogenomic predictivity testing will just constitute part of a larger scheme for "biomarker testing" comprising proteomic and/or genomic approaches (20,58). It is also foreseeable that in the near future, metabonomics might complement genomics on the way to individualized drug therapy (59).

CURRENT CHALLENGES

The euphoria associated with the human genome project and impressive investments by the pharmaceutical industry in pharmacogenomic approaches of drug discovery have triggered high, but as yet unmet, expectations (59–61). Ideally, various technology platforms (62,63) including DNA array technology, high-throughput screening systems, and advanced bioinformatics will allow the tailoring of therapeutic agents targeted for specific and genetically identifiable subgroups of the population. This would represent a shift from the current strategy of developing medications for a statistically optimized fraction of the population to a strategy that aims to provide tailored medications for genetically diverse patients and diseases states that have heterogeneous subtypes. However, much work must be completed before these future insights will have an influence on the daily practice of medicine. Non-critical attitudes and the belief that pharmacogenomics will soon lead to a new era of medicine should be greeted with a "healthy dose of scientific skepticism" (26,59,61,64). This attitude is also supported by recent reports on, for example, difficult definitions of genotypes due to imbalanced expression of SNP alleles (65,66) or on substantial variation of linkage disequilibrium patterns among human populations (67).

To date, significant information is available on the genetic variables of drug metabolism. These data are derived from single gene approaches for selected enzymes and have had a modest impact on routine drug therapy. Genetic variants of metabolic enzymes, however, tend to lead to extreme phenotypes, which is generally not the case for genetic variants involved in later steps of the dose-effect cascade. In general, pharmacological effects seldom follow extreme mono-genic traits, but, more likely, are driven by a complex and subtle interplay of several genes encoding proteins involved in multiple pathways. Studies of *ACE* polymorphisms, for example, have led to conflicting results, which may have been caused by the polygenic nature of the drug effect. To move to a more predictive level, a genomic rather than a genetic strategy must be pursued and it will become important to analyze haplotypes (25,68,69). Per defi-nition, a haplotype is a combination of alleles of closely linked loci that are found in a single chromosome and which tend to be inherited together. Recent data suggests that the average gene has 12 haplotypes, many of which are in linkage disequilibrium. In many cases, a deductive approach to the entire com-plexity of signal transduction cascades will be necessary to define rate-limiting steps. Elucidating genotype–phenotype interactions based on single candidate genes also has the disadvantage that the approach is based on current physiolog-ical knowledge of receptor cascades. Novel approaches employing "whole genome" strategies based on linkage disequilibria and expression profiling (70) appear more suitable for identifying yet unknown outcome markers suitable for forecasting drug response. Given the enormous complexity of the genome, a purely hypothesis-generating approach based on shot-gun high throughput technology will probably generate more questions than answers. Elucidation of genotype–phenotype interactions will become a crucial issue in clinical studies and can only be achieved by studies on humans because of the marked species differences in dose–response cascades in animals.

Apart from the necessity to study multiple genes, there is a need for studying gene–environment interactions. This need is underlined by the fact that there is still considerable variability in drug response in the same genotype. A particular gene or battery of genes may not always be a rate-limiting determi-nant of pharmacological response and will account for a small fraction in the variability of drug–response only. Genetically defective endothelial transporters, for example, may only lead to increased target concentrations if blood flow to the site of action is sufficient to deliver the drug. Other examples where phenotypes may differ in the same genotype involve induction phenomena. This implies that a purely genomic approach to variability in drug response will probably fail and that a multiple faceted approach incorporating physiology, variable transcription rates, and protein function will be more effective.

A number of practical aspects in the design of clinical pharmacogenomic studies deserve closer attention. One important issue is the relatively high number of poorly designed pharmacogenomic studies (39). To provide meaningful data, it will be mandatory to reduce type 2 error by appropriate sample size calculations, to set more stringent p values for declaring statistical significance in multiple hypothesis testing, and to use appropriate control groups (27,28,58,71,72). In genetic association studies, for example, it is necessary to control confounding arising from population stratification. This may be achieved by stratification for demographic factors, for example, home country, by using "genomic control" strategies, that is, data from marker loci across the genome to model the underlying population structure or by comparison of haplotype frequencies in cases and controls. The most appropriate designs for genomics trials comprise cohort studies, case-control studies, and ultimately randomized controlled clinical trials (RCT) for providing evidence that pharmacogenomic approaches improve outcome or save costs. Unfortunately, there is no example available of a large and meaningful RCT which provides evidence for the clinical usefulness of a pharmacogenomic marker, for example, in a standardized clinical study comparing the efficacy and side-effects of genotype-guided versus normal dose selection and optimization.

Another technical aspect relates to the need for collaboration. Although many genetically linked drug reactions, such as, ADRs, are rare, they may be of considerable importance in human health. To obtain adequate numbers of cases, international collaborations must be initiated. Ideally, open access to high-throughput genotyping and SNP genotyping facilities could be provided for all collaborators by a few individual centers and this would reduce costs substantially.

If these initiatives allow us to obtain meaningful clinical information and to move to "predictive-deterministic" rather than probabilistic pharmacogenomics (73), it will become necessary to deal with the issue of prediction accuracy. Given a population of one million and a genotype prevalence of 10%, a test with 95% sensitivity and specificity would give false predictions in one-third of the carriers (74). This is clearly unacceptable, as even the exposure of a low number of subjects to wrong doses may have significant consequences. At a pure genomic level, a satisfactory level of determinism may, possibly, never be achieved due to locus heterogeneity, variable penetrance and expressivity, and other reasons for non-Mendelian inheritance.

Like any genetic test, PGx approaches will be limited by several ethical considerations (75). Some core concerns in this ongoing debate relate to issues of: (*i*) confidentiality, (*ii*) resources, and (*iii*) control (76). This may be illustrated by several questions, that is, (*i*) Is it imperative to anonymize genetic data or should we allow a more open approach to connect person-specific data with data from gene banks? (*ii*) Should the opportunity be provided to patent PGx data (i.e., relevant SNPs)? Will there be obstacles to social insurances for patients with "non-responder" SNPs? (*iii*) Under which circumstances is it necessary to provide information about test results not only to the patient but also to family members?

OUTLOOK

From the patient's perspective, the concept of "pharmacogenomic drug individualization," at first glance, appears promising (77). In contrast to the psychosocial meaning of the widely used terms "personalized" or "individualized" therapy, the PGx and pharmacogenomic concepts facilitate the genotype-guided classification and stratification of patients (78). Theoretically, pharmacogenomic tools may improve drug safety and efficacy and help select optimal drugs for select patients. To fulfill its promise, however, problems of predictivity must be solved and rules must be established to move from a no/yes piece of information to quantitative dosing recommendations. Patients may also express fears about insurance and privacy issues. It is additionally to be kept in mind that providing a definitive and useful test even for a single gene is an enormous challenge and may take many years, as has been demonstrated for *BRCA1* and *BRCA2* (79).

From the perspective of an industry, besides the clear virtues of PGx in streamlining drug discovery and development, it is felt that recent drug development disasters such as rezulin, which caused severe liver damage, terfenadine, which caused cardiotoxicity or cerivastatin, which caused severer rhabdomyolyses, early after-market approval might have been avoided by more carefully selecting patients based on pharmacogenomic differences. In fact, patient selection by genomic or proteomic biomarkers may "rescue" a drug, as in the case of herceptin or abacavir. On the other hand, it was also pointed out that pharmacogenomic concepts threaten to reduce the market share by creating "orphan drugs." Instead of lumping disease entities, pharmacogenomics leads to splitting diseases into new molecular disease entities. Companies might even, for reasons of medical and product liability threats, be obliged to develop a genomic diagnostic test. Overall, pharmacogenomic testing may offer advantages, some of which may increase market share (77). But as pharmacogenomic strategies become a routine part of drug discovery and development, such models should emerge from large-scale clinical trials and follow-up of new medications. Together with the industry, public initiatives—such as the National Institutes of Health-funded Pharmacogenetics Research Network—will contribute a significant drive within the PGx sciences (80).

From a regulatory perspective, the pharmacogenomic concept is encouraging, as it might help to provide drugs with higher effectiveness and a lower safety profile (77). Currently, EMEA and FDA are working on guidance documents for PGx drug applications (81). In a recent FDA publication on the critical path in drug development, it is stated that "emerging techniques of pharmacogenomics and proteomics show great promise for contributing biomarkers to target responders, monitor clinical response, and serve as biomarkers of drug effectiveness. However, much development work and standardization of the biological, statistical, and bioinformatics methods must occur before these techniques can be easily and widely used" (82). In addition, there is a significant need for educating health professionals and the community in order to effectively move PGx into routine medicine (83).

From a third party payer's perspective, pharmacogenomic approaches are laudable, as the current situation of paying for drugs for non-responders is similar to the situation of a customer who is charged the full cost of a dysfunctional CD player in an electronics store. However, some payers may also view pharmacogenomics as a technology that will ultimately increase overall costs (77).

CONCLUSION

The opportunities created by recent conceptual and methodological advances in pharmacogenomics will probably have a significant impact on drug therapy. However, pharmacogenomics is still at the beginning with respect to its clinical application. Overall, it is estimated that pharmacogenomics will have the greatest impact on about 10–15% of the drug therapies where a single gene determines drug–response, followed by 35–40% of the cases with relevant polygenic traits (39). In about 50% of all drug therapies, the impact of pharmacogenomics will prove to be insignificant, due to lack of gene products with functional variants or because environmental influences dominate over the influence of genes (39). For the earlier two situations, it can be envisaged that a fingerprint of the patient's individual genetic profile might guide the selection of optimal drug candidates in individual patients. However, much work must still be completed before these visions will find their way into daily practice.

REFERENCES

1. Genetics White Paper. Our inheritance, our future—realising the potential of genetics in the NHS. http://www.dh.gov.uk/assetRoot/04/01/92/39/04019239.pdf (accessed June 2005).
2. Lander ES, Linton LM, Birren B, et al. Initial sequencing and analysis of the human genome. Nature 2001; 409(6822):860–921.
3. Venter JC, Adams MD, Myers EW, et al. The sequence of the human genome. Science 2001; 291(5507):1304–1351.
4. Espina V, Dettloff KA, Cowherd S, et al. Use of proteomic analysis to monitor responses to biological therapies. Expert Opin Biol Ther 2004; 4(1):83–93.
5. Kramer R, Cohen D. Functional genomics to new drug targets. Nat Rev Drug Discov 2004; 3(11):965–972.
6. Lewin DA, Weiner MP. Molecular biomarkers in drug development. Drug Discov Today 2004; 9(22):976–983.
7. Watkins SM, German JB. Metabolomics and biochemical profiling in drug discovery and development. Curr Opin Mol Ther 2002; 4(3):224–228.
8. Lindon JC, Holmes E, Nicholson JK. Metabonomics and its role in drug development and disease diagnosis. Expert Rev Mol Diagn 2004; 4(2):189–199.
9. Weinshilboum R. Inheritance and drug response. N Engl J Med 2003; 348(6): 529–537.

10. Roses AD. Pharmacogenetics and drug development: the path to safer and more effective drugs. Nat Rev Genet 2004; 5(9):645–656.

11. McGall GH, Christians FC. High-density genechip oligonucleotide probe arrays. Adv Biochem Eng Biotechnol 2002; 77:21–42.

12. Muller M. Pharmacogenomics and drug response. Int J Clin Pharmacol Ther 2003; 41(6):231–240.

13. Phillips KA, Veenstra DL, Oren E, et al. Potential role of pharmacogenomics in reducing adverse drug reactions: a systematic review. J Am Med Assoc 2001; 286(18):2270–2279.

14. Alving AS, Carson PE, Flanagan CL, et al. Enzymatic deficiency in primaquine-sensitive erythrocytes. Science 1956; 124(3220):484–485.

15. Gonzalez FJ, Skoda RC, Kimura S, et al. Characterization of the common genetic defect in humans deficient in debrisoquine metabolism. Nature 1988; 331(6155):442–446.

16. Evans WE, McLeod HL. Pharmacogenomics—drug disposition, drug targets, and side effects. N Engl J Med 2003; 348(6):538–549.

17. Psaty BM, Smith NL, Heckbert SR, et al. Diuretic therapy, the alpha-adducin gene variant, and the risk of myocardial infarction or stroke in persons with treated hypertension. J Am Med Assoc 2002; 287(13):1680–1689.

18. Lima JJ, Thomason DB, Mohamed MH, et al. Impact of genetic polymorphisms of the beta2-adrenergic receptor on albuterol bronchodilator pharmacodynamics. Clin Pharmacol Ther 1999; 65(5):519–525.

19. Sordella R, Bell DW, Haber DA, et al. Gefitinib-sensitizing EGFR mutations in lung cancer activate anti-apoptotic pathways. Science 2004; 305(5687):1163–1167.

20. Lesko LJ, Woodcock J. Translation of pharmacogenomics and pharmacogenetics: a regulatory perspective. Nat Rev Drug Discov 2004; 3(9):763–769.

21. Hoffmeyer S, Burk O, von Richter O, et al. Functional polymorphisms of the human multidrug-resistance gene: multiple sequence variations and correlation of one allele with P-glycoprotein expression and activity in vivo. Proc Natl Acad Sci USA 2000; 97(7):3473–3478.

22. Sachidanandam R, Weissman D, Schmidt SC, et al. A map of human genome sequence variation containing 1.42 million single nucleotide polymorphisms. Nature 2001; 409(6822):928–933.

23. McLeod HL, Evans WE. Pharmacogenomics: unlocking the human genome for better drug therapy. Annu Rev Pharmacol Toxicol 2001; 41:101–121.

24. Kruglyak L, Nickerson DA. Variation is the spice of life. Nat Genet 2001; 27(3):234–236.

25. Johnson GC, Esposito L, Barratt BJ, et al. Haplotype tagging for the identification of common disease genes. Nat Genet 2001; 29(2):233–237.

26. Ingelman-Sundberg M. Pharmacogenetics of cytochrome P450 and its applications in drug therapy: the past, present and future. Trends Pharmacol Sci 2004; 25(4):193–200.

27. Ingelman-Sundberg M. Genetic polymorphisms of cytochrome P450 2D6 (CYP2D6), clinical consequences, evolutionary aspects and functional diversity. Pharmacogenomics J 2005; 5(1):6–13.

28. Kirchheiner J, Brockmoller J. Clinical consequences of cytochrome P450 2C9 polymorphisms. Clin Pharmacol Ther 2005; 77(1):1–16.

29. Aithal GP, Day CP, Kesteven PJ, et al. Association of polymorphisms in the cytochrome P450 CYP2C9 with warfarin dose requirement and risk of bleeding complications. Lancet 1999; 353(9154):717–719.
30. Redman AR. Implications of cytochrome P450 2C9 polymorphism on warfarin metabolism and dosing. Pharmacotherapy 2001; 21(2):235–242.
31. Lee CR. CYP2C9 genotype as a predictor of drug disposition in humans. Methods Find Exp Clin Pharmacol 2004; 26(6):463–472.
32. Rogers JF, Nafziger AN, Bertino JS. Pharmacogenetics affects dosing, efficacy, and toxicity of cytochrome P450-metabolized drugs. Am J Med 2002; 113(9):746–750.
33. Ingelman-Sundberg M, Oscarson M, McLellan RA. Polymorphic human cytochrome P450 enzymes: an opportunity for individualized drug treatment. Trends Pharmacol Sci 1999; 20(8):342–349.
34. Kirchheiner J, Nickchen K, Bauer M, et al. Pharmacogenetics of antidepressants and antipsychotics: the contribution of allelic variations to the phenotype of drug response. Mol Psychiatry 2004; 9(5):442–473.
35. Kirchheiner J, Brosen K, Dahl ML, et al. CYP2D6 and CYP2C19 genotype-based dose recommendations for antidepressants: a first step towards subpopulation-specific dosages. Acta Psychiatr Scand 2001; 104(3):173–192.
36. Stipp D. A DNA tragedy. http://www.fortune.com/fortune/articles/0,15114,372497,00.html (accessed June 2005).
37. O'Kane DJ, Weinshilboum RM, Moyer TP. Pharmacogenomics and reducing the frequency of adverse drug events. Pharmacogenomics 2003; 4(1):1–4.
38. Guzey C, Spigset O. Genotyping as a tool to predict adverse drug reactions. Curr Top Med Chem 2004; 4(13):1411–1421.
39. Ingelman-Sundberg M. Pharmacogenetics: an opportunity for a safer and more efficient pharmacotherapy. J Intern Med 2001; 250(3):186–200.
40. Lazarou J, Pomeranz BH, Corey PN. Incidence of adverse drug reactions in hospitalized patients: a meta-analysis of prospective studies. J Am Med Assoc 1998; 279(15):1200–1205.
41. Tanigawara Y, Aoyama N, Kita T, et al. CYP2C19 genotype-related efficacy of omeprazole for the treatment of infection caused by Helicobacter pylori. Clin Pharmacol Ther 1999; 66(5):528–534.
42. Relling MV, Hancock ML, Rivera GK, et al. Mercaptopurine therapy intolerance and heterozygosity at the thiopurine S-methyltransferase gene locus. J Natl Cancer Inst 1999; 91(23):2001–2008.
43. Mallal S, Nolan D, Witt C, et al. Association between presence of HLA-B*5701, HLA-DR7, and HLA-DQ3 and hypersensitivity to HIV-1 reverse-transcriptase inhibitor abacavir. Lancet 2002; 359(9308):727–732.
44. Hetherington S, Hughes AR, Mosteller M, et al. Genetic variations in HLA-B region and hypersensitivity reactions to abacavir. Lancet 2002; 359(9312):1121–1122.
45. Siddiqui A, Kerb R, Weale ME, et al. Association of multidrug resistance in epilepsy with a polymorphism in the drug-transporter gene ABCB1. N Engl J Med 2003; 348(15):1442–1448.
46. Desmeules J, Gascon MP, Dayer P, et al. Impact of environmental and genetic factors on codeine analgesia. Eur J Clin Pharmacol 1991; 41(1):23–26.
47. Gasche Y, Daali Y, Fathi M, et al. Codeine intoxication associated with ultrarapid CYP2D6 metabolism. N Engl J Med 2004; 351(27):2827–2831.

48. Brockmoller J, Cascorbi I, Kerb R, et al. Combined analysis of inherited polymorphisms in arylamine N-acetyltransferase 2, glutathione S-transferases M1 and T1, microsomal epoxide hydrolase, and cytochrome P450 enzymes as modulators of bladder cancer risk. Cancer Res 1996; 56(17):3915–3925.

49. Israel E, Chinchilli VM, Ford JG, et al. Use of regularly scheduled albuterol treatment in asthma: genotype-stratified, randomised, placebo-controlled cross-over trial. Lancet 2004; 364(9444):1505–1512.

50. Liljedahl U, Kahan T, Malmqvist K, et al. Single nucleotide polymorphisms predict the change in left ventricular mass in response to antihypertensive treatment. J Hypertens 2004; 22(12):2321–2328.

51. Liljedahl U, Lind L, Kurland L, et al. Single nucleotide polymorphisms in the apolipoprotein B and low density lipoprotein receptor genes affect response to antihypertensive treatment. BMC Cardiovasc Disord 2004; 4(1):16.

52. Chasman DI, Posada D, Subrahmanyan L, et al. Pharmacogenetic study of statin therapy and cholesterol reduction. J Am Med Assoc 2004; 291(23):2821–2827.

53. van de Vijver MJ, He YD, van't Veer LJ, et al. A gene-expression signature as a predictor of survival in breast cancer. N Engl J Med 2002; 347(25):1999–2009.

54. van 't Veer LJ, Dai H, van de Vijver MJ, et al. Gene expression profiling predicts clinical outcome of breast cancer. Nature 2002; 415(6871):530–536.

55. Chang JC, Wooten EC, Tsimelzon A, et al. Gene expression profiling for the prediction of therapeutic response to docetaxel in patients with breast cancer. Lancet 2003; 362(9381):362–369.

56. Jansen MP, Foekens JA, van Staveren IL, et al. Molecular classification of tamoxifen-resistant breast carcinomas by gene expression profiling. J Clin Oncol 2005; 23(4):732–740.

57. Holleman A, Cheok MH, den Boer ML, et al. Gene-expression patterns in drug-resistant acute lymphoblastic leukemia cells and response to treatment. N Engl J Med 2004; 351(6):533–542.

58. Reich DE, Goldstein DB. Detecting association in a case-control study while correcting for population stratification. Genet Epidemiol 2001; 20(1):4–16.

59. Nebert DW, Vesell ES. Advances in pharmacogenomics and individualized drug therapy: exciting challenges that lie ahead. Eur J Pharmacol 2004; 500(1–3):267–280.

60. Tucker G. Pharmacogenetics—expectations and reality. Br Med J 2004; 329(7456):4–6.

61. Nebert DW, Jorge-Nebert L, Vesell ES. Pharmacogenomics and "individualized drug therapy": high expectations and disappointing achievements. Am J Pharmacogenomics 2003; 3(6):361–370.

62. Koch WH. Technology platforms for pharmacogenomic diagnostic assays. Nat Rev Drug Discov 2004; 3(9):749–761.

63. Twyman RM. SNP discovery and typing technologies for pharmacogenomics. Curr Top Med Chem 2004; 4(13):1423–1431.

64. Flockhart DA. Clinical pharmacogenetics. In: Atkinson AJ, Daniels CE, Dedrick RL, Grudzinkas CV, Markey SP, eds. Principles of Clinical Pharmacology. 1st ed. Oxford (UK): Elsevier Academic Press, 2001:157–163.

65. Lo HS, Wang Z, Hu Y, et al. Allelic variation in gene expression is common in the human genome. Genome Res 2003; 13(8):1855–1862.

66. Liljedahl U, Fredriksson M, Dahlgren A, et al. Detecting imbalanced expression of SNP alleles by minisequencing on microarrays. BMC Biotechnol 2004; 4(1):24.
67. Sawyer SL, Mukherjee N, Pakstis AJ, et al. Linkage disequilibrium patterns vary substantially among populations. Eur J Hum Genet 2005.
68. Lai E, Bowman C, Bansal A, et al. Medical applications of haplotype-based SNP maps: learning to walk before we run. Nat Genet 2002; 32(3):353.
69. Crawford DC, Nickerson DA. Definition and clinical importance of haplotypes. Annu Rev Med 2005; 56:303–320.
70. Yeoh EJ, Ross ME, Shurtleff SA, et al. Classification, subtype discovery, and prediction of outcome in pediatric acute lymphoblastic leukemia by gene expression profiling. Cancer Cell 2002; 1(2):133–143.
71. Cardon LR, Palmer LJ. Population stratification and spurious allelic association. Lancet 2003; 361(9357):598–604.
72. Meisel C, Gerloff T, Kirchheiner J, et al. Implications of pharmacogenetics for individualizing drug treatment and for study design. J Mol Med 2003; 81(3):154–167.
73. Lindpaintner K. Pharmacogenetics and the future of medical practice. J Mol Med 2003; 81(3):141–153.
74. Mansmann U, Winkelmann BR. Classification and prediction in pharmacogenetics—context, construction and validation. Pharmacogenomics 2002; 3(2):157–160.
75. Issa AM. Ethical perspectives on pharmacogenomic profiling in the drug development process. Nat Rev Drug Discov 2002; 1(4):300–308.
76. Pharmacogenetics: Ethical Issues. Nuffield Council on Bioethics 2003. http://www.nuffieldbioethics.org/go/ourwork/pharmacogenetics/introduction (accessed June 2005).
77. Bernard S. The 5 myths of pharmacogenomics. Pharmaceutical Executive 2003. http://pharmexec.mediwire.com/main/Default.aspx?P=Content&ArticleID=72796 (accessed June 2005).
78. Schmedders M, van Aken J, Feuerstein G, et al. Individualized pharmacogenetic therapy: a critical analysis. Community Genet 2003; 6(2):114–119.
79. Evans WE, Relling MV. Moving towards individualized medicine with pharmacogenomics. Nature 2004; 429(6990):464–468.
80. PharmGKB. The Pharmacogenetics and Pharmacogenomics Knowledge Base. http://www.pharmgkb.org/home/overview.jsp (accessed June 2005).
81. Guidance for Industry: Pharmacogenomic Data Submissions. FDA Draft Guidance 2003. http://www.fda.gov/cder/guidance/5900dft.pdf (accessed June 2005).
82. Innovation or Stagnation? Challenge and Opportunity on the Critical Path to New Medical Products. FDA Report 2004. http://www.fda.gov/oc/initiatives/criticalpath/whitepaper.pdf (accessed June 2005).
83. Frueh FW, Gurwitz D. From pharmacogenetics to personalized medicine: a vital need for educating health professionals and the community. Pharmacogenomics 2004; 5(5):571–579.
84. Vandel P, Haffen E, Vandel S, et al. Drug extrapyramidal side effects. CYP2D6 genotypes and phenotypes. Eur J Clin Pharmacol 1999; 55(9):659–665.
85. Scordo MG, Spina E, Romeo P, et al. CYP2D6 genotype and antipsychotic-induced extrapyramidal side effects in schizophrenic patients. Eur J Clin Pharmacol 2000; 56(9–10):679–683.

86. Schillevoort I, de Boer A, van der Weide J, et al. Antipsychotic-induced extrapyramidal syndromes and cytochrome P450 2D6 genotype: a case-control study. Pharmacogenetics 2002; 12(3):235–240.

87. Bertilsson L, Dahl ML, Dalen P, et al. Molecular genetics of CYP2D6: clinical relevance with focus on psychotropic drugs. Br J Clin Pharmacol 2002; 53(2):111–122.

88. Brandolese R, Scordo MG, Spina E, et al. Severe phenytoin intoxication in a subject homozygous for CYP2C9*3. Clin Pharmacol Ther 2001; 70(4):391–394.

89. Ninomiya H, Mamiya K, Matsuo S, et al. Genetic polymorphism of the CYP2C subfamily and excessive serum phenytoin concentration with central nervous system intoxication. Ther Drug Monit 2000; 22(2):230–232.

90. Schwarz UI. Clinical relevance of genetic polymorphisms in the human CYP2C9 gene. Eur J Clin Invest 2003; 33(suppl 2):23–30.

91. Goldstein JA. Clinical relevance of genetic polymorphisms in the human CYP2C subfamily. Br J Clin Pharmacol 2001; 52(4):349–355.

92. Shon JH, Yoon YR, Kim KA, et al. Effects of CYP2C19 and CYP2C9 genetic polymorphisms on the disposition of and blood glucose lowering response to tolbutamide in humans. Pharmacogenetics 2002; 12(2):111–119.

93. Kirchheiner J, Bauer S, Meineke I, et al. Impact of CYP2C9 and CYP2C19 polymorphisms on tolbutamide kinetics and the insulin and glucose response in healthy volunteers. Pharmacogenetics 2002; 12(2):101–109.

94. Lee AY, Kim MJ, Chey WY, et al. Genetic polymorphism of cytochrome P450 2C9 in diphenylhydantoin-induced cutaneous adverse drug reactions. Eur J Clin Pharmacol 2004; 60(3):155–159.

95. Mukae S, Itoh S, Aoki S, et al. Association of polymorphisms of the renin-angiotensin system and bradykinin B2 receptor with ACE-inhibitor-related cough. J Hum Hypertens 2002; 16(12):857–863.

96. Mukae S, Aoki S, Itoh S, et al. Bradykinin B(2) receptor gene polymorphism is associated with angiotensin-converting enzyme inhibitor-related cough. Hypertension 2000; 36(1):127–131.

97. Kouwaki M, Hamajima N, Sumi S, et al. Identification of novel mutations in the dihydropyrimidine dehydrogenase gene in a Japanese patient with 5-fluorouracil toxicity. Clin Cancer Res 1998; 4(12):2999–3004.

98. van Kuilenburg AB, Haasjes J, Richel DJ, et al. Clinical implications of dihydropyrimidine dehydrogenase (DPD) deficiency in patients with severe 5-fluorouracil-associated toxicity: identification of new mutations in the DPD gene. Clin Cancer Res 2000; 6(12):4705–4712.

99. Gross E, Ullrich T, Seck K, et al. Detailed analysis of five mutations in dihydropyrimidine dehydrogenase detected in cancer patients with 5-fluorouracil-related side effects. Hum Mutat 2003; 22(6):498.

100. Lerer B, Segman RH, Fangerau H, et al. Pharmacogenetics of tardive dyskinesia: combined analysis of 780 patients supports association with dopamine D3 receptor gene Ser9Gly polymorphism. Neuropsychopharmacology 2002; 27(1):105–119.

101. Carlsson LE, Santoso S, Baurichter G, et al. Heparin-induced thrombocytopenia: new insights into the impact of the FcgammaRIIa-R-H131 polymorphism. Blood 1998; 92(5):1526–1531.

102. Martin AM, Nolan D, Gaudieri S, et al. Pharmacogenetics of antiretroviral therapy: genetic variation of response and toxicity. Pharmacogenomics 2004; 5(6):643–655.

103. Watson ME, Pimenta JM, Spreen WR, et al. HLA-B*5701 and abacavir hypersensitivity. Pharmacogenetics 2004; 14(11):783–784.
104. Priori SG, Barhanin J, Hauer RN, et al. Genetic and molecular basis of cardiac arrhythmias: impact on clinical management. Parts I and II. Circulation 1999; 99(4):518–528.
105. Priori SG, Napolitano C, Schwartz PJ, et al. Association of long QT syndrome loci and cardiac events among patients treated with beta-blockers. J Am Med Assoc 2004; 292(11):1341–1344.
106. Huang YS, Chern HD, Su WJ, et al. Polymorphism of the N-acetyltransferase 2 gene as a susceptibility risk factor for antituberculosis drug-induced hepatitis. Hepatology 2002; 35(4):883–889.
107. Ohno M, Yamaguchi I, Yamamoto I, et al. Slow N-acetyltransferase 2 genotype affects the incidence of isoniazid and rifampicin-induced hepatotoxicity. Int J Tuberc Lung Dis 2000; 4(3):256–261.
108. McLeod HL, Siva C. The thiopurine S-methyltransferase gene locus—implications for clinical pharmacogenomics. Pharmacogenomics 2002; 3(1):89–98.
109. Evans WE. Pharmacogenetics of thiopurine S-methyltransferase and thiopurine therapy. Ther Drug Monit 2004; 26(2):186–191.
110. Nagasubramanian R, Innocenti F, Ratain MJ. Pharmacogenetics in cancer treatment. Annu Rev Med 2003; 54:437–452.
111. Sanderson J, Ansari A, Marinaki T, et al. Thiopurine methyltransferase: should it be measured before commencing thiopurine drug therapy? Ann Clin Biochem 2004; 41(4):294–302.
112. Lecomte T, Ferraz JM, Zinzindohouc F, et al. Thymidylate synthase gene polymorphism predicts toxicity in colorectal cancer patients receiving 5-fluorouracil-based chemotherapy. Clin Cancer Res 2004; 10(17):5880–5888.
113. Marsh S, McLeod HL. Pharmacogenetics of irinotecan toxicity. Pharmacogenomics 2004; 5(7):835–843.
114. Ieiri I, Takane H, Otsubo K. The MDR1 (ABCB1) gene polymorphism and its clinical implications. Clin Pharmacokinet 2004; 43(9):553–576.
115. Sakaeda T, Nakamura T, Okumura K. Pharmacogenetics of drug transporters and its impact on the pharmacotherapy. Curr Top Med Chem 2004; 4(13):1385–1398.
116. Elbein SC, Sun J, Scroggin E, et al. Role of common sequence variants in insulin secretion in familial type 2 diabetic kindreds: the sulfonylurea receptor, glucokinase, and hepatocyte nuclear factor 1alpha genes. Diabetes Care 2001; 24(3):472–478.
117. Ortlepp JR, Hanrath P, Mevissen V, et al. Variants of the CYP11B2 gene predict response to therapy with candesartan. Eur J Pharmacol 2002; 445(1–2):151–152.
118. Daigo S, Takahashi Y, Fujieda M, et al. A novel mutant allele of the CYP2A6 gene (CYP2A6*11) found in a cancer patient who showed poor metabolic phenotype towards tegafur. Pharmacogenetics 2002; 12(4):299–306.
119. Furuta T, Shirai N, Sugimoto M, et al. Pharmacogenomics of proton pump inhibitors. Pharmacogenomics 2004; 5(2):181–202.
120. Chong E, Ensom MH. Pharmacogenetics of the proton pump inhibitors: a systematic review. Pharmacotherapy 2003; 23(4):460–471.
121. Schwartz GL, Turner ST. Pharmacogenetics of antihypertensive drug responses. Am J Pharmacogenomics 2004; 4(3):151–160.

122. Mattison LK, Soong R, Diasio RB. Implications of dihydropyrimidine dehydrogen-ase on 5-fluorouracil pharmacogenetics and pharmacogenomics. Pharmacogenomics 2002; 3(4):485–492.

123. Marsh S, McLeod HL. Cancer pharmacogenetics. Br J Cancer 2004; 90(1):8–11.

124. Donald PR, Sirgel FA, Venter A, et al. The influence of human N-acetyltransferase genotype on the early bactericidal activity of isoniazid. Clin Infect Dis 2004; 39(10):1425–1430.

125. Humma LM, Terra SG. Pharmacogenetics and cardiovascular disease: impact on drug response and applications to disease management. Am J Health Syst Pharm 2002; 59(13):1241–1252.

126. Cascorbi I, Paul M, Kroemer HK. Pharmacogenomics of heart failure—focus on drug disposition and action. Cardiovasc Res 2004; 64(1):32–39.

127. Cusi D, Barlassina C, Azzani T, et al. Polymorphisms of alpha-adducin and salt sen-sitivity in patients with essential hypertension. Lancet 1997; 349(9062):1353–1357.

128. Mason DA, Moore JD, Green SA, et al. A gain-of-function polymorphism in a G-protein coupling domain of the human beta1-adrenergic receptor. J Biol Chem 1999; 274(18):12670–12674.

129. Borjesson M, Magnusson Y, Hjalmarson A, et al. A novel polymorphism in the gene coding for the beta (1)-adrenergic receptor associated with survival in patients with heart failure. Eur Heart J 2000; 21(22):1853–1858.

130. Small KM, Wagoner LE, Levin AM, et al. Synergistic polymorphisms of beta1- and alpha2C-adrenergic receptors and the risk of congestive heart failure. N Engl J Med 2002; 347(15):1135–1142.

131. Mialet Perez J, Rathz DA, Petrashevskaya NN, et al. Beta 1-adrenergic receptor polymorphisms confer differential function and predisposition to heart failure. Nat Med 2003; 9(10):1300–1305.

132. Siest G, Jeannesson E, Berrahmoune H, et al. Pharmacogenomics and drug response in cardiovascular disorders. Pharmacogenomics 2004; 5(7):779–802.

133. Liggett SB, Wagoner LE, Craft LL, et al. The Ile164 beta2-adrenergic receptor poly-morphism adversely affects the outcome of congestive heart failure. J Clin Invest 1998; 102(8):1534–1539.

134. Wagoner LE, Craft LL, Singh B, et al. Polymorphisms of the beta(2)-adrenergic receptor determine exercise capacity in patients with heart failure. Circ Res 2000; 86(8):834–840.

135. Liggett SB. Polymorphisms of beta-adrenergic receptors in heart failure. Am J Med 2004; 117(7):525–527.

136. Liggett SB. Polymorphisms of adrenergic receptors: variations on a theme. Assay Drug Dev Technol 2003; 1(2):317–326.

137. Hingorani AD, Jia H, Stevens PA, et al. Renin–angiotensin system gene polymorph-isms influence blood pressure and the response to angiotensin converting enzyme inhibition. J Hypertens 1995; 13(12 Pt 2):1602–1609.

138. Schunkert H, Hense HW, Gimenez-Roqueplo AP, et al. The angiotensinogen T235 variant and the use of antihypertensive drugs in a population-based cohort. Hyperten-sion 1997; 29(2):628–633.

139. Miller JA, Thai K, Scholey JW. Angiotensin II type 1 receptor gene polymorphism predicts response to losartan and angiotensin II. Kidney Int 1999; 56(6):2173–2180.

140. Baudin B. Angiotensin II receptor polymorphisms in hypertension. Pharmacogenomic considerations. Pharmacogenomics 2002; 3(1):65–73.

141. Ginsberg G, Smolenski S, Hattis D, et al. Population distribution of aldehyde dehydrogenase-2 genetic polymorphism: implications for risk assessment. Regul Toxicol Pharmacol 2002; 36(3):297–309.

142. Gerdes LU, Gerdes C, Kervinen K, et al. The apolipoprotein epsilon4 allele determines prognosis and the effect on prognosis of simvastatin in survivors of myocardial infarction: a substudy of the Scandinavian simvastatin survival study. Circulation 2000, 101(12):1366–1371.

143. Evans RM, Hui S, Perkins A, et al. Cholesterol and APOE genotype interact to influence Alzheimer disease progression. Neurology 2004; 62(10):1869–1871.

144. van Venrooij FV, Stolk RP, Banga JD, et al. Common cholesteryl ester transfer protein gene polymorphisms and the effect of atorvastatin therapy in type 2 diabetes. Diabetes Care 2003; 26(4):1216–1223.

145. Kuivenhoven JA, Jukema JW, Zwinderman AH, et al. The role of a common variant of the cholesteryl ester transfer protein gene in the progression of coronary atherosclerosis. The Regression Growth Evaluation Statin Study Group. N Engl J Med 1998; 338(2):86–93.

146. Carlquist JF, Muhlestein JB, Horne BD, et al. The cholesteryl ester transfer protein Taq1B gene polymorphism predicts clinical benefit of statin therapy in patients with significant coronary artery disease. Am Heart J 2003; 146(6):1007–1014.

147. Siffert W. G protein polymorphisms in hypertension, atherosclerosis, and diabetes. Annu Rev Med 2005; 56:17–28.

148. Harvey L, Reid RE, Ma C, et al. Human genetic variations in the 5HT2A receptor: a single nucleotide polymorphism identified with altered response to clozapine. Pharmacogenetics 2003; 13(2):107–118.

149. Angiolillo DJ, Fernandez-Ortiz A, Bernardo E, et al. PlA polymorphism and platelet reactivity following clopidogrel loading dose in patients undergoing coronary stent implantation. Blood Coagul Fibrinolysis 2004; 15(1):89–93.

150. Quinn MJ, Topol EJ. Common variations in platelet glycoproteins: pharmacogenomic implications. Pharmacogenomics 2001; 2(4):341–352.

151. Blons H, Gad S, Zinzindohoue F, et al. Matrix metalloproteinase 3 polymorphism: a predictive factor of response to neoadjuvant chemotherapy in head and neck squamous cell carcinoma. Clin Cancer Res 2004; 10(8):2594–2599.

152. Hollopeter G, Jantzen HM, Vincent D, et al. Identification of the platelet ADP receptor targeted by antithrombotic drugs. Nature 2001; 409(6817):202–207.

153. Piccart M, Lohrisch C, Di Leo A, et al. The predictive value of HER2 in breast cancer. Oncology 2001; 61(suppl 2):73–82.

154. Petricoin EF, Ardekani AM, Hitt BA, et al. Use of proteomic patterns in serum to identify ovarian cancer. Lancet 2002; 359(9306):572–577.

155. Duggan BJ, Gray S, Johnston SR, et al. The role of antisense oligonucleotides in the treatment of bladder cancer. Urol Res 2002; 30(3):137–147.

156. Duggan BJ, Maxwell P, Kelly JD, et al. The effect of antisense Bcl-2 oligonucleotides on Bcl-2 protein expression and apoptosis in human bladder transitional cell carcinoma. J Urol 2001; 166(3):1098–1105.

157. Kelly JD, Dai J, Eschwege P, et al. Downregulation of Bcl-2 sensitises interferon-resistant renal cancer cells to Fas. Br J Cancer 2004; 91(1):164–170.

158. Bischoff JR, Kirn DH, Williams A, et al. An adenovirus mutant that replicates selectively in p53-deficient human tumor cells. Science 1996; 274(5286):373–376.
159. Khuri FR, Nemunaitis J, Ganly I, et al. a controlled trial of intratumoral ONYX-015, a selectively-replicating adenovirus, in combination with cisplatin and 5-fluorouracil in patients with recurrent head and neck cancer. Nat Med 2000; 6(8):879–885.
160. Seemann S, Maurici D, Olivier M, et al. The tumor suppressor gene TP53: implications for cancer management and therapy. Crit Rev Clin Lab Sci 2004; 41(5–6):551–583.
161. Lynch TJ, Bell DW, Sordella R, et al. Activating mutations in the epidermal growth factor receptor underlying responsiveness of non-small-cell lung cancer to gefitinib. N Engl J Med 2004; 350(21):2129–2139.
162. Heinrich MC, Corless CL, Demetri GD, et al. Kinase mutations and imatinib response in patients with metastatic gastrointestinal stromal tumor. J Clin Oncol 2003; 21(23):4342–4349.
163. Debiec-Rychter M, Dumez H, Judson I, et al. Use of c-KIT/PDGFRA mutational analysis to predict the clinical response to imatinib in patients with advanced gastrointestinal stromal tumours entered on phase I and II studies of the EORTC Soft Tissue and Bone Sarcoma Group. Eur J Cancer 2004; 40(5):689–695.
164. The International HapMap Consortium. The International HapMap Project. Nature 2003; 426(6968):789–796.
165. Cargill M, Altshuler D, Ireland J, et al. Characterization of single-nucleotide polymorphisms in coding regions of human genes. Nat Genet 1999; 22(3):231–238.
166. Sullivan-Klose TH, Ghanayem BI, Bell DA, et al. The role of the CYP2C9-Leu359 allelic variant in the tolbutamide polymorphism. Pharmacogenetics 1996; 6(4):341–349.
167. Crespi CL, Miller VP. The R144C change in the CYP2C9*2 allele alters interaction of the cytochrome P450 with NADPH:cytochrome P450 oxidoreductase. Pharmacogenetics 1997; 7(3):203–210.
168. Scordo MG, Pengo V, Spina E, et al. Influence of CYP2C9 and CYP2C19 genetic polymorphisms on warfarin maintenance dose and metabolic clearance. Clin Pharmacol Ther 2002; 72(6):702–710.
169. Greenblatt DJ, von Moltke LL. Interaction of warfarin with drugs, natural substances, and foods. J Clin Pharmacol 2005; 45(2):127–132.
170. Chu K, Wu SM, Stanley T, et al. A mutation in the propeptide of Factor IX leads to warfarin sensitivity by a novel mechanism. J Clin Invest 1996; 98(7):1619–1625.
171. Oldenburg J, Quenzel EM, Harbrecht U, et al. Missense mutations at ALA-10 in the factor IX propeptide: an insignificant variant in normal life but a decisive cause of bleeding during oral anticoagulant therapy. Br J Haematol 1997; 98(1):240–244.
172. D'Ambrosio RL, D'Andrea G, Cappucci F, et al. Polymorphisms in factor II and factor VII genes modulate oral anticoagulation with warfarin. Haematologica 2004; 89(12):1510–1516.

9

Optimal Dose Finding in Drug Development: Approaches and Regulatory Perspectives[a]

Jogarao V. S. Gobburu

Pharmacometrics, Office of Clinical Pharmacology and Biopharmaceutics, United States Food and Drug Administration, Silver Spring, Maryland, U.S.A.

Mathangi Gopalakrishnan

Department of Mathematics and Statistics, University of Maryland, Baltimore, Maryland, U.S.A.

INTRODUCTION

Dose–response (effectiveness and toxicity) relationships aid in optimizing the use of drugs. These relationships can also form the basis for drug approval or refusal. Several regulatory initiatives emphasize the need for better dose finding and individualization of drug therapy (1,2). A recent article reported that 21% of the new molecular entities approved by the FDA during 1980–1999 underwent a dose-related labeling change (3). Of those, 80% of the changes represented net reductions in the dosing regimen. It was suggested that the frequency might be less than 21%, if the definition of "dose change" is more appropriate (4). Nevertheless, it was generally accepted that the current dose-finding paradigm is not optimal. It was concluded that the pivotal trials tend to study relatively high-end doses after inadequate dose-finding efforts.

---

[a]The views expressed in this chapter are those of the authors and do not necessarily reflect the official views of the FDA.

The primary focus of this chapter is on dose finding during clinical drug development. This chapter first describes the dose–response nomenclature, and the regulatory initiatives and presents some motivations for good dose–response. Later, the chapter deals with the various clinical trial designs and quantitative methods for investigating dose–response, followed by discussion on dose adjustments in special populations. The chapter ends by providing future perspectives on good dose–response in drug development.

NOMENCLATURE

Probably due to the diverse group of experts who contribute to drug development, such as clinicians, clinical pharmacologists, and biostatisticians, the nomenclature used to describe dose–response is quite varied. Dose finding is often used to describe the process for identifying the optimal dosing strategy. This includes recommendations on a starting dose, a strategy for titration if applicable, and stopping criteria. For the purposes of this chapter, the term dose finding is not limited to "dose" per se, but is also equally applicable to finding a target exposure (concentration) for eliciting a target effect. Perhaps "dose finding" is in wider use because of the fact that, ultimately, a dose is prescribed.

The terms dose–response, exposure–response, concentration–effect, and pharmacokinetic–pharmacodynamic (PK–PD) relationships are used interchangeably. The term exposure–response will be used in this chapter. Exposure includes any measure of drug in the body, such as dose and concentration in biological fluids. Response includes a broad range of endpoints, including biomarkers (e.g., receptor occupancy), a presumed mechanistic effect (e.g., ACE inhibition), a potential or accepted surrogate (e.g., effects on BP), and the full range of short- or long-term clinical effects (e.g., mortality) related to either effectiveness or safety.

The terminology pertaining to the drug development phases (e.g., Phase I, Phase IIb), together with the learn-confirm paradigm (5), has led to some confusion about the roles of different clinical trials. Dose ranging trials, typically called the Phase II trials, which collect the relevant endpoint data in target patients, can be used as the evidence of effectiveness (confirm). On the other hand, dose ranging should be continued during the so-called Phase III trials (learn). For these reasons, in the current chapter those trials, which provide primary evidence of effectiveness and safety, will be called pivotal trials (can also be called registration trials).

CURRENT LEGAL REQUIREMENTS AND
REGULATORY EXPECTATIONS

The legal requirements that dictate the approval or refusal of a new drug application (NDA) are listed in the Code of Federal Regulations (CFR). Section 314.105 deals with the requirement for approval, §314.125 deals with refusal, and §314.126 describes an adequate, well-controlled trial. Direct reference to the type of study designs, endpoints, analyses, and quality of exposure–response information required for approval is not made in these regulations. However, §314.125 states that "there is insufficient information about the drug to determine whether the product is safe for use under the conditions prescribed, recommended, or suggested in its proposed labeling as a basis for refusal." Although there is no clear consensus, this statement could be interpreted as requiring good dose–response. Importantly, the following FDA guidances to the industry clarify the need for collecting good exposure–response information pre-marketing:

1. Exposure–response relationships: study design, data analysis, and regulatory applications (1).
2. Dose–response information to support drug registration (2).
3. Providing clinical evidence of effectiveness for human drug and biological products (6).
4. Pre-marketing risk assessment (7).

There are several others, such as the guidance on PK in patients with impaired renal function—study design, data analysis, and regulatory applications (8) and the guidance on drug metabolism/drug interaction studies in drug development process—studies in vitro (9) that describe the Agency's expectations on evaluating the need for dose adjustments.

The proceedings of the Cardiovascular and Renal Advisory Committee meeting held on October 20, 2000 are worth noting (10–12). Based on a retrospective analysis presented by the FDA on 10 approved antihypertensive drugs, it was suggested that frequently optimum dose finding is not performed, which could affect many regulatory decisions. The main outcome of the meeting was the emphasis on determining exposure–response relationships using model-based analysis and use of innovative designs to allow frequentist and Bayesian methods of analysis.

In general, the FDA expects sponsors to characterize the exposure–response reasonably well, where applicable.

THE NEED FOR BETTER DOSE-FINDING STUDIES

In addition to the legal requirements and other regulatory initiatives, the current attrition rate and motivating case studies emphasize the need for good exposure–response information pre-marketing. Poor dose finding is probably an important cause of late attrition. Also, from a good clinical practice and patient perspective, lack of optimal dosing guidelines could lead to sub-optimal therapeutic advantage.

Late Attrition

Recent surveys suggest that the average cost of discovering and developing a new drug is in excess of US $800 million (13). These spiraling costs threaten to make the development of new drugs increasingly unaffordable to both manufacturers

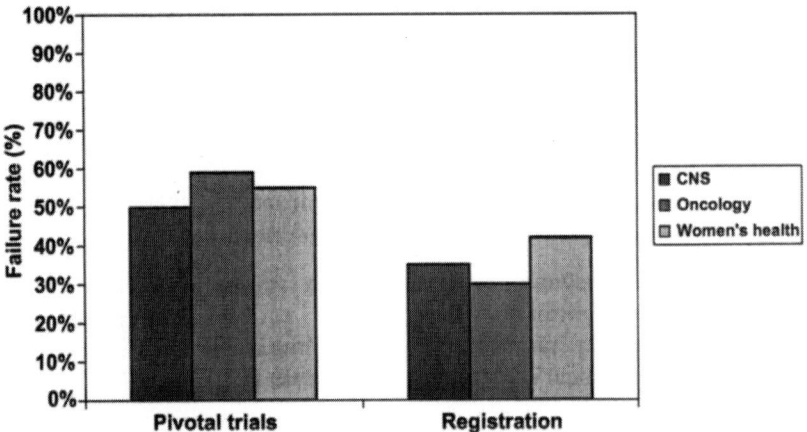

Figure 1   Success rate by the phase of development and by the therapeutic area. The percentages indicate the failure rate in that phase of development. For example, out of 100 molecules which are tested in pivotal trials, 59% fail to show utility. *Source*: Adapted from Ref. 14.

and consumers. The mammoth amount spent in developing a drug does not guarantee its entry into the market as a medicine. The drug development paradigm is supposed to filter out poor drug candidates early on, and to be economically viable. However, the rate of failures in pivotal trials and rejection by regulatory authorities have been reported to be discouragingly high, especially in the therapeutic areas like oncology (59%) and women's health (42%), respectively (Fig. 1) (14).

　　While clear reasons have not been identified, it is reasonable to consider poor dose selection as one of the important factors for the high attrition. Early and better dose-finding studies might be able to reduce this attrition rate.

Case Studies

Nesiritide

The original new drug application (NDA) for nesiritide was submitted for the treatment of acute decompensated coronary heart failure (CHF) in April 1998. The changes in pulmonary capillary wedge pressure (PCWP) at 6 hours in 0.015, 0.03, and/or 0.05 μg/min/kg groups are compared with that in the placebo group. During that review, the FDA recommended the sponsor to develop an exposure–response model relating concentrations and PCWP, and blood pressure (BP) to facilitate regulatory decision-making. Nesiritide was discussed at the Cardiorenal Advisory Committee on January 29, 1999. From a clinical viewpoint, the maximum desired effect at a given dose does not occur instantaneously and the desired effects cannot be achieved without the undesired effects. The fact that the hypotension occurs at a later time than changes in PCWP limits the ability for titration to take effect. Taking all these factors into consideration, plus input from the Advisory Committee, the sponsor was recommended to optimize the dosing regimen, such that the desired effect occurs instantaneously and the hypotension is minimized. In April 1999, the Agency issued a non-approval letter to the sponsor. Among other concerns, the Agency identified the need to better understand the onset and offset characteristics of symptomatic hypotension and to optimize the dosing regimen to achieve faster decrease in PCWP and minimize undesired hypotension.

The developed exposure–response model was used to explore various alternative dosing scenarios. A bolus dose followed by a maintenance infusion would allow faster achievement of the desired effect. Evidently, a 2 $\mu g/kg$ bolus followed by 0.01 $\mu g/min/kg$ infusion over 48 hours seems to offer a reasonable benefit-risk profile. This dosing regimen was selected for further investigation in the VMAC (vasodilation in the management of acute CHF) trial. The effects predicted by the model are in close agreement with those observed in the VMAC trial. In May 2001, the sponsor submitted the results of the VMAC study in support of a revised dosing regimen. The Agency approved nesiritide for acute CHF in May 2001.

Drug for Symptomatic Effect

One of the case studies presented at the recent Advisory Committee meetings demonstrated the need for a more optimal dosing regimen by means of an exposure–response analysis (15). The drug was indicated for a symptomatic benefit and the sponsor had proposed a once-a-day dosing regimen, which meant a sustained effect over 24 hours. Though evidence of effectiveness was obtained, exposure–response analysis suggested inadequacy of the once-a-day dosing regimen. The effect was not sustained for 24 hours because of the short half-life of the drug. Simulations suggested that twice daily or three times a day dosing regimen could provide sustained effect. For better compliance, a modified release formulation could serve the purpose of maintaining a sustained effect. The Agency decided that the NDA was approvable pending optimization of the dosing regimen, among other aspects.

Antiretroviral Therapy

Potent combination of antiretroviral regimens has led to profound decrease in morbidity and mortality associated with HIV-1 infection. The traditional practice in antiretroviral therapy is to administer the combination drugs at fixed dose regimens. Fixed dose regimens are reported to lead to higher rate of virological failures in clinical trials (16), which is attributed to the variability in response caused by high interpatient variability in systemic or intracellular concentrations achieved (17). Studies have related systemic or intracellular concentrations to anti-HIV effect (18). A recently published article compared the responses between a concentration-controlled approach and a conventional fixed dose combination antiretroviral therapy (19). The trial was a prospective, randomized

52-week open-label trial. Zidovudine, lamivudine, and indinavir were administered as fixed doses for two weeks to all patients and then patients were randomized to receive either fixed dose therapy or concentration-controlled therapy. The primary endpoint was the proportion of patients with HIV-RNA levels below 50 copies/ml at 52 weeks. The concentration-controlled approach resulted in a greater proportion of patients ($\sim$100%) having undetectable HIV-RNA levels than fixed dosing strategy ($\sim$50%) at the end of the trial. The results of the study support the notion that good dosing strategies, to accommodate interpatient variability, can improve therapeutic outcome.

Anticancer Therapy

It was reported that systemic clearance of anticancer agents differs up to 3–10 times in children with acute lymphoblastic leukemia (ALL) (20). It was seen that the outcome was significantly worse among children with ALL who had low plasma concentrations of methotrexate due to rapid clearance than among those with slower clearance. Based on these findings, a prospective study compared the outcome between a fixed dosing approach, based on body surface area, and individualized dosing based on clearance (21). Individualized dosing of methotrexate improved the five-year rate of continuous complete remission (76% vs. 66%) in children with B-lineage ALL.

The first two case studies presented demonstrate that inadequate dose selection could lead to increased drug development time. The latter case studies highlight the importance, from a public health point of view, of the need for tailoring doses for an individual. In both these cases, the ultimate endpoint is mortality and, thus, it becomes critical for drug developers to make dose individualization a priority.

APPROACHES FOR FINDING OPTIMAL DOSE

Conceptual Basis for Dosing

The conceptual basis for dosing requires knowledge of three aspects of exposure–response to derive optimal dosing strategies. They are: (*i*) shape of the exposure–response (desired/undesired) curve (steep or shallow), (*ii*) type of response (reversibility of the disease, time of occurrence of disease event, and seriousness of the adverse events), and (*iii*) variability between and within patients. Each of the aspects is described in detail in the following.

Shape of the Exposure–Response Curve

Figure 2 shows a hypothetical exposure–response curve for the desired and undesired effects. This curve provides information on the starting dose, highest effective dose given the corresponding safety and the step-size for titration of the dose. If sufficient exposure–response information is available for a drug, dosing recommendations in special populations could also be provided, if certain assumptions can be made.

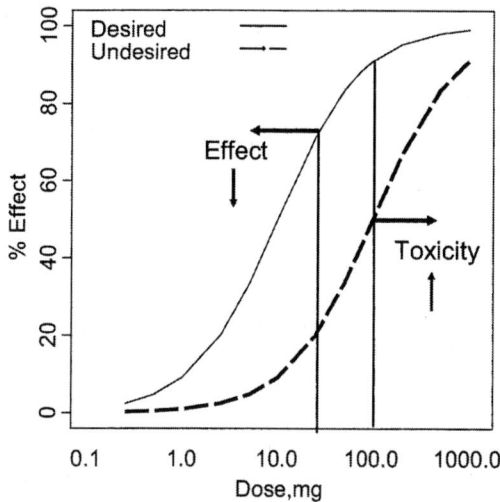

Figure 2   The exposure–response (desired and undesired) relationships of a hypothetical drug.

Population vs. individual exposure–response curves: The shape and location of the population (average) exposure–response curves are helpful in choosing the starting dose for a drug. Study designs that allow estimation of individual dose–response curves are useful in guiding titration. Certain amount of caution needs to be exhibited when estimating population exposure–response curves from individual exposure–response information. Let us consider a few individual dose–response curves with steep exposure–response relationships. The population (simple average) exposure–response curve is flatter than the individual curves, which is a statistical artifact. This typically leads to titration in step-sizes much more than optimal, which is an often ignored phenomenon. Figure 3 shows individual exposure–response curves for five subjects along with population exposure–response curves.

Type of Response

Three different aspects need to be considered based on the type of responses to optimize dosing strategy.

Reversibility of the disease state: The assessment of the need for dosing adjustment depends on whether the response variable is reversible (symptom/sign-related benefit) or irreversible (morbidity/mortality benefit). For example, Metoprolol (Toprol-XL) is indicated for use in high BP (reversible), and heart failure (irreversible). For treatment of high BP, dosing starts at 50–100 mg daily and could be increased to 400 mg daily depending on how the patient responds. The label recommends following the patient to decide the need for

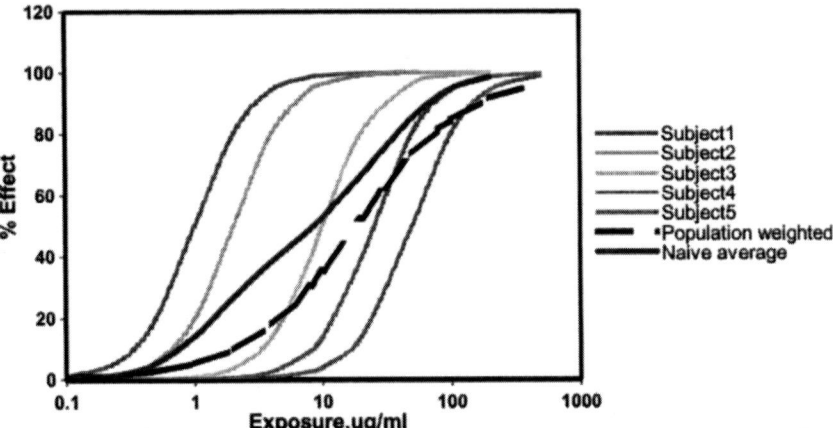

Figure 3   Population (weighted average and naïve average) and individual exposure–response curves. The graph shows that the population curves are not truly representative of the individual curves.

titration. But for a patient with heart failure, the recommended starting dose of the same drug is 25 mg daily for two weeks. The dose may be doubled every two weeks until dose-limiting toxicities occur. Generally, for drugs that decrease mortality and/or morbidity rates, the maximum tolerated doses are administered.

Time of occurrence of the disease event: The decision of which "surrogate" to employ for dosing decisions partly depends on the relative timing of the event. If the PD response occurs fairly soon after dosing, then dose adjustments could be based on that response. The time of occurrence of the disease event or toxicity could be much later than the initiation of therapy. For example, gentamicin trough concentrations greater than 2 µg/ml are associated with renal toxicity, which occurs upon chronic administration of the drug. Creatinine clearance (CL_{CR}) explains a majority of the variability in gentamicin, and the dose should be adjusted based on CL_{CR}, so that trough concentrations are maintained below 2 µg/ml. In this case, the trough concentrations serve as a surrogate to adjust doses. Another example would be the risk of bleeding events during warfarin therapy. Dose adjustments are constantly made based on international normalized ratio of prothrombin time (INR), which signifies the ability of the blood to form clots.

Seriousness of the adverse events: Optimal dose can be derived based on the seriousness of the adverse events, which influences the utility of a therapy. Briefly, utility of the therapy is the net effect of not taking the therapy to the benefit obtained by taking the therapy, given the adverse events of the therapy, as described by the equation that follows (22):

$$\text{Utility} = f(\text{Cost[No Therapy]}, \text{Benefit}, \text{Cost[Toxicity]})$$

For example, the utilities of a drug treating stroke and another treating migraine, but both causing nausea, are different. In the case of stroke, benefit from the therapy outweighs no therapy, even though associated with nausea. Although subjective for migraine, which might need daily treatment, the inconvenience from nausea might be weighted differently.

There are two types of utilities—population and individual utilities. The population utility is determined from an epidemiological perspective, whereas the individual utility is determined by the patient. For example, the LIFE (Losartan Intervention For Endpoint reduction in hypertension) (23) study showed that, out of 9222 patients, 11% of the patients receiving losartan and 13% receiving atenolol had death due to cardiovascular event, myocardial infarction, or stroke ($p = 0.021$). These results indicate that not every patient who received losartan or atenolol benefited, however, epidemiologically, the 2% difference in the losartan arm might translate to millions of patients overall (population utility), given the risks of not treating at all and the drug-related toxicity. This is the typical benefit-risk assessment regulatory bodies and health management organizations employ. On the other hand, a particular patient might consider nausea to be much worse in return for migraine relief as against another patient who might not. This type of benefit-risk evaluation might be considered by marketing departments in pharmaceutical companies to project sales. Several approaches to evaluate the individual utilities from the pivotal trials are available (24), but seldom employed prospectively in drug development.

Sources of Variability

Patient populations are heterogeneous, and characteristics, such as age, body size, genetic status, and disease status, vary from one patient to another. These aspects often lead to variations in the response to a drug. The widely used "one dose fits all" paradigm is clearly not suitable for most disease settings. Optimizing dosing regimen involves four important aspects to be taken into account, namely PK variability, PD variability, the shape of exposure–response (steep or shallow) relationship, and clinical practice. Variability includes both inter- and intrasubject variability.

If the intersubject variability in PK is the rate-limiting factor, then by therapeutic drug monitoring (TDM), the variability in response (desired/undesired) can be controlled. A recent article on antiretroviral therapy provided a scientific basis of individualizing therapy by means of a concentration-controlled trial, which resulted in a greater proportion of patients ($\sim$100%) with undetectable HIV-RNA, as compared with a fixed dose trial ($\sim$50%) (18). The intrinsic variability between patients in virological, immunological, behavioral, and pharmacological factors was controlled by means of monitoring concentrations. If the intrasubject variability in PK is relatively high, then TDM cannot completely control the response.

On the other hand, if the response is highly variable (high inter- and intrasubject PD variability), for example, BP measurement (25) monitoring of concentrations or response would not be able to control variations in drug effect. While continuous monitoring of BP in each patient increases the precision, clinical practice often includes monthly or more infrequent visits to the doctor.

Role of Biomarkers

The utility of biomarkers towards improving the efficiency of drug development is widely recognized (26), and specifically in the selection of suitable dose (or regimen) range for pivotal trials. Depending on the type of indication, an exposure–biomarker relationship can be used in rational dose finding. Several examples on the role of biomarkers for optimizing dosing are outlined here.

Symptom/Sign-Related Benefits

Clinical trials of drugs that are developed for symptom/sign-related benefits (e.g., antidepressants, antiarrhymics, analgesics) are shorter and the magnitudes of drug effect are relatively larger. Studying several doses in the pivotal trials is possible. Use of an exposure–biomarker in such a case could narrow down the choice of dose ranges or doses to be studied in pivotal trials. For example, the effect on QT prolongation for Class-III antiarrhythmics, like dofetilide, which are intended to maintain normal sinus rhythm, is useful to narrow down the doses to be studied in the pivotal trials. An effect on exercise-induced heart rate in healthy subjects is helpful in guiding the choice of doses/regimens for beta-blockers that are intended for use in angina.

Mortality/Morbidity Benefits

Establishing an exposure–biomarker relationship for mortality/morbidity benefit (e.g., treatment of cancer and CHF) is challenging primarily due to a large unexplained variability and/or small effect size. Defining an exposure–response relationship for such an indication, given the effect size and cost, is impractical. But if the effect size is relatively large, then the assessment of an exposure–response is pragmatic for these indications as well.

Challenges in the Use of Biomarkers

Unclear biomarker–clinical endpoint relationships could be because of multiple or putative mechanisms of action (AchE activity in Alzheimer's disease), high unexplained variability in clinical endpoint, and/or small effect size. Then selection of a dose to be tested in pivotal trials based solely on biomarker data would be misleading. As long as a biomarker has a reasonable mechanistic basis, there are several important contributions of biomarker(s) towards improving the efficiency of drug development, irrespective of whether the relationship with the clinical outcome(s) is formally established or not. Specifically, biomarkers can aid in the selection of suitable dose (or exposure) range for pivotal trials, identification of sub-populations with important differences in the drug effects, accelerated approval of drugs for life-threatening diseases, approval of new formulations, extension of a drug's use to new populations, and to assess product quality.

Choice of Dosing Regimen

As compared with the selection of doses, choice of dosing regimens to be studied in pivotal trials is more challenging. Often, no clear exposure–response-based rationale for choice of the dosing regimen is provided, except for some areas like anti-infectives where the in vitro activity is routinely considered. The time course of the effects on biomarkers should be considered in making decisions regarding optimal dosing regimens. For example, dutasteride, used to treat benign prostratic hypertrophy, was administered at a dose of 0.5 mg daily in a pivotal trial, when it was seen that dihydrotestosterone (5-alpha reductase inhibition) levels return to baseline after 14–28 days after initiation of therapy (27). Here the time course of the biomarker (dihydrotestosterone) was ignored when deciding the once-a-day regimen. One of the most frequently quoted reasons for such a choice is compliance. Patients are believed to be more compliant to daily treatments when compared with once in two- or three-day regimens. While that might be true, non-compliance can also emerge from undesired toxicity, particularly if the drug needs to be taken daily. Further, innovative methods to formulate drugs are now available, which can lead to more compliant dosage forms. Another approach could be to sequence drug and placebo pills according to regimen and yet dose daily. One potential concern of that could be the cost of the placebo pills and who pays for it.

Experimental Designs and Analysis

The choice of the experimental study design and the study population in exposure–response trials depends upon the phase of the development, therapeutic indication, and the severity of disease in the patient population of interest. The strengths and limitations of specific trial designs are provided in the following.

Parallel, Fixed Dose

In parallel design (23), patients are randomized to receive one of the several treatments (placebo, test dose 1, test dose 2). This design could be applied when the study endpoint or adverse effect is delayed, persistent, or irreversible (e.g., stroke or heart attack prevention, asthma prophylaxis, arthritis treatments with late onset response, survival in cancer, treatment of depression). The study need not be placebo-controlled, since a positive slope in the exposure–response implies evidence of effectiveness. But a placebo control could salvage a study where most of the doses chosen are in the flat portion of the exposure–response curve by showing that all doses were superior to the placebo. The design provides group mean (population-average) dose responses, not the distribution or shape of individual dose response. The advantage of such a design is the lack of confounding factors, such as time (carry-over effects) and design-dependent outcomes.

Cross-Over, Fixed Dose

According to a cross-over design (28), each patient would receive more than one possible treatment. The design is suitable when the effect develops rapidly and patients return to baseline conditions quickly after cessation of therapy, if responses are not irreversible (cure, death) and if patients have reasonably stable disease. If the ultimate aim is to estimate the distribution of individual exposure–response curves, such a design is very powerful. Potential problems of the design could be uncertainty of carry-over effects, baseline comparability after the first period, period-by-treatment interactions. Such data are best analyzed by sophisticated data analysis (linear or non-linear mixed effects modeling).

Titration Design

Mostly, titration designs are designed to titrate the dose to safety events (e.g., cancer). Toxicity-guided dose-finding approaches do not provide optimal dosing for effectiveness. On the other hand, titration to effect or effectiveness guided dose-finding approach provides optimal effective dose along with safety information. Following are the two types of commonly followed titration designs.

Forced titration: In a forced titration design (29), all patients are randomized to move through a series of rising doses. The design is similar in concept and limitations, to a randomized multiple cross-over design, except that assignment to dose levels is ordered, not random. A reasonable approximation of both population-average exposure–response and the distribution of individual exposure–response relationships can be obtained if the time-dependent drug effect is minimal and the number of treatment withdrawals is not excessive. A critical limitation of this design is that, by itself, the study cannot distinguish response to an increased dosage from response to an increased time of therapy, or a cumulative drug dosage effect.

Optional titration (placebo-controlled titration to endpoint):   In an optional titration design (30), the patients are titrated until they reach a well-characterized favorable or unfavorable response as expressed in the protocol. The design is suitable for conditions where response is prompt and not an irreversible event like stroke or death. A crude analysis of such studies could lead to misleading inverted "U-shaped" curve, as the patients who are less sensitive to the drug need higher doses of the drug, making it appear as if the response decreases after a certain dose. However, mixed effects modeling approaches can provide valid exposure–response information. The design confounds time and dose effects, and therefore poses problems in safety assessment.

Randomized Concentration-Controlled Trial (RCCT)

According to the RCCT design (31,32), patients are randomized to defined target concentrations or concentration ranges (rather than doses). These target concentration levels are selected based on the PK–PD relationship characterized in previous trials. The design is particularly efficient for drugs with high intersubject variability in PK. Both group concentration response curves and individual curves (if cross-over) could be obtained. Potential difficulties associated with this design include defining target concentrations, intrasubject variability in PK over time, uncertainty in the most appropriate concentration measure for intermittent dose administration (e.g., peak, average or trough concentration), availability of suitable assays and PK expertise, blinding issues, and PD variability (33). A special case of RCCT is the PK-modified design. According to the PK-modified design (34), patients will be dosed based on a covariate. For example, the dose of an exclusively renally cleared drug could be adjusted a priori for CL_{CR}. It is very important to note that for this design to be useful in characterizing the exposure–response, a dose range is still required. Trials that investigate only one dose which is adjusted for some key prognostic factor are perhaps the most uninformative trials, in terms of exposure–response.

Randomized Effect-Controlled Trial (RECT)

In a RECT (35), the subjects are randomly assigned to a set of pre-specified target effect levels. This design is specifically suitable when there is a pronounced PD variability in addition to the PK variability and when sparse sampling is done. Prerequisites of RECT are that drug response must be reversible without any pronounced pharmacodynamic hysteresis or time dependency. Unlike RCCT, determination of drug concentrations can be performed at convenient times.

Randomized Withdrawal Design

In a randomized withdrawal design (36), patients initially receive open treatment with the test drug and then they are randomized to receive test drug or placebo (withdrawal of active treatment). Any difference that emerges between groups receiving continued treatment and placebo would demonstrate effectiveness of the active treatment. The pre-randomization period could be any length (can establish long-term effectiveness) and the post-withdrawal observation period could be any fixed duration or early escape or time to any event. The randomized withdrawal approach is suitable in several situations. It may be suitable for drugs that appear to resolve an episode of recurring illness (e.g., antidepressants) and where a placebo-controlled trial would be difficult (hypertension, CHF, chronic pain), especially in pediatrics. Potential advantages of the design are: (*i*) the trial is enriched with responders, therefore large placebo-drug difference (clear evidence of effectiveness), (*ii*) ideal for use in pediatrics, as placebo phase could be shortened, and (*iii*) exposure–response relationship could be assessed after an initial placebo-controlled titration design.

Methods of Data Analysis

Essentially data analysis can be either confirmatory or exploratory. These two types of analyses differ in the data and testing criteria employed to make inferences.

Confirmatory analysis: Confirmatory analysis is expected to be the most unbiased inference of a hypothesis testing that is prespecified. Data from all patients are required to be included in such analysis. Missing data are imputed, most frequently using the last observation carried-forward principle (LOCF) (37). The hypothesis testing is expected to preserve the typical 5% type 1 error (false-positive) rate. The most widely tested hypothesis is whether the change from baseline at a prespecified single point in time in the control and test treatment groups is different. Other endpoints include the number of patients with a prespecified change in the response (e.g., patients with 50% reduction in seizures), time of the event (time to first myocardial infarction or time to death), and so on. The most important requirement for comparing two or more groups is randomization of treatments. That is, patients should have received, say, placebo or the active drug randomly, irrespective of their baseline characteristics.

Exploratory analysis: Exploratory analysis can generate hypotheses that can be confirmed in future trials. Most importantly, exploratory analysis can serve as and has been used to provide supportive evidence for regulatory decision-making (38). By definition, exploratory analysis cannot be prespecified, as new hypotheses are proposed after inspecting patterns in the observations. Almost all of the safety analyses are exploratory, as clinical trials are seldom powered to test safety hypotheses. Such analysis is critical to assess the benefit-risk and labeling.

An exploratory analysis could lead to building probabilistic models relating outcomes, exposure, and prognostic factors. These models allow projecting optimal dosing strategies. Table 1 compares the various features of confirmatory and exploratory analyses.

Table 1 Features of Confirmatory and Exploratory Analysis

Features	Confirmatory analysis	Exploratory analysis
Analysis plan	Prespecified	Not prespecified
Analysis type	Predominantly change from baseline	Mostly model-based
Analysis outcome	Primary evidence of effectiveness	Can provide supportive evidence of effectiveness
Inferences	Unbiased	Biased
Prior knowledge	Required if stratifying	Required
Compliance	Ignores	Can account
Time course of response	Ignores	Can account
Patient heterogeneity	Ignores	Can account
Explain observations	Cannot	Can
Dose	Ignores	Can account
Imputing missing data	Fixed	Can be explored
Improve future trials	Not intended	Can

Dosing in Special Populations

Well-established exposure–response knowledge can be used for dosing recommendations in special populations (pediatrics, organ function impaired, geriatrics).

Pediatrics

The FDA has proposed a pediatric decision tree (Fig. 4), which provides a general idea for proposing labeling changes in the pediatric population. This decision tree is generally applicable to all special populations. According to the pediatric decision tree, if the disease is similar in adults and pediatrics and if a biomarker is available, then pediatric studies measuring concentrations and effects can be used to propose dosing recommendations in pediatrics. Availability of a reliable biomarker is very useful for a pediatric indication, as clinical outcome-based studies are difficult to be conducted in pediatrics.

Few examples are provided where appropriate use of exposure–response relationships developed in adults is used to recommend dosing adjustments in pediatrics. BUSULFEX® (Busulfan) injection is indicated for use in combination with cyclophosphamide as a conditioning regimen prior to allogeneic hematopoietic progenitor cell transplantation for chronic myelogenous leukemia in adults. It was approved in pediatrics by matching exposures in adults and

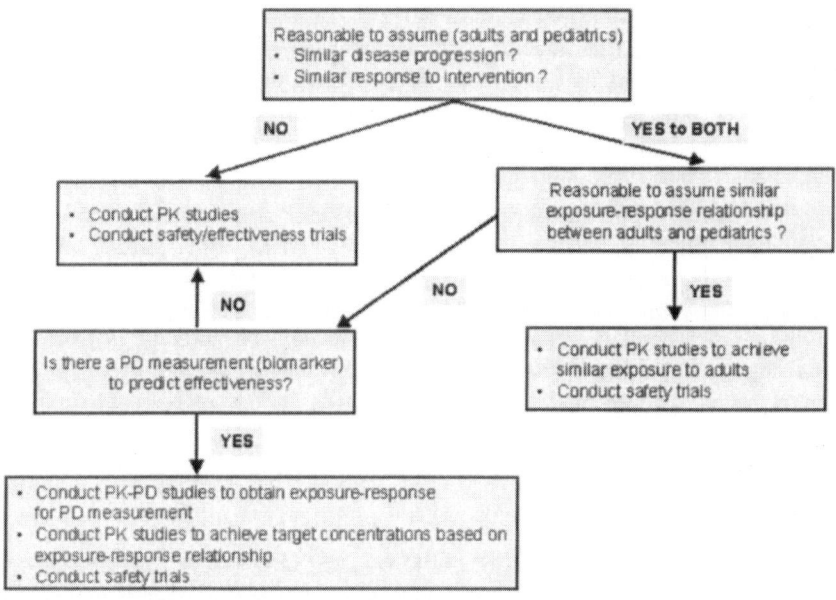

Figure 4 Pediatric decision tree (1). *Source*: Adapted from the Guidance to Industry. Courtesy of U.S. Food and Drug Administration.

pediatrics by conducting a PK study, as disease and response to intervention were similar (39). Another example would be d,l sotalol hydrochloride. Sotalol is originally approved in adults to treat life-threatening ventricular fibrillation, tachycardia, and maintenance of sinus rhythm in patients with symptomatic atrial fibrillation and flutter. A clinical study assessing the antiarrthymic and beta-blocking effects of sotalol in pediatrics on QTc and heart rate in pediatrics was used for approval (40).

Sub-Populations Based on Prognostic Factors

As part of the NDA, frequently, dose-finding and bridging studies are submitted. The dose-finding and other large "pivotal" clinical trials allow the clinical pharmacologists to describe the exposure–response relationship and thereby to select an appropriate dose/regimen for a given patient (41). The bridging studies evaluate the influence of various prognostic factors (e.g., food, smoking, hepatic/renal impairment, concomitant drugs, and so on). The bridging studies seldom assess the effectiveness and (long-term) safety, although short-term safety is assessed in all clinical studies routinely. The drug sponsors and the regulators would like to seek answers to "what-if" questions like: "What is the effect of co-administering an interacting drug on the performance (say, effectiveness) of the new drug?" or "Is it necessary to alter dosing if given to a patient with renal insufficiency? If so, by how much?" With respect to dosage adjustment, the results from the bridging studies can be used in at least two ways: (*i*) always adjust the dose to match the reference population, or (*ii*) use the exposure–response relationship to judge the clinical relevance. Clearly, the first option may lead to unnecessarily complicated dosing recommendations and, practically, might be a costly endeavor. Based on prognostic factors like age, body weight, diet, smoking, drug interactions, demographics, renal, or hepatic impairment etc., exposure–response relationships can support dose adjustments in these subpopulations. For instance, if exposure–response relationship is established previously, a PK study in smaller number of patients with varied renal function (normal, mild, moderate, severe) could suggest dosing adjustments in terms of exposure in renal impaired patients (42). Judicious use of biomarkers could also suggest dosing adjustments in sub-populations. Since enrollment of adequate number of target patients with varying degrees of renal/hepatic impairment could be difficult, the biomarker relationship in the general target patients and exposure differences in the special populations could be used for recommending dosing adjustments.

FUTURE CONSIDERATIONS

The legal requirements, regulatory initiatives, and their active implementation are critical to institutionalize good dose finding. Currently good dose finding is not considered as a requirement. Hopefully, the motivating examples and the technological advances in effect measurements (biomarkers including imaging) will lead to the requiring of good dose finding. Also, from a pharmaceutical sponsors' perspective, the root cause analysis for the high attrition rates is crucial for proposing effective solutions. We believe poor dose finding will be found as one of the drivers of the high attrition rate. To efficiently address the late phase attrition, the FDA has recently proposed end-of-phase IIa (EOP2A) meetings. EOP2A meetings occur following the completion of the first set of exposure–response studies in patients, and before the beginning of the pivotal clinical studies. At such meetings, issues pertaining to the overall development strategy needed to support drug dosing and NDA approval could be discussed.

The current confirmatory trials are lagging behind the advances in quantitative techniques. Innovative designs and methods of analysis could be incorporated, which could improve the efficiency of drug development process and lead to more meaningful labeling instructions. Enrichment design (43) is an innovative design methodology where the trial is performed in responders, who are identified after a treatment run-in phase. Such design demonstrates clearer evidence of effectiveness, and a more precise estimate of the effect size, and thus increases the study power to detect drug effects and select doses. The main idea of this design is that if patients cannot respond to the main pharmacologic effect of the drug, they cannot be expected to show a clinical response, and such patients would dilute the drug effect if included in the trial. Such a design could also be useful in situations where effectiveness is hard to demonstrate, as only few patients respond to treatment. Examples would be motility-modifying agents in gastro-esophageal reflux disease or antiasthmatic drugs other than steroids and beta-agonists. The tacrine trials (44) employed an enrichment design, where the initial phase was a cross-over, dose titration phase to determine responsiveness and best dose.

Conventionally, regulatory decisions have been based on change from baseline at some pre-specified time for the control and test treatments. All data between baseline and that time are ignored. Innovative data analysis methodologies like longitudinal data analysis could be more powerful in assessing evidence of effectiveness, as entire data generated is utilized. Because of increased power, more optimal dose finding could be performed. Longitudinal data analysis could also provide less biased estimates of effect size and intersubject variability, as this method offers reasonable ways of handling missing data as opposed to the LOCF approach.

We strongly believe that drug developers and regulatory agencies should better exploit the vast information accrued from the hundreds of clinical trials for a given indication. To the best of our knowledge, no systematic data mining methods are in place to learn from successes and failures, and for designing more efficient future trials. Institutions should invest in infrastructures that enable standard storage of data, and tools that translate information into knowledge. Modeling could play a useful role in integrating knowledge across drug development programs. A related area which requires immediate attention regards labeling updates. Currently, scientists continue to investigate the dosing strategies of drugs post-approval. For example, the "Antiretroval Therapy" section of this chapter exemplifies such a study post-approval. If targeting a particular concentration could achieve therapeutic success in 100% of the HIV patients, instead of 50%, one is left to wonder why the clinical practice ignores it. There has to be a mechanism to systematically review such study results and update labeling if appropriate. Pharmaceutical sponsors should be expected to take an initiative.

Pharmacological endpoints or biomarkers require invasive sampling of body fluids and tissues. Innovative non-invasive procedures, such as functional or molecular imaging techniques, are shown to be of great importance in linking together all the events from the administration of the drug through its activity and modulation on the molecular target to the clinical outcome. Identifying improved pharmacological endpoints could modernize drug design and development, especially in oncology (45).

While deriving optimal dosing instructions is the first step towards optimal therapy, implementing the instructions effectively in practice is critical. Review of literature revealed that prescribing errors are a common occurrence in hospital in-patients (46,47). Most of the prescribed errors are reported as human errors occurring at various stages of administering a treatment, like ordering, errors in dosing, route, or frequency (47). Current technological advances should be exploited to develop tools for accurate prescription of doses. Such electronic tools should be able to efficiently integrate patient information, such as demographics and current medications, and up-to-date labeling.

REFERENCES

1. U.S Department of Health and Human Services. Guidance for industry: exposure–response relationships: study design, data analysis and regulatory applications. http://www.fda.gov/cder/guidance/4614dft.pdf. (Access date January 31, 2005).
2. International Conference on Harmonisation. Guidance for Industry: dose–response information to support drug registration. http://www.fda.gov/cder/guidance/iche-4.pdf. (Access date January 31, 2005).
3. Cross J, Lee H, Westelinck A, Nelson J, Grudzinskas C, Peck C. Postmarketing drug dosage changes of 499 FDA-approved new molecular entities, 1980–1999. Pharmacoepidemiol Drug Saf 2002; 11(6):439–446.
4. Temple RJ. Defining dose decrease. Pharmacoepidemiol Drug Saf 2003; 12(2): 151–152.
5. Sheiner LB. Learning versus confirming in clinical drug development. Clin Pharmacol Ther 1997; 61(3):275–291.
6. Guidance for industry: providing clinical evidence of effectiveness for human drug and biological products. http://www.fda.gov/cder/guidance/1397fnl.pdf. (Access date January 31, 2005).
7. Guidance for industry: premarketing risk assessment. http://www.fda.gov/cber/gdlns/premarkrisk.pdf. (Access date January 31, 2005).

8. Guidance for industry: pharmacokinetics in patients with impaired renal function—study design, data analysis and regulatory applications. http://www.fda.gov/cder/guidance/1449fnl.pdf. (Access date January 31, 2005).

9. Guidance for industry: drug metabolism–drug interactions studies in drug development process—studies in vitro. http://www.fda.gov/cder/guidance/clin3.pdf. (Access date January 31, 2005).

10. Gobburu JVS, Lipicky RJ. 2000. Dose–response characterization in current drug development: do we have a problem? Part I: Inferences from animal/human data. http://www.fda.gov/ohrms/dockets/ac/00/backgrd/3656b2a.pdf. (Access date January 31, 2005).

11. Sheiner LB. 2000. Dose finding—What do we want to know? ed. Cardiovascular and Renal Drug Products Advisory Committee Meeting (FDA). Bethesda, October 20, 2000. http://www.fda.gov/ohrms/dockets/ac/00/transcripts/3656t2b.pdf. (Access date February 1, 2005).

12. Peck CC. 2000. Does the currently drug development find the right-dose, ed., Cardiovascular and Renal Drug Products Advisory Committee Meeting (FDA). Bethesda, October 20, 2000. http://www.fda.gov/ohrms/dockets/ac/00/transcripts/3656t2a.pdf. (Access date February 1, 2005).

13. DiMasi JA, Hansen RW, Grabowski HG. The price of innovation: new estimates of drug development costs. J Health Econ 2003; 22(2):151–185.

14. Kola I, Landis J. Can the pharmaceutical industry reduce attrition rates? Nat Rev Drug Discov 2004; 3(8):711–715.

15. Gobburu JVS. 2003. Could an EOP2A meeting shorten drug development time? http://www.fda.gov/ohrms/dockets/ac/03/slides/3998S1_06_Gobburu_files/frame.htm. (Access date February 10, 2005).

16. Ledergerber B, Egger M, Opravil M, et al. Clinical progression and virological failure on highly active antiretroviral therapy in HIV-1 patients: a prospective cohort study. Swiss HIV Cohort Study. Lancet 1999; 353(9156):863–868.

17. Fletcher CV, Acosta EP, Henry K, et al. Concentration-controlled zidovudine therapy. Clin Pharmacol Ther 1998; 64(3):331–338.

18. Fletcher CV, Kawle SP, Kakuda TN, et al. Zidovudine triphosphate and lamivudine triphosphate concentration–response relationships in HIV-infected persons. Aids 2000; 14(14):2137–2144.

19. Fletcher CV, Anderson PL, Kakuda TN, et al. Concentration-controlled compared with conventional antiretroviral therapy for HIV infection. Aids 2002; 16(4):551–560.

20. Rodman JH, Relling MV, Stewart CF, et al. Clinical pharmacokinetics and pharmacodynamics of anticancer drugs in children. Semin Oncol 1993; 20(1):18–29.

21. Evans WE, Relling MV, Rodman JH, Crom WR, Boyett JM, Pui CH. Conventional compared with individualized chemotherapy for childhood acute lymphoblastic leukemia. N Engl J Med 1998; 338(8):499–505.

22. Gobburu JVS. Population pharmacokinetic and pharmacodynamic analyses in new drug application: regulatory and scientific principles for clinical pharmacology and biopharmaceutics. In: Sahajwalla C, ed. Marcel Dekker, 2001.

23. Dahlof B, Devereux RB, Kjeldsen SE, et al. Cardiovascular morbidity and mortality in the Losartan Intervention For Endpoint reduction in hypertension study (LIFE): a randomised trial against atenolol. Lancet 2002; 359(9311):995–1003.

24. Sheiner LB, Beal SL, Dunne A. Analysis of nonrandomly censored ordered categorical longitudinal data from analgesic trials. J Am Stat Assoc 1997; 92(440):1235–1244.

25. Pickering TG. The role of ambulatory monitoring in reducing the errors associated with blood pressure measurement. Herz 1989; 14(4):214–220.

26. Jadhav PR, Mehta MU, Gobburu JVS. How biomarkers can improve drug development. Am Pharm Rev 2004; 7(3):62–64.

27. Gisleskog PO, Hermann D, Hammarlund-Udenaes M, Karlsson MO. A model for the turnover of dihydrotestosterone in the presence of the irreversible 5 alpha-reductase inhibitors GI198745 and finasteride. Clin Pharmacol Ther 1998; 64(6):636–647.

28. de Visser SJ, van der Post JP, Nanhekhan L, Schoemaker RC, Cohen AF, van Gerven JM. Concentration–effect relationships of two rilmenidine single-dose infusion rates in hypertensive patients. Clin Pharmacol Ther 2002; 72(4):419–428.

29. Charbonnel B, Dormandy J, Erdmann E, Massi-Benedetti M, Skene A. The prospective pioglitazone clinical trial in macrovascular events (PROactive): can pioglitazone reduce cardiovascular events in diabetes? Study design and baseline characteristics of 5238 patients. Diabetes Care 2004; 27(7):1647–1653.

30. White WB, Saunders E, Noveck RJ, Ferdinand K. Comparative efficacy and safety of nisoldipine extended-release (ER) and amlodipine (CESNA-III study) in African American patients with hypertension. Am J Hypertens 2003; 16(9 Pt 1):739–745.

31. Sanathanan LP, Peck CC. The randomized concentration-controlled trial: an evaluation of its sample size efficiency. Control Clin Trials 1991; 12(6):780–794.

32. Holford N, Black P, Couch R, Kennedy J, Briant R. Theophylline target concentration in severe airways obstruction—10 or 20 mg/L? A randomised concentration-controlled trial. Clin Pharmacokinet 1993; 25(6):495–505.

33. Grahnen A, Karlsson MO. Concentration-controlled or effect-controlled trials: useful alternatives to conventional dose-controlled trials? Clin Pharmacokinet 2001; 40(5):317–325.

34. STRATTERA (Atomoxetine) Label. http://www.fda.gov/cder/pediatric/labels/Atomoxetine.pdf. (Access date February 1, 2005).

35. Ebling WF, Levy G. Population pharmacodynamics: strategies for concentration-and effect-controlled clinical trials. Ann Pharmacother 1996; 30(1):12–19.

36. Schick EC Jr, Liang CS, Heupler FA Jr, et al. Randomized withdrawal from nifedipine: placebo-controlled study in patients with coronary artery spasm. Am Heart J 1982; 104(3):690–697.

37. Little R, Yau L. Intent-to-treat analysis for longitudinal studies with drop-outs. Biometrics 1996; 52(4):1324–1333.

38. Gobburu JV, Marroum PJ. Utilisation of pharmacokinetic–pharmacodynamic modelling and simulation in regulatory decision-making. Clin Pharmacokinet 2001; 40(12):883–892.

39. BUSULFEX (Busulfan) Label. http://www.fda.gov/cder/pediatric/labels/busulfan.pdf. (Access date January 26, 2005).

40. BETAPACE (d,l sotalol hydrochloride) label. http://www.fda.gov/cder/pediatric/labels/sotalol.pdf. (Access date January 26, 2005).

41. Gobburu JVS, Sekar V. Application of modeling and simulation to integrate clinical pharmacology knowledge across a new durg application. Int Clin Pharmacol Ther 2001; 40(7):281–288.

42. Jonsson S, Karlsson MO. A rational approach for selection of optimal covariate-based dosing strategies. Clin Pharmocol Ther 2003; 73(1):7–19.

43. Robert Temple. 2004. Where protocol design has been a critical factor for success or failure. DIA Annual Meeting, June 2004. www.fda.gov/cder/present/DIA2004/ Temple.ppt. (Access date February 1, 2005).
44. Davis KL, Thal LJ, Gamzu ER, et al. A double-blind, placebo-controlled multicenter study of tacrine for Alzheimer's disease. The Tacrine Collaborative Study Group. N Engl J Med 1992; 327(18):1253–1259.
45. Seddon BM, Workman P. The role of functional and molecular imaging in cancer drug discovery and development. Br J Radiol 2003; 76 Spec No 2:S128–S138.
46. Dean B, Schachter M, Vincent C, Barber N. Causes of prescribing errors in hospital inpatients: a prospective study. Lancet 2002; 359(9315):1373–1378.
47. Fortescue EB, Kaushal R, Landrigan CP, et al. Prioritizing strategies for preventing medication errors and adverse drug events in pediatric inpatients. Pediatrics 2003; 111(4 Pt 1):722–729.

10

Optimal Dose Selection in Drug Development: Role of Population Pharmacokinetics in Phase III

Willi Weber and Diether Rueppel

Global Metabolism/Pharmacokinetics, Sanofi-Aventis Deutschland GmbH, Frankfurt, Germany

INTRODUCTION

The Goal of Drug Development

The pharmaceutical industry seeks to meet medical needs of drug treatment by developing new drug applications (NDA). The final step in drug development is to confirm that the NDA significantly improves the disease state in a population of the target patients.

In a confirmatory design of a Phase III study, the test group is assigned a dose regimen that achieves the maximum response possible without toxicity, while the control group is assigned the least effective ethically acceptable alternative treatment without the test drug (1,2).

Using large doses will maximize the benefit magnitude, whereas zero dose minimizes new drug-related benefit. The major task in drug development is to find the optimal dose, which will show sufficient evidence of efficacy in a placebo- or comparator-controlled double-blind clinical trial without unacceptable adverse events. The dose finding requires understanding of the disease and learning the functional relationship between dosages, prognostic variables (like body size and kidney function), and clinical outcome. A list of acronyms is presented in an Appendix at the end of this chapter.

Why Is Population Pharmacokinetics (PopPK) Useful in Drug Development?

We often look at the occurrence of events critical for a disease as clinical endpoint in a RCT (randomized clinical trial). This type of data is recorded as binary data (3), that is, either yes or no, typically coded as 1 or 0, respectively. Similarly, drug treatment may successfully suppress or fail to suppress harmful events. The success or failure of a drug treatment again can be coded as 1 or 0, respectively. Behind the binary outcome is our model for the continuous probability between 0 and 1 to observe or not to observe a certain event.

To model the relationship between the probability of success and drug concentration, we use either the Hill equation or the logistic equation. The empirical Hill model:

$$\text{Prob(success}|C) = \frac{C^s}{\text{EC}_{50}^S + C^S} \tag{1}$$

can be transformed into the logistic equation:

$$\text{logit(success}|C) = -S \log \text{EC}_{50} + S \log C = \beta_0 + \beta_1 \log C \tag{2}$$

$$\text{Prob(success}|C) = \frac{e^{\text{logit}}}{1 + e^{\text{logit}}} \tag{3}$$

Both equations 1 and 3 describe the transition from no drug effect at all to a condition of a full drug effect at sufficient high concentrations. EC_{50} corresponds to the concentration at half-maximal effect (Prob $= 0.5$) and S to the Hill-exponent. A large S $\gg 1$ value describes a steep relationship between concentration and effect. In terms of a logistic distribution, the location parameter $\log \text{EC}_{50} = \mu$ is the mean and the shape parameter $1/S$ defines the variance $\pi^2/3S^2$.

EC_{50} and S will vary between patients and are elements of a random vector drawn from a multi-variate PDF (probability density function) defined by a mean vector and a covariance matrix. The concentration C expected in a patient is a function of the given dose and the random vector of the individual PK (pharmacokinetics) parameters like CL_{tot} (total clearance) and V_{ss} (volume of distribution at steady-state). Optimizing the probability of clinical success is crucial in drug development. The expectation value for the probability of observing a clinical success in a patient is given as a function of the dose and the random variables EC_{50}, S, CL_{tot}, and V_{ss}. To minimize the risk of failure in drug development, we want to predict the probability of observing a clinical success for a given dose as precisely as possible. Therefore, we need to know the *mean and variability* of the critical random variables linking the probability of success with dose. The appropriate method for estimating the mean and the variance of the random variables EC_{50}, S, CL_{tot}, and V_{ss} is the PopPK (population pharmacokinetics) approach.

Population PK/PD (relationship between pharmacokinetics and pharmacodynamics) modeling and simulation can provide a vital aid to the drug development process by providing reliable predictions of the individualized dose–exposure–effect relationship (where effect refers to both efficacy and toxicity), which is key to successful therapy (4,5).

THE LEARNING AND CONFIRMING CONCEPT

What Is Learning and Confirming in Drug Development?

Sheiner (1) introduced the learning and confirming concept into the science of the drug development process. The development of a new chemical entity (NCE) to a new drug application (NDA) is described as an information gathering process that can be thought of as two successive learning–confirmation cycles, which are linked by a decision point.

The first cycle (traditional Phase I and Phase IIa) addresses the question of whether benefit in terms of efficacy and safety can reasonably be expected over existing therapies. It involves learning (Phase I) what is the largest short-term dose that may be administered to humans without causing harm, and then testing (Phase IIa) whether that dose induces some measurable short-term benefit in patients for whom the drug is intended to be therapeutic.

An affirmative answer at this first cycle provides the justification for a more elaborate second cycle (traditionally, Phase IIb and Phase III). The aim of this second cycle is to first learn (Phase IIb) what is a good, if not optimal, dosage regimen to achieve useful clinical value (i.e., an acceptable benefit–risk ratio), and then to perform several formal clinical trials (in Phase III) of that regimen versus a comparator to confirm a clinical value of the drug.

In summary:

- First learning and confirming cycle
  Phase I: What is the largest short-term dose that may be administered to humans without causing harm?
  Phase IIa: Confirm that this dose has promise of efficacy in a selected group of patients.
- Decision: Is there a sufficiently positive indication of efficacy and lack of toxicity to justify investment in the future development of the drug?
- Second learning and confirming cycle
  Phase IIb, dose finding: What is a good, if not optimal, dosage regimen to achieve useful clinical value (i.e., an acceptable benefit–risk ratio)?
  Phase III, approval: Confirm in a randomized clinical trial in a large representative patient population that when using the selected dose regimen an acceptable benefit–risk ratio is achieved.

At the confirmatory stage, the most credible analyses are those that make as few assumptions as possible. A confirmatory design is optimized to reveal rejection of the H0-hypothesis, which is, in general, that the drug shows no effect. A confirmatory design chooses a homogeneous set of patients, that is, one type of patients likely to show the expected benefit are selected.

In a learning design, doses are spread out from not effective to intermediate and maximum effective, to reveal the whole dose–response curve, not just two extreme points. Furthermore, to learn as much as possible about the influence of prognostic factors, patients with a broad range of prognostic factors are enrolled in the learning studies.

In this chapter, we describe the learning and confirming cycles in the development of cariporide.

Clinical PK data obtained in drug development, often sparse and unbalanced repeated observations, are appropriate for using mixed effect modeling. The hierarchical PopPK approach is the method of choice for this type of data.

Clinical PD data is typically a single observation of success or failure obtained in a subject. In cases where repeated observations are available, the information content is often insufficient to estimate the intersubject variability of the PD parameters. The functional relationship between concentration and effect is often not hierarchical. The PK/PD method is the method of choice for this type of data. If the PD data contains enough rich information, the mixed effect modeling approach can also successfully be applied in the PK/PD analysis (3).

In the area of modeling and simulation (M&S), both the hierarchical PopPK and the non-hierarchical PK/PD methods are combined.

Use of PopPK and M&S in Learning and Confirming Steps

Figure 1 illustrates the typical learning and confirming steps during the drug development. M&S is always involved during the learning steps.

Phase I, the first learning step: Normally PK and efficacy data from animals are available when starting the first-in-man study. They can tentatively be combined to a PK/PD model in man. Simulations with this first model will help to decide on the first dose in man. The PK part of the model can continously be improved when PK data in man become avaliable. In Phase I of the drug development, safety and tolerability within a broad dose range are investigated. Phase I studies are designed to generate rich data and balanced PK information in each individual.

Phase IIa, the first confirming step: A PopPK meta-analysis of the pooled Phase I data leads to a population PK model including fixed effects and random effects (Eq. 18). In general special populations like renally impaired patients, men and women and elderly subjects are included. The first PK/PD model contains information about human PK and, typically, information about

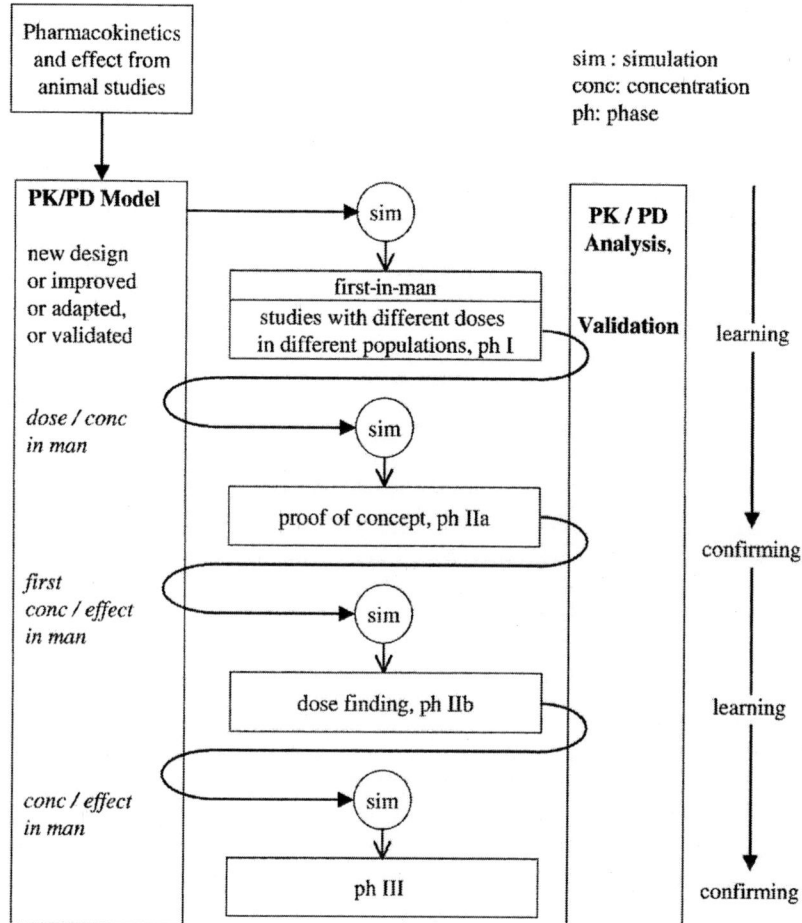

Figure 1 PK/PD modelling and simulation. *Abbreviations*: PK, pharmacokinetics; PD, pharmacodynamics; ph, phase.

the relationship between the concentration and the effect observed in animals. Simulations will be performed to find a dose which probably will show the desired effect in man.

In Phase IIa, most often, learning while confirming happens simultaneously. The primary objective is to confirm the proof of the concept. For the learning step, concentrations are observed using a sparse and unbalanced sampling schedule. Once the proof of the concept is confirmed, the relationship between the concentration and the effect is analyzed. Now the findings in humans will be incorporated into the PK/PD model. Given that PK is linear, we can use the PopPK model to optimize the dose in a way that, for example, 95% of the patients will achieve an exposure to the drug that leads to a successful clinical outcome.

Phase IIb, the second learning step: In Phase IIb, you want to improve your learning about variation in PK and PD in the target patient population. Simulations using the PopPK and PK/PD model will again help to design a variety of dose-finding studies, which elucidate the dose/concentration/effect relationship. Simultaneous observations of the exposure and the effect are analyzed to improve the models describing the PopPK and the PK/PD relationship. Using the improved models of PopPK and PK/PD for simulations, an optimized dose for the confirming Phase III study can be proposed. Of course it will be cross-checked with all safety and tolerability data to achieve an optimal benefit/risk ratio in Phase III.

Phase III, the second confirming step: Phase III combines confirming efficacy and learning about toxicity in the target patient population. Phase III hopefully confirms the desired efficacy without learning too much about toxicity.

There are good reasons to include a sparse sampling design which is applied in a small satellite group and supports us with exposure data. The main reason to prepare further learning is because sometimes confirming efficacy fails. The lesson is not that the drug does not work, but only that the present Phase III study does not allow rejection of the NULL hypothesis, which states that the drug does not work. Why did confirmation fail? Using the data obtained in the satellite group, we can validate our PopPK model. Using the information on influential covariates like body size, kidney function, and disease status, we can predict the most probable exposure in the total study population. Using the predicted concentrations and the observed clinical outcome, we can revalidate our PK/PD model. Simulation studies based on the updated models may change the dose recommendation and a new Phase III may be designed to finally confirm the efficacy.

When Phase III confirmed efficacy, we would also use the satellite group data to update our models. Simulations may investigate the unobserved clinical outcome after potential studies using a broader range of dose regimens. Such simulation studies may help in discussions with the authorities about special populations or adjustments in the dose regimen to be indicated in the drug label.

DEVELOPMENT OF A CARDIOPROTECTIVE DRUG

Can Cariporide Protect Acute Ischemic Patients?

Medical Need

Ischemic heart disease is the leading cause of morbidity and mortality in all industrialized nations (6). The goal of the cariporide project is to protect the heart from ischemia and reperfusion injury to avoid myocyte death, arrhythmias, and contractile dysfunction.

How can we construct our disease model? In our disease model, an event was attributed to either a chronic low risk related to the underlying CHD (coronary heart disease) or attributed to an acute high risk related to a risk situation of the CHD patient like a CABG (coronary artery bypass graft surgery). Counts of events per day are observed as clinical outcome of a RCT and need to be predicted by the disease model. In a time-to-event analysis, the time for the occurrence of the first event in a patient was used as dependent variable.

The contribution of events by both the acute and the chronic risk source is reflected in a mixture probability model for the time-to-event random variable T. Which event belongs to the acute risk source and which to the chronic risk source cannot be decided. Let T be a non-negative random variable representing the event time for an individual from a mixture of two homogeneous populations. The mixture probability model for T was constructed using a mixture of two Weibull distributions (7), given as follows:

$$P_{\text{mix}}(T|\alpha, \tau) = \sum_{i=1}^{2} p_i P_{\text{Weibull}}(T|\alpha_i, \tau_i) \qquad (4)$$

and the weighting factors:

$$p_1 = P(\text{event}|\text{drug, acute high risk situation of CHD}) \text{ and} \qquad (5)$$

$$p_2 = P(\text{event}|\text{chronic low risk of CHD}) = 1 - p_1 \qquad (6)$$

The probability that a time-to-event (T) is less or equal to time t is given by the cumulative distribution function $P_{\text{mix}}(T \leq t)$. The probability that T is less or equal to a value t, conditional on the parameter estimates, α and τ, of the time-to-event analysis and given the mixture probability density function (Eq. 4), can be calculated as:

$$P_{\text{mix}}(T \leq t|\alpha, \tau) = \sum_{i=1}^{2} p_i \left(1 - e^{-(t/\tau_i)^{\alpha_i}}\right) \qquad (7)$$

where α_i (location of the i-th Weibull distribution) and τ_i (shape of the i-th Weibull distribution) are the location and shape parameters of the i-th Weibull distribution.

The target study population comprised acute ischemic patients with either UAP (unstable angina pectoris), PCI (percutaneous coronary intervention), or patients undergoing CABG surgery. The treatment with cariporide targeted to reduce the acute risk of the occurrence of a combined event of either MI (myocardial infarction) or death, given as p_1 in equation 5. The treatment may be limited to a maximum effect when the probability of success for the drug is approaching unity, Prob(success|drug) $\rightarrow$ 1, and a minimum effect under placebo when Prob(success|drug) = 0.

$$p_1 = p_{1,\text{placebo}}(1 - \Delta_{\text{Acute risk}}\text{Prob(success|drug)}) \qquad (8)$$

In Equation 8, the term $p_{1,\text{placebo}}$ corresponds to the placebo treatment when $p_1 = \text{Prob(success|placebo)}$.

$$\Delta_{\text{Risk}} = \frac{P_{\text{mix}}(T \leq t|\text{placebo}) - P_{\text{mix}}(T \leq t|\text{drug})}{P_{\text{mix}}(T \leq t|\text{placebo})} \tag{9}$$

The observed clinical outcome is related to the combined risk, P_{mix}, and the target drug effect, judged as clinically relevant, is a relative risk reduction of $\Delta_{\text{Risk}} = 25\%$ of the total event rate at $t = 36$ days. Simulation of the clinical outcome and the effect of a successful drug treatment is shown in Figure 2. The ratio of the event rates following placebo and cariporide treatment is shown in Figure 3. To observe 25% and 21% Δ_{Risk} (relative risk reduction) of the total event rate on day 5 and day 36, respectively, $\Delta_{\text{Acute risk}}$ (relative reduction of the acute risk) = 30% of the acute risk p_1 is required.

What sample size is required?   When designing a clinical study, one of the first questions that arises is about sample size necessary to confirm efficacy. The sample size depends upon the minimum detectable difference of interest, the acceptable probability of rejecting a true NULL hypothesis ($\alpha = 0.05$), the

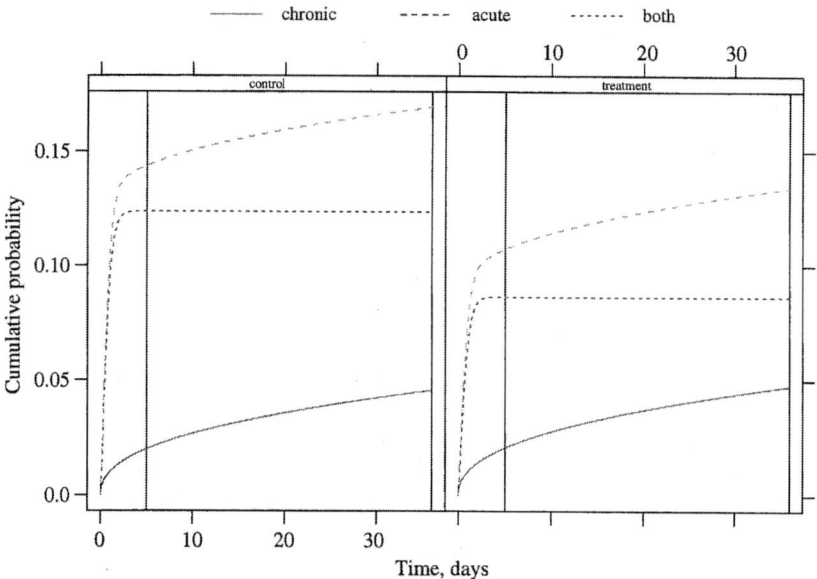

Figure 2   Probability of myocardial infarction or death. The total risk (*broken lines*) of the occurrence of an event is the sum of the acute risk and the chronic risk observed during the study. The acute high risk (*dotted lines*) is related to CABG surgery, chronic low baseline risk (*solid lines*) related to the coronar syndrome, *left panel*: placebo observation, *right panel*: cariporide reduces the acute risk within the first day by 30%. No further additional effect of cariporide at later times.

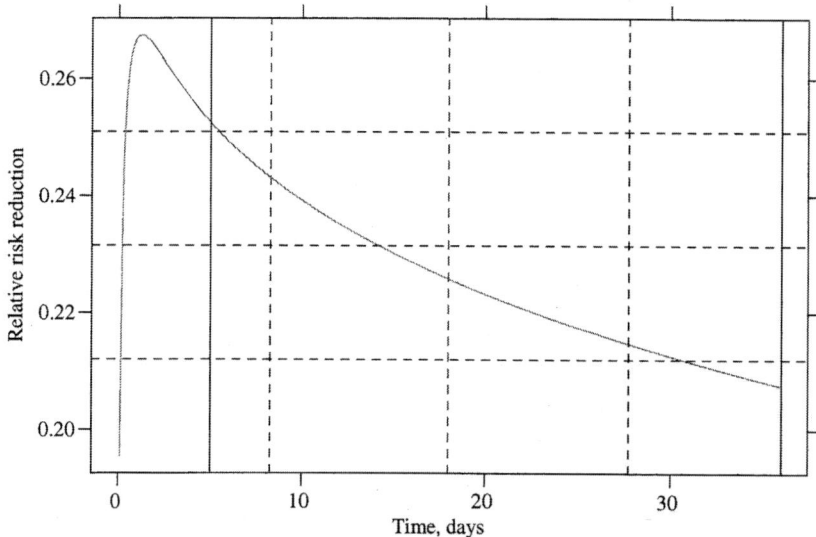

Figure 3   Relative risk reduction over time. A minimum relative risk reduction of 30% for the acute risk related to CABG surgery was estimated (Fig. 2). Due to the increasing cumulative chronic risk, the observable relative total risk reduction shows its maximum on day 1 and is continuously decreasing with time afterwards. The observable relative risk reduction is 25% on day 5 and 21% on day 36, respectively. *Abbreviation*: CABG, coronary artery bypass graft.

desired probability of correctly rejecting a false null hypothesis (power = 0.80), and the variability within the population(s) under study (8).

The NULL hypothesis simply assumes that there is no drug effect at all. If there is no drug action, there is no place for modeling any drug effect. In the alternative hypothesis, we assume that the drug responses have an effect. The size of the effect should be significantly different from no effect and at least should be clinically relevant. A larger effect can be detected using a smaller sample size. Sample size calculation is based on the size of the effect, which may be achieved by an unknown dose of the new drug. The difficult task remains to select an appropriate dose regimen to achieve the target effect. Now modeling a relationship between dose and effect size becomes important for optimizing the dose selection.

The target product profile (TPP) required to show evidence for a clinically relevant effect of at least 25% relative risk reduction of the event rate observed 36 days after the patient was enrolled into the study. In low risk patients with a placebo event rate of approximately 2–5% on day 36, a sample size of more than 20,000 patients would be needed to show a 25% relative risk reduction of the event rate ($\alpha = 0.05$ and power $= 0.8$). The investment in time and money would be much too high for such a large proof of concept study (Phase IIa).

Seeking the proof of concept in a high-risk population with a 15% risk on day 36, a 25% relative risk reduction would require a sample size of 2650 patients. Such a large sample size is typically used in a Phase III trial, but still too expensive for a Phase IIa proof of concept study. We gave up confirming proof of concept in man and continued with a high-risk development of cariporide of combining Phase IIa, Phase IIb, and Phase III in a single big clinical study [GUARDIAN (9)].

What Dose Can Achieve the Target Effect?

The goal of learning in drug development is to attribute outcome differences to variation in actual dose regimens. Drug exposure or its surrogate, plasma concentration, is the most important covariate to predict outcome.

A relationship between dose and clinical outcome is usually split into first defining a relationship between dose and concentration and then defining a relationship between concentration and clinical outcome.

Inhibitors of sodium/hydrogen (Na/H) exchange like cariporide have been shown to protect the ischemic myocardium in cardiac surgery of animals. In pharmacologic experiments in pigs using cariporide, the outcome was successful in all ischemic experiments with drug concentrations above a threshold of 0.2–0.4 mg/L. So, the relationship between concentration and clinical outcome is approximated as a step function where any concentration above the observed threshold should show the maximum probability of a successful outcome. The threshold concentration referred to is almost full NHE (sodium–hydrogen type 1 exchanger) inhibition. Concentrations have been above the threshold before the start of ischemia and were prolonged until the end of reperfusion.

The relationship between concentration and NHE inhibition in human thrombocytes was determined [Fig. 4 and Ref. (10)] and used to link the animal data to hypothesized effects in man. Human plasma concentrations above 0.2 mg/L–0.4 mg/L translate to more than 80% NHE inhibition. We hypothesized that 80% NHE inhibition will also be achieved in the ischemic area of the heart and 80% NHE inhibition will show the target cardioprotective effect in man.

With this assumption, the question of what dose regimen may achieve maximum response in man could be replaced with the question of what dose regimen achieves concentration above the minimum effective threshold concentration of 0.2 mg/L in the majority of the patients. To answer this question we need a PopPK model predicting the concentration time course for a given dose regimen. Using M&S, we are looking for a dose regimen leading in the majority of patients to a mean drug concentration during the period of a high risk for the event, which is above the hypothesized minimum effective threshold concentration.

How to Predict the Exposure Using PopPK?

The PopPK approach relies on a hierarchical model describing random effects at the intrapatient and interpatient levels.

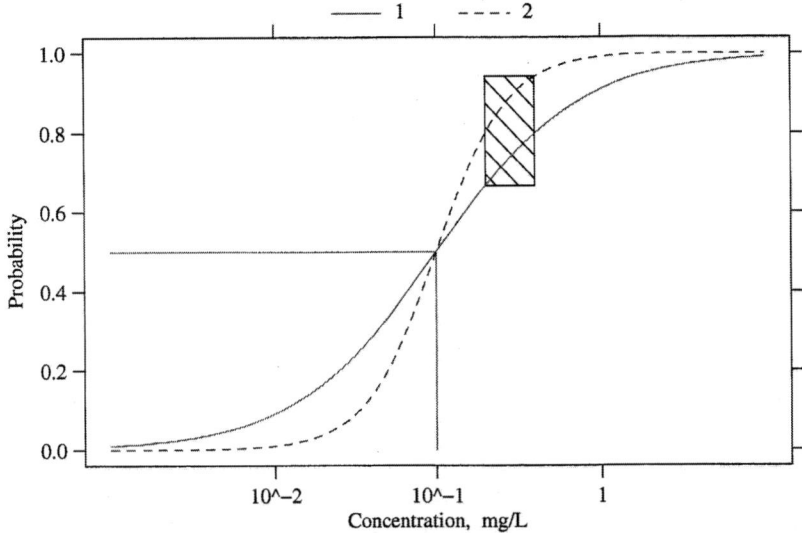

Figure 4 The relationship between the probability of NHE inhibition and cariporide concentration (log scale) was estimated using the NHE inhibition assay applied on human thrombocytes. Estimates for EC_{50} were between 0.06 mg/L and 0.09 mg/L and Hill coefficient was approximately 1.7. Approximating as $EC_{50} \approx 0.1$ mg/L, we expect 80% of the maximum NHE inhibition at 0.4 mg/L and 0.2 mg/L when we assume a Hill coefficient S of 1 and 2, respectively. Depending on the true S our expectation about the probability of NHE inhibition is marked as the *polygon area*. *Abbreviation*: NHE, sodium–hydrogen exchanger.

Intrapatient level: The rich and balanced data observed in Phase I was fitted separately for each subject and than the summary statistics were reported. PK following bolus injections was best described by a 3-compartment (cmt) PK model. The concentration observed for one subject at time t_i is predicted as:

$$C_i = f_{3cmt}(\text{dose}, t_i, \theta) + \epsilon_i \qquad (10)$$

The 3-cmt model f_{3cmt} is built using the following parameter vector $\vec{\theta}$:

$$\vec{\theta} = \{CL, Vss, V_2, V_3, Q_1, Q_2\} \qquad (11)$$

and a residual error is modeled as proportional to the model-predicted concentration.

$$SD(\epsilon_i) = \sigma f_{3cmt}(\text{dose}, t_i, \theta) \qquad (12)$$

Interpatient level: Describing the PopPK of a group of subjects, the individual parameter vector θ_j of the j-th subject can be viewed as a random vector drawn from a multivariate distribution, describing the joint probability of all possible individual parameter vectors. The individual parameter vector θ_j of the j-th subject is assumed to be drawn from a multi-variate PDF with a typical mean $\vec{\theta}$ and a between subject variability Ω. The between subject variability is modeled as a log normal distribution. For the j-th patient a vector would be drawn as:

$$\vec{\theta}_j = \vec{\theta}e^{\eta_j}; \ \eta_j \sim N(0, \Omega) \tag{13}$$

Part of the interpatient variability can be explained by differences between subjects in the body characteristics like size and kidney function.

Describing the demographics of a group of subjects, the individual demographic parameter vector Z_j of the j-th subject can be viewed as a random vector drawn from a multivariate distribution, describing the joint probability of all possible individual demographic parameter vectors. Again, the multivariate PDF describes the demographic distribution, for example, of AGE (age of subject), BW (body weight), and HT (body height), conditional on GENDER (gender of a subject) with a typical mean $\vec{Z}$ and an intersubject variability τ.

$$\vec{Z}_k = \{\overline{AGE}, \overline{BW}, \overline{HT}, \overline{SCREA}\}|GENDER_k \tag{14}$$

We summarized body size either to LBM (lean body mass) or to IBW (ideal body weight) and the kidney function to CL_{CR} (creatinine clearance) and normalized on a typical demographic vector:

$$\vec{Z} = \left\{\frac{\overline{CL}_{CR}}{100\,ml/min}, \frac{\overline{LBM}}{50\,kg}, \frac{\overline{IBW}}{70\,kg}\right\} \tag{15}$$

which is no longer conditional on GENDER. The individual demographic parameter vector Z_j of the j-th subject is drawn from the joint probability of all possible individual demographic parameter vectors:

$$\vec{Z}_j = \vec{Z}e^{z_j}; \quad z_j \sim N(0, \tau) \tag{16}$$

When no influential demographic variables are used in the parameter model, then the $\vec{\theta}$ is calculated for a subject with the mean demographic properties given in equation 15.

$$\vec{\theta} = \begin{pmatrix} \theta_{CLR} \\ \theta_{CL_{NR}} \\ \theta_{V_{SS}} \\ \theta_{V_2} \\ \theta_{V_3} \\ \theta_{Q_2} \\ \theta_{Q_3} \end{pmatrix}; \vec{Z}_\theta = \begin{pmatrix} Z_{CL_{CR}} \\ Z_{IBW} \\ Z_{LBM} \\ Z_{LBM} \\ Z_{LBM} \\ Z_{LBM} \\ Z_{LBM} \end{pmatrix}; z_{\vec{\theta}_j} = \begin{pmatrix} z_{CL_{CR}} \\ z_{LBM} \\ z_{LBM} \\ z_{LBM} \\ z_{LBM} \\ z_{LBM} \\ z_{LBM} \end{pmatrix}; \vec{\eta}_j = \begin{pmatrix} \eta_{CLR} \\ \eta_{CL_{NR}} \\ \eta_{V_{SS}} \\ \eta_{V_2} \\ \eta_{V_3} \\ \eta_{Q_2} \\ \eta_{Q_3} \end{pmatrix} \tag{17}$$

$$\vec{\theta}_j = \vec{\theta} \, \vec{Z}_\theta \, e^{z_{\theta_j} + \eta_j} \tag{18}$$

The typical patient is described by the mean demographic parameters, that is, $z_{\vec{\theta}_j} = 0$, and the mean PopPK parameters, that is, $\vec{\eta}_j = 0$. Part of the variability given as $\mathrm{Var}(\vec{\eta}_j)$ in equation 13 is explained in equation 18 by differences in CL_{CR}, IBW, and LBM.

NONMEM analysis of pooled Phase I data: For a specific subpopulation of healthy subjects defined by an LBM of 50 kg, IBW of 70 kg, and CL_{CR} of 100 ml/min, we found the following typical parameter vector:

$$\vec{\theta} = \left\{ \begin{array}{c|c|c|c|c|c|c} CL_{Ren} & CL_{Non.ren} & V_{ss} & V_2 & V_3 & Q_2 & Q_3 \\ 180 & 86 & 88 & 46 & 31 & 52.4 & 215 \\ \mathrm{ml/min} & \mathrm{ml/min} & \mathrm{L} & \mathrm{L} & \mathrm{L} & \mathrm{L/hr} & \mathrm{L/hr} \end{array} \right\} \tag{19}$$

$$CV = \sqrt{\mathrm{diag}\ \Omega} = \{18.6, 39.8, 13.8, \ldots, 20.5, 21.7\}\%, \quad \sigma = 20\% \tag{20}$$

CL_{CR} as surrogate for the kidney function has the greatest influence on cariporide pharmacokinetics. The relationship between the typical CL_{Ren} (renal clearance) for a sub-population with a specific CL_{CR} can be calculated as follows:

$$CL_{Ren}[\mathrm{mL/min}] = 180\left(\frac{CL_{CR}}{100\,\mathrm{mL/min}}\right); \quad CV = 18.6\% \tag{21}$$

IBW has only a weak influence on $CL_{Non.ren}$. The relationship between $CL_{non.ren}$ and IBW can be described as follows:

$$CL_{Non.ren}[\mathrm{mL/min}] = 86\left(\frac{\mathrm{IBW}}{70\,\mathrm{kg}}\right); \quad CV = 39.8\% \tag{22}$$

The relationship between total $CL_{tot} = CL_{Ren} + CL_{Non.ren}$ and CL_{CR} is shown in Figure 5.

LBM has a strong influence on the volume of distribution at steady-state (V_{ss}). The relationship between V_{ss} and LBM can be described as follows:

$$V_{ss}[\mathrm{L}] = 88\left(\frac{\mathrm{LBM}}{50\,\mathrm{kg}}\right); \quad CV = 13.8\% \tag{23}$$

The relationship between V_{ss} versus LBM is shown in Figure 6.

Dose selection for Phase II/III: Combined use of PopPK and M&S revealed that a dose of 120 mg t.i.d. was required to predict concentrations above the assumed threshold concentration of 0.2 mg/L for longer than 80% of the dose interval in more than 80% of patients. As observed in animal experiments, we expected the maximum cardioprotective effect above this threshold concentration. To get a better understanding of the relationship between dose and clinical outcome, we also included the lower doses of 20 mg and 80 mg of cariporide every 8 hours in the Phase II/III GUARDIAN study (Fig. 7).

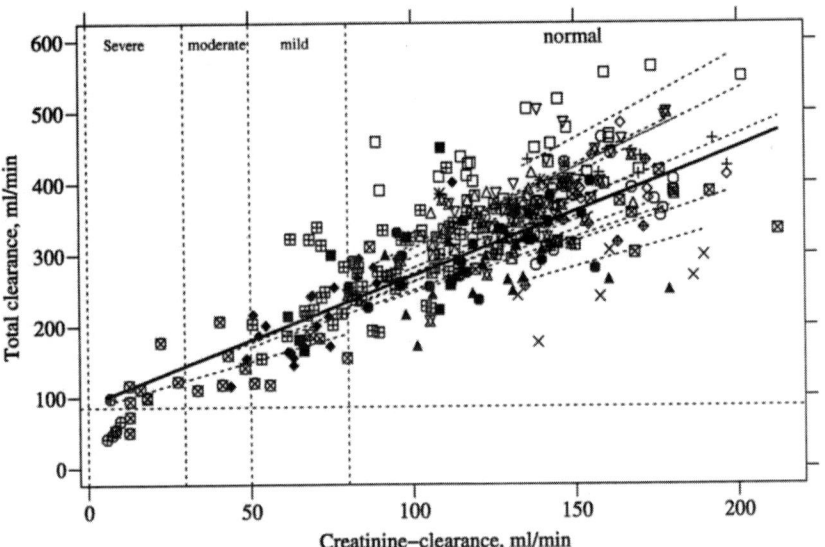

Figure 5 Total clearance versus creatinine clearance from a pooled Phase I analysis. *Symbols* correspondent to different trials. The *horizontal line* corresponds to the contribution of the non-renal part of the clearance. Clearance is linearly increasing with creatinine clearance, *dotted lines* are individual fits for the different trials. Limits for normal kidney function and also for mild, moderate, and severe renal impairments are indicated. *Source*: From Ref. 10.

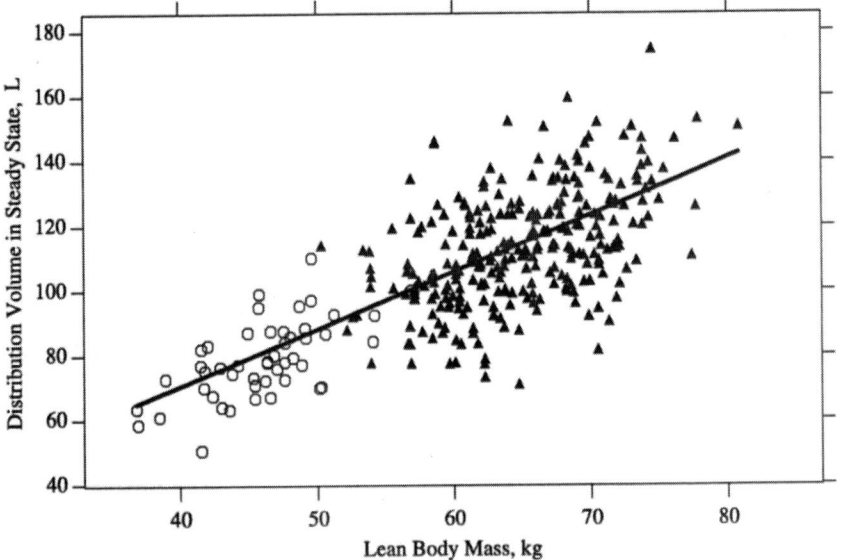

Figure 6 Distribution volume at steady-state versus lean body mass in the pooled Phase I analysis. *Circles* correspond to females, *triangles* to male volunteers. *Source*: From Ref. 10.

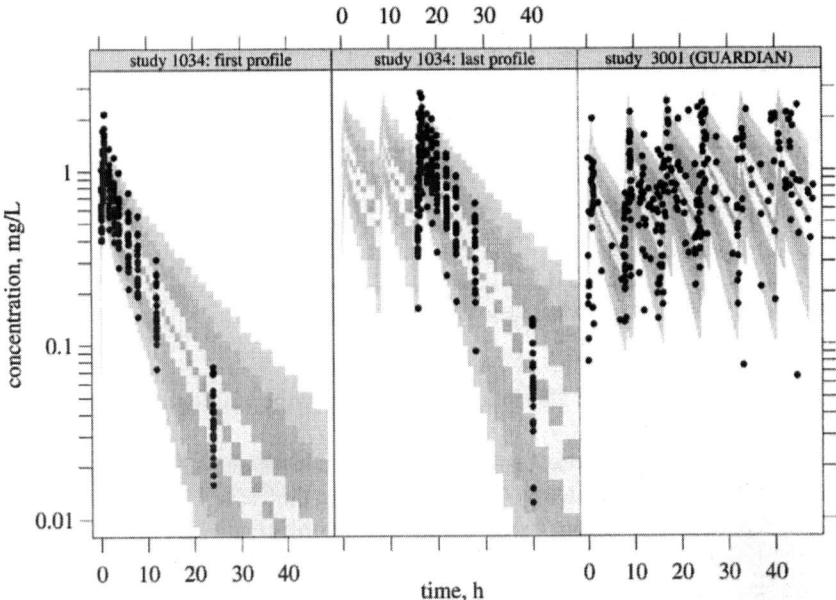

Figure 7 Concentration versus time courses observed in a Phase I study and in the PPK sub-study of the GUARDIAN study after 120 mg t.i.d. cariporide. The *dots* correspond to individual observations. The *grey areas* indicate the prior predictions with 98%, 95%, 50%, and 10% percentiles. *Left panel*: Phase I single dose; *middle panel*: Phase I last three doses; *right panel*: PK data observed on the first 2 days in UAP and PCI patients enrolled in the PPK sub-study. *Abbreviations*: UAP, unstable angine pectoris; PCI, percutaneous coronary intervention; PK, pharmacokinetics.

Proof of Concept in CABG Patients

Is there a dose–effect relationship? In the Phase II/III GUARDIAN study, a total of 11,590 patients with unstable angina or non-ST elevation MI or undergoing high-risk percutaneous or surgical revascularization were randomized to receive placebo or 20, 80 or 120 mg doses of cariporide every 8 hours for at least 2 days and up to a maximum of 7 days. The Phase II/III study failed with respect to the Phase III part to confirm benefit of cariporide over placebo on the primary endpoint of MI or death assessed after 36 days. There were no increases in clinically serious adverse events.

A post hoc analysis of the GUARDIAN data confirmed the proof of concept (Phase IIa part) in the sub-population of CABG patients. Pretreatment with 120 mg t.i.d. of the NHE inhibitor cariporide resulted in a significant reduction in the primary endpoint. No effect was seen on mortality. No effects existed at the 20- and 80-mg doses, whereas a 25% reduction in MI or death was present with the 120-mg dose of cariporide ($p = 0.027$). The event rate of MI or death

Table 1   Time Course of the Clinical Benefit Observed as Relative Risk
Reduction (Δ_{Risk}) of the Combined Event of MI or Death in CABG
Patients Enrolled in the 120 mg t.i.d. Group of the GUARDIAN Study (9)

Time (days)	Δ_{Risk} (%)	p value
5	32.3	0.007
10	28.5	0.016
36	25	0.027
183	19.3	0.033

Abbreviation: CABG, coronary artery bypass graft.

at 36 days was 16.2% and 12.1% in the placebo and the 120 mg t.i.d. cariporide
group, respectively.

With 120 mg t.i.d. dose, benefit was observed in patients undergoing bypass
surgery as relative risk reduction (Δ_{Risk}) as shown in the Table 1. Because the drug
effect reduces only the acute risk ($\Delta_{Acute\ risk}$) occuring on the first day and is less
pronounced on the second day, the observed relative risk reduction Δ_{Risk}
decreases due to the continuing contributions of events by the chronic risk. As
shown in Figure 8, the observed events were clustered mainly on the first day
showing that the acute high risk is related to CABG surgery. The observed low
event rate after the third day reflects the chronic low risk of the underlying CHD.

**Is there a relationship between concentration and clinical
outcome?**   In Figure 8, we see a clustering of the events as a result of an
acute high risk period limited between the start of the anesthesia and the end
of surgery. Only the number of events observed at this initial peak is large
enough to observe any beneficial effect of the drug in the given sample size.
The observed target effect of reducing the event rate by Δ_{Risk} % will depend
only on the cariporide concentration during this initial period of the acute high
risk. Due to the increasing contribution of the chronic risk to the observed
event rate, the observed relative risk reduction is always smaller than the drug-
related reduction of the acute risk, that is $\Delta_{Risk} < \Delta_{Acute\ risk}$.

$$p_1 = p_{1,\bar{c}=0}(1 - \Delta_{Acute\ risk}\text{Prob}(\text{success}|\bar{C})) \qquad (24)$$

In Equation 24, the term $p_{1,\bar{c}=0}$ corresponds to the placebo treatment when
$\text{Prob}(\text{success}|\bar{C} = 0) = 0$.

A relationship between concentration and clinical outcome was constructed
correlating the weight of the acute risk p_1 in the time-to-event risk probability
(given in Eq. 5) to the mean plasma concentration during the acute high risk
period of CABG surgery $\bar{C}$ (Eq. 24).

Let us approach the important question: Whether there is a relationship
between concentration and clinical outcome? The situation after a RCT is
often that we observe the clinical outcome in a large study population but miss

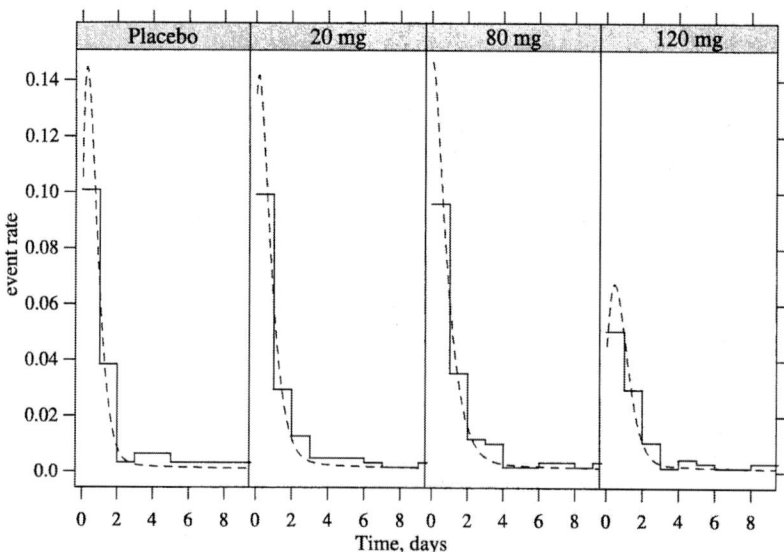

Figure 8 Event rate (relative count of events per day) versus time after start of treatment. *Step solid lines*: experimental data; *dotted lines*: predicted event rate using a mixture probability model. *Source*: From Ref. 11. Courtesy of American Society of Clinical Pharmacology and Therapeutics.

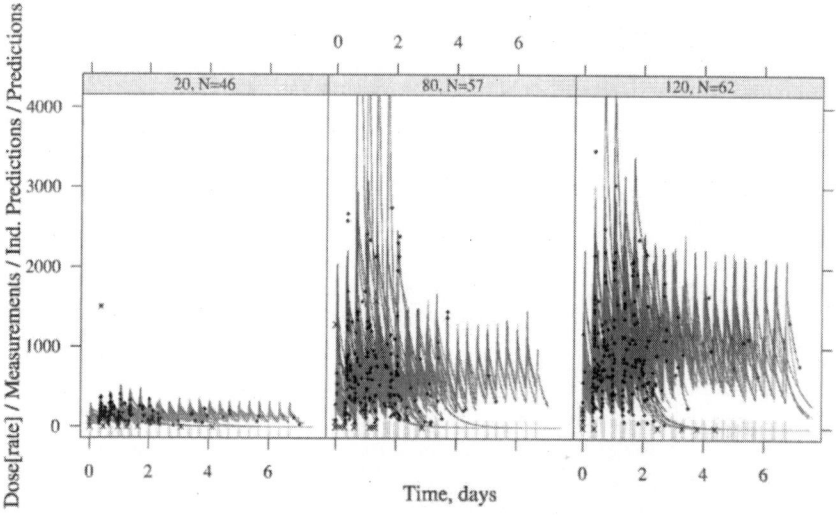

Figure 9 Concentration time courses in UAP and PCI patients enrolled in the PPK substudy of the GUARDIAN study. *Black dots*: observed concentrations; *grey lines*: post hoc predictions using the PPK model obtained from pooled Phase I data; *left panel*: 20 mg t.i.d., *middle panel*: 80 mg t.i.d. and *right panel*: 120 mg t.i.d. *Abbreviations*: UAP, unstable angina pectoris; PCI, percutaneous coronary interventions.

any information on exposure to the drug in most or all of the patients. Within the GUARDIAN study, we included a PopPK sub-study. Plasma samples were collected in a small satellite group of 377 out 11,590 patients using a sparse sampling design. Discarding the patients on placebo, at least some PK information for validation of the known PopPK model was available in 269 patients of the small satellite group. However, most of the patients were enrolled for indications other than CABG. We assumed that the PK is comparable between the observed group of UAP and PCI patients and the group of CABG patients for whom the predictions are required. The concentration–time courses sampled in the UAP and PCI patients enrolled in the PopPK sub-study are shown in Figure 9.

PopPK analysis of the pooled Phase I data revealed that body size and kidney function were powerful predictors of the PK parameters V and CL, respectively (Figs. 5 and 6). The clinical outcome was observed in almost 2840 CABG patients. The missing PK information in these CABG patients was predicted using the PopPK model and M&S, incorporating their dose history and their influential demographic information on body size and kidney function.

The most important role of the PopPK approach was learning about the unobserved PK in the major study population from a small satellite group of patients with sparse sampling data. The small amount of PK information obtained from a satellite group is, in general, sufficient to validate an *a priori* known PopPK model for the target population. The missing PK data necessary for a concentration–effect analysis in the target population is simply predicted using the PopPK model, the influential demographic patient information, and the M&S technique. In the cariporide project, the mean concentration during the period of surgery $\bar{C}$ (mean concentration during the priod of acute risk) was predicted and used as a predictor of the drug effect in a time-to-event analysis including all CABG patients with observed information on clinical outcome.

The concentration–efficacy analysis revealed a steep onset of reduction in the risk of MI or death with cariporide plasma concentration above a minimum effective threshold concentration of 0.55 mg/L [Fig. 10 and Ref. (11)]. The threshold concentration in man is approximately twice the threshold concentration found in animal experiments. The exposure achieved with 120 t.i.d. seems just to cover the lower range of efficacy. At concentrations distinctly higher than the minimum effective threshold concentration, the number of patients exposed was too low to precisely evaluate the maximum therapeutic potential. Nevertheless, due to its clinical importance, a rough estimate of the maximum effect revealed that for the observed event rate of 16% in placebo-treated patients the relative risk reduction $\Delta_{\text{Acute risk}}$ should be at least 30% or higher. Such reduced acute risks would translate to at least 25% and 21% (Δ_{Risk}) lower event rates on day 2 and day 36, respectively.

As shown in Figure 11, the minimum effective threshold plasma levels found in man were reached in none of the patients who received the 20-mg dose, in 24% of those who received the 80-mg dose, and in 69% of those who received the 120-mg

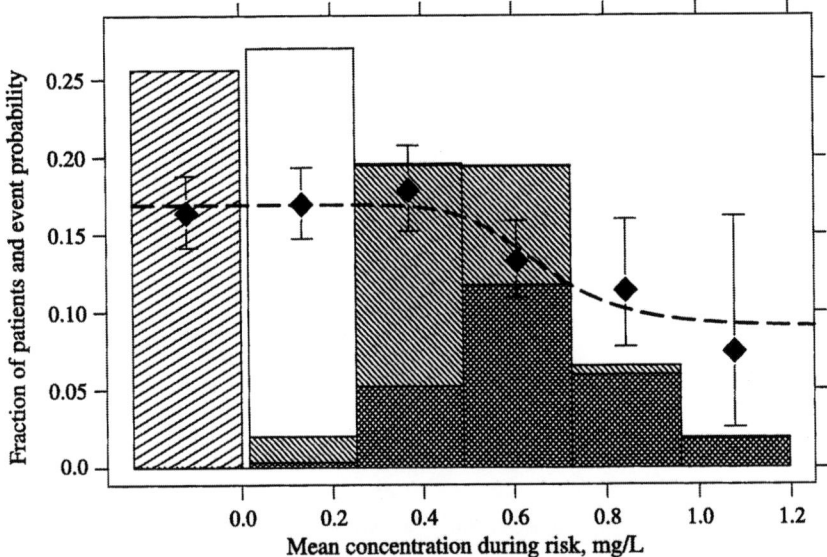

Figure 10 Relationship between event rate and cariporide concentration. *Bar histogram:* fraction of 2840 patients with a predicted concentration within the limits of the individual bar. Placebo is shown as the bar with negative concentrations. Intersections on the other bars show the fraction corresponding to each dose group: 20 mg (*wide hatching*), 80 mg (*narrow hatching*), and 120 mg (*no hatching*). The probability of an event, $P_{mix}(T \leq 36$ days), given in equation 4 is shown using the Hill model (equation 1, *solid line*) to describe the concentration dependency of the drug effect described in equation 24. The *filled diamonds* with error bars represent the observed event rate, that is, the sum of acute and chronic risk events, in each concentration box and their 5% and 95% percentiles. The event probability contributed by the chronic risk was 0.045. *Source*: From Ref. 11. Courtesy of American Society of Clinical Pharmacology and Therapeutics.

dose, suggesting that higher dosages and/or dosing modifications that achieve exposure above the minimum effective threshold during the period of risk in most of the patients could improve the efficacy of cariporide.

How to optimize the dose: The secondary goal of the GUARDIAN study (the Phase IIb part) was to attribute outcome differences to variation in actual regimens and find an optimized dose regimen for future clinical use.

In the GUARDIAN study most patients were operated between 2 and 9 hours after start of the t.i.d. treatment with cariporide. As a consequence of the chosen t.i.d. regimen, the cariporide concentrations declined during the dose interval below the minimum effective threshold concentration within the period of increased risk. Using a constant infusion regimen instead of a t.i.d. treatment could avoid such decline of the cariporide concentration below the minimum effective threshold concentration during the CABG surgery.

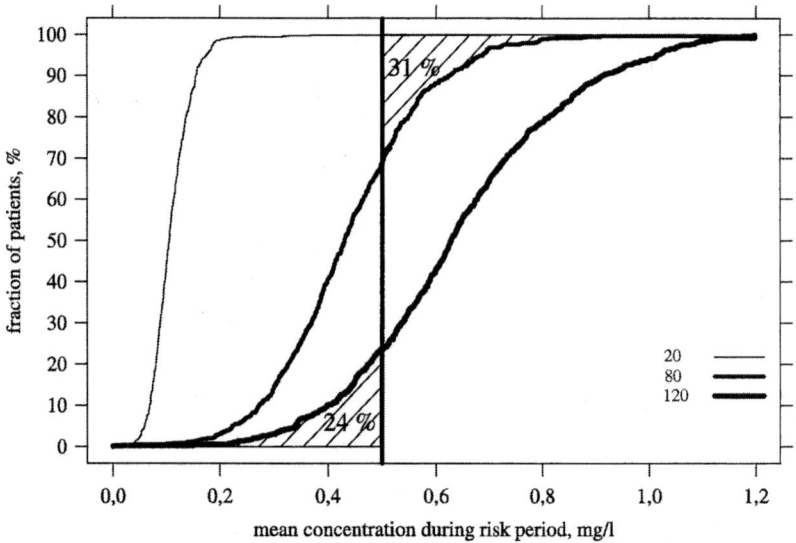

Figure 11 Distribution of mean cariporide concentration under CABG surgery for each dose group. The *vertical line* marks the threshold concentration of 0.5 mg/L. In the 80 mg dose group only 31% of the patients reached mean concentrations above this minimal effective concentration, whereas in the 120 mg dose group, 76% are above. *Abbreviation*: CABG, coronary artery bypass graft.

Cardioprotection is required only on the first day when the acute risk related to CABG surgery is high and is less important on the second day.

The learning step in a new Phase IIb study aimed to find an optimized infusion dose regimen, which constantly exposed 95% of the patients on the day of the CABG surgery and the day after to concentrations above the minimum effective threshold concentration without exceeding the range of concentrations observed in the GUARDIAN trial.

What infusion regime covers exposure of 120 mg t.i.d. in CABG patients?—120 mg t.i.d. sums up to a daily dose of 360 mg cariporide or to a mean infusion rate of 15 mg/hr. To quickly obtain the concentration range above the minimum effective threshold concentration, we decided to start with the initial 1 hour infusion of 120 mg. To avoid the decline of the cariporide concentrations, we could continue with a 15 mg/hr maintenance infusion. Such 120 mg/15 mg/hr approach would achieve the mean concentration time course of the 120 mg t.i.d. dose regimen without any fluctuation of exposure. As clinical trial simulations revealed, an increase of the 15 mg/hr maintenance infusion to a 20 mg/hr maintenance infusion would still achieve concentrations below the peak concentrations of the 120 mg t.i.d. approach and, at the same time, would increase exposure to such an extent that more than 95% of the patients would achieve concentrations above the minimum effective threshold concentration during surgery. Therefore, a 120 mg loading infusion administered within 1 hour and followed by a 20 mg/hr maintenance infusion given for a further 48 hours was expected to cover the exposure of 120 mg t.i.d. and was the first dose regimen investigated in a new Phase IIb study.

What infusion regime constantly exceeds 1 mg/L in the majority of patients? The second target of the Phase IIb study aimed to explore the safety and tolerability in the concentration range above 1 mg/L, where the PK/PD model obtained from the GUARDIAN data potentially predicts additional efficacy. Our second target aims to investigate such a high concentration range well above the peak concentrations observed in the GUARDIAN study, which was never investigated in humans. As clinical trial simulations revealed, an increase of the 1 hour loading infusion of 120 mg to an 1 hour loading infusion of 180 mg and simultaneously increasing the 20 mg/hr maintenance infusion to a 40 mg/hr maintenance infusion would mean that more than 95% of the patients would achieve concentrations above twice the minimum effective threshold concentration during surgery (Fig. 12). To limit the risk with safety and tolerability in this unexplored range of exposure, we decided to increase the dose step-wise from 120 mg/20 mg/hr to 180 mg/30 mg/hr and continue with 180 mg/40 mg/hr only if no issues with safety and tolerability occurred.

To validate our PopPK model for the use of the higher than previously used dose regimen, we compared the PK data expected and observed in the Phase IIb study. The available PopPK model predicted the concentration time course suffciently well to optimize the dose regimen.

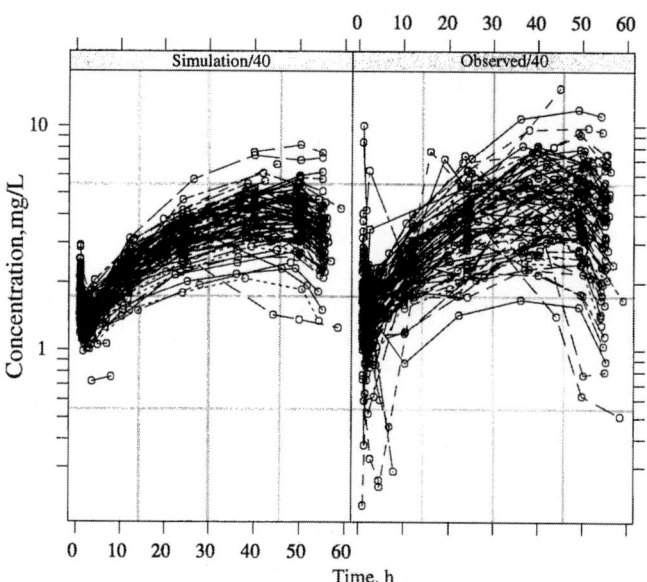

Figure 12   Concentration versus time in a Phase IIb study with 180 mg/hr loading dose and 40 mg/hr maintenance dose. Observations are shown on the right, simulations with the population PK model on the *left side. Abbreviation*: PK, pharmacokinetics.

Designing the confirmatory Phase III study: Continuously administered intravenous (IV) cariporide for up to 48 hours in subjects undergoing CABG surgery was safe and well tolerated at all three dose levels tested in this study. Exploratory analysis of the combined incidence of MI or death demonstrated a reduction in the occurrence of this endpoint with cariporide compared with placebo, which was most pronounced in the high-dose cariporide group. The findings of this study support the continued investigation of optimal continuous IV cariporide dosing in patients undergoing CABG surgery.

As the three dose levels tested exhibited a similar safety profile, the ultimate selection of a dose regimen for further studies was based upon the results of the PopPK analyses (12) and M&S. In Figure 13, we compared the outcome for the mean concentration during the risk period between 100 simulations of the Phase IIb study and the observed study results.

The results of the PopPK analysis of the dose-finding Phase IIb study are summarized as follows:

- Using doses of 120/20 mg/hr and 180/40 mg/hr we achieved the target exposure during CABG surgery of concentrations above 0.5 mg/L and above 1 mg/L, respectively in 95% of the patients.

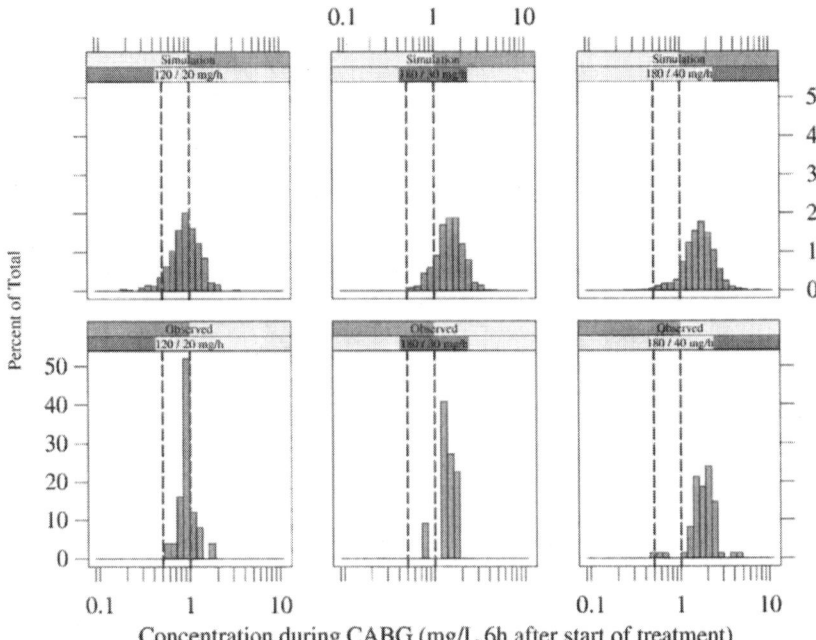

Figure 13 Simulated and observed concentrations during CABG for three dosing regimens (120/20 mg/hr, 180/10 mg/hr, 180/40 mg/hr) in a Phase IIb study. *Abbreviation*: CABG, coronary artery bypass graft. *Source*: From Ref. 12.

- Because no dose-limiting adverse events occurred, 180/40 mg/hr was found appropriate to be tested in a new clinical trial; 120/20 mg/hr may serve as a back-up dose option.
- Due to the considerably lower risk of suffering an event on the second treatment day (Fig. 8), the observed higher concentrations on day 2 probably will not add additional benefit to the patient. Therefore, the modified infusion regimen of 180/40/20 mg/hr, consisting of 180 mg/40 mg/hr infusion on the first treatment day and half the maintenance infusion (20 mg/hr) on the second day was recommended.

Simulations using the demographics of the Phase IIb CABG population and the 180/40/20 mg/hr dose regimen are shown in Figure 14. Assuming that we achieve maximum relative risk reduction $\Delta_{Acute\,risk}$ when using the 180/40/20 mg/hr dose regimen, the expected event probability curves for placebo and maximum treatment effect are shown in Figure 15.

What was the Role of PopPK in the Development Process? (Table 2)

The development started with animal experiments, showing that in all clamp experiments the heart was successfully protected against ischemic injury above a threshold concentration.

The question was how to translate the successful treatment in animals to cardioprotection in ischemic diseases in man. The threshold concentration

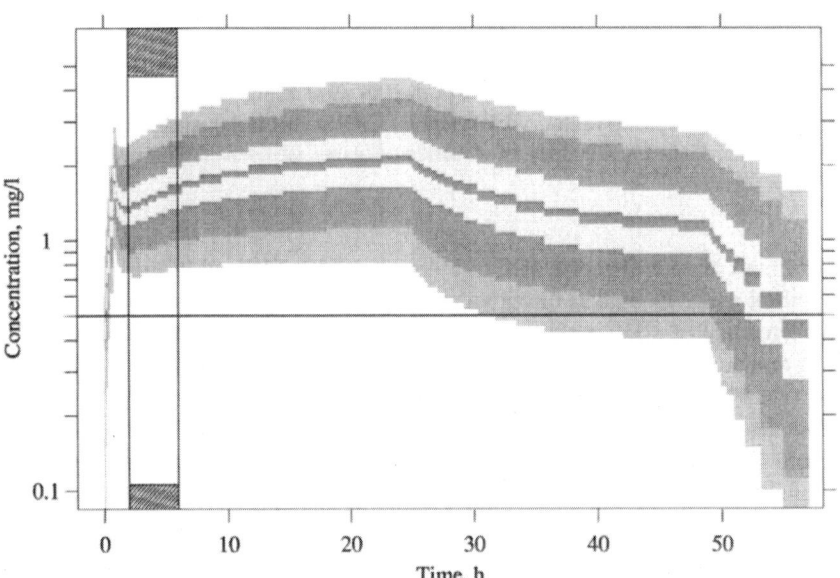

Figure 14 Simulation of the concentration–time course in CABG patients. The dosing is 180 mg/hr for 1 hr, 40 mg/hr for 24 hours, 20 mg/hr for 24 hours. *Abbreviation*: CABG, coronary artery bypass graft. *Source*: From Ref. 12.

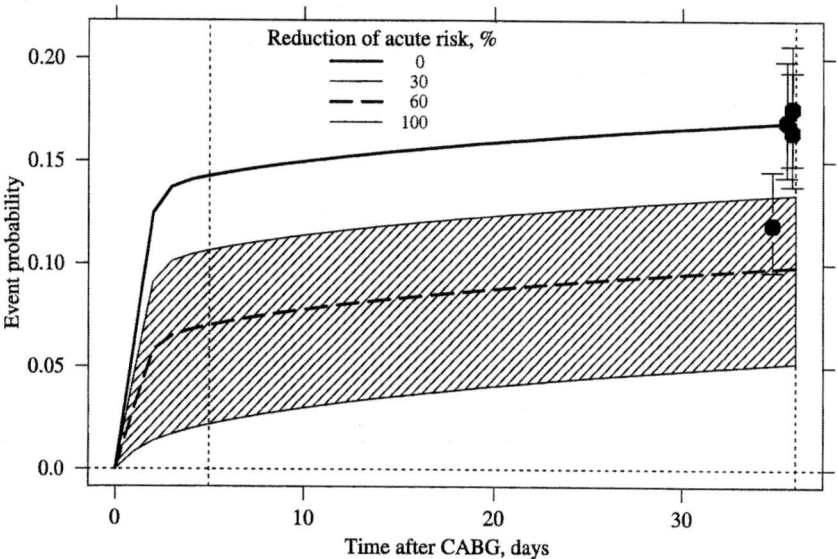

Figure 15 Expected event probability curves for placebo and maximum treatment effect, $\Delta_{\text{Acute risk}}$, calculated using equation 7. $\Delta_{\text{Acute risk}}$ was estimated as 60% (95% confidence interval: 30–100%) relative reduction of the acute risk of an event, which is assumed to be directly related to the CABG surgery. The *lowest curve*, that is, 100% reduction, corresponds to the chronic risk of an event, which is assumed not to be related to the CABG surgery. The event rates of 0.164, 0.169, 0.176, and 0.119 observed in patients enrolled in the GUARDIAN trial and treated per protocol with placebo, 20, 80, and 120 mg cariporide t.i.d., respectively, are shown as *filled circles* with 95% confidence intervals. The *vertical dotted lines* mark day 5 and day 36 after beginning of treatment as the discussed days of observation. *Abbreviation*: CABG, coronary artery bypass graft. *Source*: From Ref. 11. Courtesy of American Society of Clinical Pharmacology and Therapeutics.

determined in animals correlated to more than 80% NHE inhibition. The NHE inhibition assay in human thrombocytes led to plasma threshold concentration correlated to 80% NHE inhibition in human. We assumed that the NHE inhibition in thrombocytes correlates with the NHE inhibition in the ischemic myocard. Our first PK/PD relationship was a simple step function describing no effect below the threshold concentration and the full effect above the threshold concentration. However, cardioprotection in animals was always observed above the threshold concentration. We decided to design a confirmatory study to detect a 25% difference between the event rate in placebo and cariporide treatment. Knowledge of the wide range of placebo responses in patients with ischemic diseases was found in the literature. To limit the sample size of the clinical study, we decided to investigate only high-risk patient groups with an event rate between 10% and 20%. When the type I error α and the power $1 - \beta$ are given for the

Table 2 Use of PopPK Preparing Phase III of the Cariporide Development

Question	Experiment	Result	Phase
Reduction of infarct size with cariporide?	Clamping and reperfusion in pigs	Above 0.2 mg/L reduced	Preclin., Pigs
NHE effect in humans?	Human thrombocyte test, NON/MEM	80% inhibition of NHE exchanger for conc > 0.2–0.4 mg/L	Preclin., in vitro
For which dose concentration > 0.2 mg/L?	Pooled Phase I, PopPK, simulation	120 mg t.i.d.	I
Proof of concept and confirming?	GUARDIAN study	Proof of concept: yes, confirming in a large patient population: no	IIa, III
Dose response?	GUARDIAN	25% reduction for CABG patients at 120 mg t.i.d., no reduction at 80 mg t.i.d.	IIb
Concentration response in CABG patients?	GUARDIAN, PopPK for 269 patients satellite logistic regression for 2116 patients	Yes, minimum effective threshold 0.55 mg/L	IIb
High-risk period in CABG?	GUARDIAN	Time of CABG surgery	IIb
Dose for concentration above a threshold of 0.55 mg/L?	Study in CABG patients, PopPK, simulation	Infusion 120 mg/hr for 1 hr + 20 mg/hr for 47 hours	IIb
Safety concerns?	GUARDIAN, study in CABG patients	no safety concerns	IIb
Dose for concentration above 2 times threshold?	Study in CABG patients, PopPK, simulation	Infusions of 180 mg/hr for 1 hr, 40 mg/hr for one day, 20 mg/hr for the following days	IIb

Abbreviations: NHE, sodium–hydrogen exchanger; CABG, coronary artery bypass graft.

sample size calculation, you need only to decide about the minimal detectable, but still clinically relevant, effect size i.e., the expected event probability and the Δ_{Risk} (8).

The challenging question was: Which dose regimen is necessary to achieve at least the minimal detectable effect size? From the animal experiments, we learnt that a simple step function may serve as a first estimate of the relationship between concentration and effect. So our hypothesis was that all doses leading to concentrations above the threshold concentration will at least achieve the target effect size. With this assumption, the dose we are looking for could be found if a PopPK model for cariporide would be available for M&S.

The PopPK model was built retrospectively using the NONMEM approach and the pooled data obtained in Phase I. Our PopPK model was then used to simulate the concentration–time courses of all further future studies, which always included a sparse sampling strategy. After completion of the studies, the PopPK model was validated by comparing the predicted concentration–time courses with the concentration–time courses observed in the following study.

The GUARDIAN study failed to confirm efficacy over all patient groups. However, there was a strong effect found in a sub-group analysis in CABG patients receiving the largest dose amounts. Plasma concentrations were measured only in a small satellite group of patients using a sparse sampling design. PK information was only available in a small satellite group of patients and most of them with indications other than CABG. The clinical outcome was observed in almost 3000 CABG patients. The PK information required to estimate the relationship between concentration and clinical outcome was taken from predicting the PK using the PopPK model. M&S incorporated the dose history and the influential demographic information on body size and kidney function, which were powerful predictors of the PK parameter V and CL, respectively. The most important role of the PopPK approach was learning about the PK in the major study population from small satellite groups of patients. The missing PK data necessary for a PK/PD analysis is simply predicted using the PopPK model and M&S. The predicted mean concentration during the period of surgery was used as a predictor of the drug effect in a time-to-event analysis including all patients with observed information on clinical outcome.

The resulting PK/PD model was used to predict the PK and clinical outcome for a variety of dose regimens. Three dose regimens were selected to investigate their safety and tolerance in a following Phase IIb study. Validation of the PopPK model in the target population of CABG patients was our second objective in this Phase IIb study. A sparse sampling design was applied in all CABG patients enrolled in this study. Optimizing the design of future studies, especially dose finding for Phase III studies, is an important role of the PopPK approach.

All three dose regimens were safe and tolerable. The PopPK model was validated by comparing predicted and observed plasma concentrations. We updated the PopPK model parameter estimates using the PK data obtained in the Phase IIb study. Using the updated model we simulated the PK and clinical outcome for slightly modified dose regimens. The finally chosen dose regimen was investigated in the final Phase III trial. The outcome of this Phase III study was summarized by Bolli et al. (6) as follows: The NHE inhibitor "cariporide has been shown to be cardioprotective in high-risk CABG patients." Unfortunately, Bolli et al. continued with "but its neurologic effects preclude its use at the present time." The sad result of the cariporide development is that the demonstrated beneficial cardioprotective effects were offset by unexpected neurologic side effects. The good news is that PopPK combined with simulation techniques was successfully applied in the learning and confirming steps about efficacy in drug development.

CONCLUSION

When designing any experimental study, we always have a model about our experimental unit in mind supporting us with expectations of the outcome of the study. When optimally designing a Phase III study, we need a model for predicting the outcome with respect to the dose/concentration/effect relationship in our experimental unit, that is, the population of target patients.

Drug development is a sequence of learning and confirming steps gathering the information necessary to optimize the pivotal Phase III study, which hopefully confirms the efficacy of the new drug. The role of PopPK and PK/PD modeling is summarizing available data into a predictive model. The hypothesis concerning the functional relationship between dose, concentration and effect, the selection of physiological variables as influential covariates, and the parameter estimates were incorporated into the model and tested against our available experimental data.

Modeling and simulation helps in general to structure the drug development process and to ask question about what is already known or where we have only vague ideas and where we require more information for making qualified decisions. Putting things into equations of a model needs to decide on each parameter and think about possible influential covariates.

The value of a model is given by its usefulness to answer specific drug development questions. Our PopPK model was useful to answer important questions related to the design of our Phase III study, such as:

- What dose regimen achieves in 95% of the target patients' plasma concentration constantly above a minimum effective threshold concentration?
- How to obtain reliable predictions on missing concentration data required for PK/PD modeling?

We used the PopPK approach combined with M&S for all the learning steps to acquire the information needed for decision-making and for planning efficient confirmatory clinical studies.

ACKNOWLEDGMENTS

We wish to acknowledge Dr. Andreas Jessel, Sanofi-Aventis, and Dr. Lutz Harnisch, now with GlaxoSmithKline, for their contributions, fruitful discussions, and excellent cooperation.

APPENDIX: LIST OF ACRONYMS

AGE	age of subject; year
CABG	coronary artery bypass graft surgery
$\bar{C}$	mean concentration during the period of acute risk
CHD	coronary heart disease
CL_{tot}	total clearance; L/hr
CL_{CR}	creatinine clearance; L/hr
$CL_{Non.ren}$	non-renal clearance; L/hr
CL_{Ren}	renal clearance; L/hr
EC_{50}	concentration at half maximum effect; mg/L
GENDER	gender of a subject; 1 = male and 2 = female
HT	body height; cm
IBW	ideal body weight; kg
IV	intravenous
LBM	lean body mass; kg
α_i	location of the i-th Weibull distribution
M&S	modeling and simulation
MI	myocardial infarction
Ω	Covariance matrix describing the between subject variability
NHE	sodium–hydrogen type 1 exchanger
NONMEM	nonlinear mixed-effects modeling
PCI	percutanous coronary intervention
PDF	probability density function
PK	pharmacokinetics
PK/PD	relationship between pharmacokinetics and pharmacodynamics
PopPK	population pharmacokinetics
Q	intercompartment clearance
RCT	randomized clinical trial
Δ_{Risk}	relative risk reduction
$\Delta_{Acute\ risk}$	relative reduction of the acute risk
SCREA	serum creatinine concentration
τ_i	shape of the i-th Weibull distribution
S	Hill coefficient
UAP	unstable angina pectoris
V_{ss}	volume of distribution at steady-state; L
BW	body weight; kg

REFERENCES

1. Sheiner LB. Learning versus confirming in clinical drug development. Clin Pharmacol Ther 1997; 61:275–291.
2. Sheiner LB, Steimer J-L. Pharmacokinetic/pharmacodynamic modeling in drug development. Annu Rev Pharmacol Toxicol 2000; 40:67–95.
3. Collett D. Modelling Binary Data. 2nd ed. Chapman and Hall, 2003.
4. FDA. Guidance for Industry: Population Pharmacokinetics, February 1999. CP1.
5. Sheiner L, Wakefield J. Population modelling in drug development. Stat Methods in Med Res 1999; 8:183–199.
6. Bolli R, Becker L, Gross G, Mentzer R Jr, Balshaw D, Lathrop DA. Myocardial protection at crossroads: the need for translation into clinical therapy. Therapies for protecting the heart from ischemia. Circ Res 2004; 95(2):125–134.
7. Gelman A, Carlin JB, Stern HS, Rubin DB. Bayesian Data Analysis. Chapman and Hall, 1995.
8. MathSoft, ed. S-PLUS 6.0 for UNIX Guide to Statistics, Volume I, October 2000.
9. Theroux P, Chaitman BR, Danchin N, Erhardt L, Meinertz T, Schroeder JS, Tognoni G, White HD, Willerson JT, Jessel A. Inhibition of the sodium-hydrogen exchanger with cariporide to prevent myocardial infarction in high-risk ischemic situations. Main results of the Guardian trial. Circulation 2000; 102:3032–3038.
10. Weber W, Harnisch L. Population pharmacokinetics of cariporide (HOE642) in healthy volunteers and patients with renal impairment: Phase I, Appendix C: NHE inhibition as surrogate effect. Technical Report, Hoechst Marion Roussel, March 1999. Doc.No.: 8235A.
11. Weber W, Harnisch L, Jessel A. Lessons learned from a phase III population pharmacokinetic study of cariporide in coronary artery bypass graft surgery. Clin Pharmacol Therap 2002; 71(6):457–467.
12. Weber W, Rueppel D. Population pharmacokinetics of cariporide (HOE642) administered intravenously. Analysis of study HOE642a/2008 (coronary artery bypass graft): placebo-controlled, randomized, doubleblind, sequential groups study. Technical Report, Aventis Pharma, 2003.

11

Dose Optimization Strategy for Strattera®, a CYP2D6 Substrate

Jennifer W. Witcher and Stephan Chalon
Lilly Research Laboratories, Eli Lilly & Company, Indianapolis, Indiana, U.S.A.

John-Michael Sauer
Elan Pharmaceuticals, Inc., South San Francisco, California, U.S.A.

INTRODUCTION

The development of atomoxetine hydrochloride (Strattera®) involved several important factors. In addition to demonstrating efficacy in attention-deficit/hyperactivity disorder (ADHD), key aspects of development included the polymorphic metabolism of atomoxetine by cytochrome P450 2D6 (CYP2D6) and the primary target population being children. Dose optimization was a critical part of the successful development of atomoxetine and employed phase-appropriate development strategies. Earlier clinical studies focused on dose optimization related to the safety and tolerability of atomoxetine, and also defining the impact of the CYP2D6 polymorphism on the general disposition of the molecule. Later clinical studies focused on dose optimization of atomoxetine related to efficacy measures, and the potential necessity of individualizing dosing based on genotype. This chapter presents only a subset of the data available for Strattera, and, therefore, complete safety, efficacy, and dosing information should be obtained from the current package insert.

BACKGROUND

Atomoxetine is a potent inhibitor of the presynaptic norepinephrine (NE) transporter with lower affinity for other monoamine transporters or receptors (1–5). The efficacy of atomoxetine has been demonstrated for the treatment of ADHD in children, adolescents, and adults (6–9). As the first FDA approved nonstimulant pharmaceutical treatment for ADHD, atomoxetine represents a significant advance in the treatment of this disease. Furthermore, due to its mechanism of action, atomoxetine does not share the abuse potential associated with psychostimulant drugs (10).

In vitro studies demonstrate that atomoxetine has potent nanomolar to subnanomolar affinity for the rat and human NE transporters and minimal affinity for serotonin and dopamine transporters, and also other receptors and ion channels (1). A number of preclinical in vivo studies have characterized the potency of atomoxetine as an inhibitor of NE reuptake at both central and peripheral sites (2,3,11). Furthermore, microdialysis measurement of rat brain extracellular monoamines has helped to define the central effects of atomoxetine (12). In these studies, atomoxetine increased extracellular NE in the prefrontal cortex threefold, but did not alter serotonin. Atomoxetine also increased dopamine concentrations in the prefrontal cortex threefold, but did not alter dopamine in the striatum or nucleus accumbens. In contrast to the psychostimulant methylphenidate, atomoxetine does not increase dopamine in the striatum or nucleus accumbens nor does it increase locomotor activity, suggesting it would have less potential for motoric or drug abuse liabilities. This conclusion is further supported by the finding that atomoxetine did not substitute for cocaine in monkeys that self-administered cocaine (13,14).

PK AND METABOLISM, INFLUENCE OF PHARMACOGENETICS

The most interesting feature of atomoxetine disposition is its metabolism and the influence of pharmacogenetics. Three oxidative metabolic pathways are involved in the systemic clearance of atomoxetine: aromatic ring-hydroxylation, benzylic hydroxylation, and *N*-demethylation (15). Aromatic ring-hydroxylation results in the formation of the primary oxidative metabolite of atomoxetine, 4-hydroxyatomoxetine, which is subsequently glucuronidated and excreted in urine. The formation of 4-hydroxyatomoxetine is primarily mediated by the polymorphically expressed enzyme, CYP2D6 (16). Therefore, alterations in the catalytic activity of CYP2D6 due to genetic polymorphism have a profound effect on the clearance of atomoxetine. This results in two distinct populations of individuals: those exhibiting active metabolic capabilities (CYP2D6 extensive metabolizers, EMs) and those exhibiting poor metabolic capabilities due to mutations or deletion of the *CYP2D6* gene (CYP2D6 poor metabolizers, PMs) for atomoxetine (17,18). The PM trait, which is known to be inherited as an autosomal recessive characteristic, is an important source of intersubject variability in metabolism for a number of drugs (17,19,20). This genetic mutation is most prevalent in Caucasians, in which approximately 7% of the population can be genetically classified as PMs (21). Although the compromised ability to metabolize CYP2D6 substrates is principally mediated by the genetic polymorphism associated with CYP2D6, the phenotypic manifestation of this condition can result from exposure to chemical inhibitors of this metabolic pathway.

The EM population can be subdivided into two additional groups based on the number and intrinsic catalytic activity of functional alleles. These subpopulations are identified as ultra-rapid metabolizers (UM) and intermediate metabolizers (IM). The UM genotype results from gene duplication of functional *CYP2D6* alleles (*CYP2D6*2XN*) and has been associated with greater CYP2D6 catalytic activity (22). The UM genotype accounts for approximately 3–7% of the overall EM population (23). Individuals that are defined as IMs possess two compromised *CYP2D6* alleles (*CYP2D6*10, CYP2D6*17*) that have decreased activity due to genetic mutation (24,25). Although the enzyme produced from these alleles is functional, its catalytic activity is lower than that associated with fully functional alleles (*CYP2D6*1*).

In PMs, multiple cytochrome P450 enzymes are capable of forming 4-hydroxyatomoxetine and secondary pathways become more dominant (benzylic hydroxylation and *N*-demethylation) (15,16). Therefore, should one or more of these multiple routes of metabolism be affected due to drug–drug interactions or due to interindividual differences in the activity of cytochrome P450 enzymes, changes in the overall clearance of atomoxetine in PMs are not expected.

PK in Adult Subjects

The clinical pharmacokinetic (PK) and metabolic properties of atomoxetine have been well characterized in children, adolescents, and adults (for review, see Ref. 26). Atomoxetine has high aqueous solubility and biological membrane permeability that facilitates its rapid and complete absorption after oral administration. Absolute oral bioavailability ranges from 63% in EMs to 94% in PMs, which is governed by the extent of the first-pass metabolism. The oral bioavailability and clearance of atomoxetine are influenced by the activity of CYP2D6; nonetheless, plasma PK parameters are predictable in both EM and PM patients. After single oral doses, atomoxetine reaches maximum plasma concentration in about 1–2 hours after dosing. In EMs atomoxetine has a half-life of 5.2 hours, while in PMs atomoxetine has a plasma half-life of 21.6 hours. The systemic plasma clearance of atomoxetine is 0.35 and 0.03 L/hr/kg in EMs and PMs, respectively. Correspondingly, the mean steady-state plasma concentrations are approximately 10-fold higher in PM compared with EM subjects. Upon multiple dosing, there is plasma accumulation of atomoxetine in PMs, but very little accumulation in EMs. The volume of the distribution is 0.85 L/kg, indicating that atomoxetine is distributed in total body water in both EMs and PMs. Atomoxetine is highly bound to plasma albumin (approximately 99% bound in plasma) (15).

Although steady-state concentrations of atomoxetine in PMs are higher than those in EMs following the administration of the same mg/kg/day dose, there are only modest differences observed in tolerability which do not appear to have marked effects on overall clinical outcomes (27).

In Figure 1, the mean steady-state plasma concentration-time profiles (normalized to a 1-mg/kg dose of atomoxetine) are shown for atomoxetine, *N*-desmethylatomoxetine, and 4-hydroxyatomoxetine. In both EM and PM subjects, *N*-desmethylatomoxetine and 4-hydroxyatomoxetine are the principal oxidative metabolites of atomoxetine found in the plasma. In EM subjects at steady state, plasma concentrations of both *N*-desmethylatomoxetine and 4-hydroxyatomoxetine are relatively low compared with atomoxetine. The plasma concentrations ($C_{ss,avg}$) of *N*-desmethylatomoxetine were about 5% of atomoxetine, while 4-hydroxyatomoxetine plasma concentrations were about 1% of atomoxetine. In PM subjects, steady-state 4-hydroxyatomoxetine concentrations ($C_{ss,avg}$)

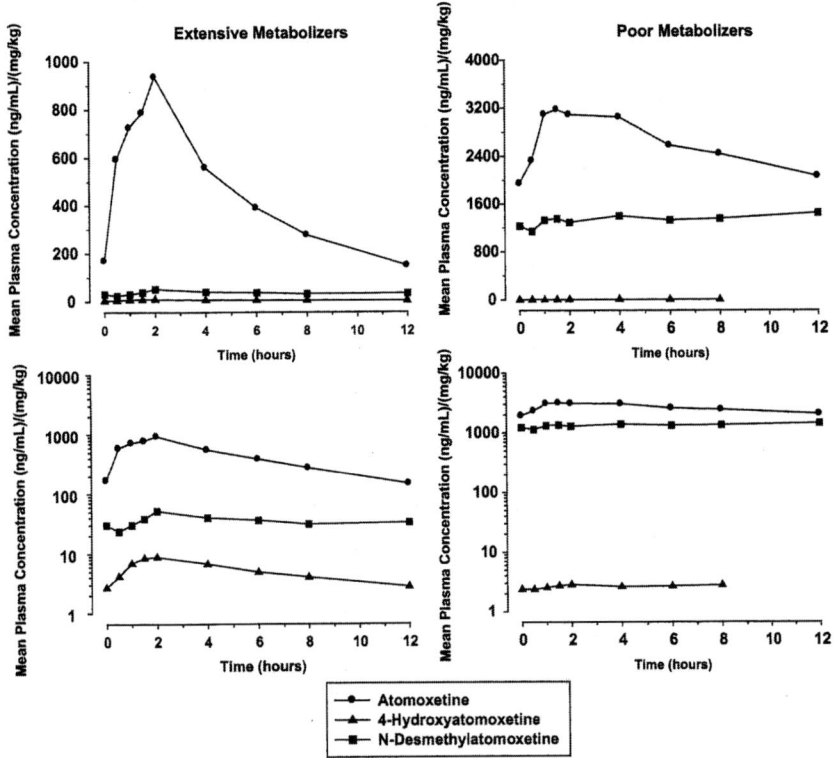

Figure 1   Mean steady-state concentration (normalized to a 1-mg/kg dose) versus time profiles for extensive and poor metabolizer subjects.

are relatively low compared with atomoxetine (about 0.1%). However, plasma concentrations of *N*-desmethylatomoxetine were approximately 45% of atomoxetine in the PM subjects (Strattera package insert).

With regard to the genetically defined subgroups present in the overall EM population (UM and IM genotypes), the PK differences observed with atomoxetine are relatively minor. A great deal of overlap in the PK of atomoxetine is observed, suggesting that neither the UM or IM genotype are distinct phenotypic populations, in contrast to the substantial PK differences observed overall between the EM and PM individuals (data on file at Lilly Research Laboratories).

PK in Pediatric Patients

The PK in children and adolescents were fully evaluated in more than 400 patients and shown to be similar to adults, after adjustment for body weight (28–30). Based on the marked effect of body weight on the clearance of atomoxetine, it was decided early in development that a weight-based dosing regimen would be used for pediatric patients.

DEVELOPMENT STRATEGY FOR A CYP2D6 SUBSTRATE

In addition to demonstrating efficacy in ADHD, key aspects of development included the polymorphic metabolism of atomoxetine by cytochrome P450 2D6 (CYP2D6), and the primary target population being children. Phase I study initially revealed the effect of the CYP2D6 polymorphism on the disposition of atomoxetine, and, therefore, this attribute was known during the development of atomoxetine for ADHD. This characteristic increased the complexity of clinical drug development because there were several additional safety and PK aspects to explore. One question to be answered was whether individuals lacking CYP2D6 activity, who have higher atomoxetine plasma concentrations than the majority of the population, would tolerate the same doses as EMs. Depending on the safety and tolerability of atomoxetine in the PMs, patients may need to be phenotypically or genotypically characterized for CYP2D6 status in order to receive the appropriate dosage. Another interesting subset of the population, the UMs, needed to be explored in order to understand if they may have subtherapeutic plasma concentrations, and, therefore, lack of efficacy. These questions were addressed during clinical development and the appropriate dosing regimen and labeling for the drug was determined.

The clinical development of atomoxetine followed a thorough and stepwise progression in the understanding of the PK, safety, tolerability, and efficacy in PMs, and also the population as a whole. Clinical pharmacology studies dosed healthy adult subjects without regard to genotype in order to fully understand the safety, tolerability, and PK over the dose range of interest. Early efficacy trials in adults dosed atomoxetine at lower doses without regard to genotype. In initial efficacy trials in children and adolescents, patients were dosed in accordance with their genotype, such that PMs received lower doses than EMs (data on file at Lilly Research Laboratories). Another feature of these initial clinical trials in pediatric patients was that the dosing regimens were very flexible, with the aim of titrating doses slowly based on the individual's response and tolerability to the drug. These individualized titration design studies allowed for a more conservative approach in early trials and also provided much information about the doses that physicians found useful (31). After demonstrating a very broad therapeutic index in these initial safety and tolerability studies, later clinical trials in both pediatric and adult patients dosed atomoxetine without regard for genotype (32,33). Another strategy to further optimize dosing was a large clinical trial which allowed investigators to titrate doses as they would in the clinical setting, while blinded to the patient's CYP2D6 genotype (data on file at Lilly Research Laboratories). This provided information on whether PM patients would have sufficient efficacy at lower doses, or whether investigators would increase their doses similar to EMs because their response was not substantially different. The clinical trial results and safety comparisons between EMs and PMs are discussed later in this chapter.

Biomarkers, Clinical, and Safety Endpoints

Atomoxetine being an NE reuptake inhibitor, several possible biomarkers were considered to support dose finding in the early drug development process. No human-validated PET ligand for the NE transporter was available when Phase I studies were conducted with this compound. Other tools described in the literature to document pharmacodynamic (PD) effects of NE reuptake inhibitors in humans include the tyramine pressor test (34), pupillary diameter (35), and measurements of catecholamines in plasma, urine, and CSF (36,37). While some of these evaluations were conducted in small Phase I inpatient studies (38), none of them were considered suitable for large outpatient Phase II and III trials. Therefore, focus was made on the primary clinical endpoint for efficacy, as well as on cardiovascular effects, which are both easy to measure and are believed to reflect the increased availability of NE induced by atomoxetine.

In pediatric populations, the primary efficacy variable was the Attention-Deficit/Hyperactivity Disorder Rating Scale-IV-Parent Version: Investigator Administered and Scored (ADHDRS-IV-Parent:Inv) total score including hyperactive/impulsive and inattentive subscales (39). The scale consists of 18 items used to diagnose ADHD as defined in the *Diagnostic and Statistical Manual of Mental Disorders, Fourth Edition* (DSM-IV) (40). The total score is the sum of the scores for each of the 18 items, with each symptom rated from 0 to 3 with a total score ranging from 0 to 54. The primary efficacy analysis is based on baseline, last-observation-carried-forward (LOCF) endpoint, and change from baseline to endpoint in ADHDRS-IV-Parent:Inv total score.

In adults, signs and symptoms of ADHD were evaluated using the investigator administered CAARS (Conners Adult ADHD Rating Scale Screening Version), employing the 18 items that correspond to the ADHDRS scale (41). Since NE reuptake inhibitors are expected to interfere with the regulation of cardiovascular function via increased availability of NE (42), blood pressure and heart rate were closely monitored across all the clinical studies as a safety endpoint. In clinical studies, increases in pulse and blood pressure were small and of little, if any, clinical significance (for review, see Ref. 43).

The method for determining CYP2D6 status in clinical efficacy studies was typically by obtaining a blood sample for determining the CYP2D6 genotype for selected defective alleles (*CYP2D6 *3, *4, *5, *6, *7, *8*). This method was shown to be adequate for predicting the phenotype. In clinical pharmacology studies, typically a genotype and phenotype test (using dextromethorphan as the probe substrate) were obtained in order to show concordance.

EFFICACY AND SAFETY STUDIES

The safety and effectiveness of atomoxetine in the treatment of ADHD was established in randomized double-blind placebo-controlled trials in both pediatric patients and adults who met DSM-IV criteria for ADHD (data on file at Lilly Research Laboratories) (8,43,44). Since differences in CYP2D6 genotype and phenotype could potentially affect the patient's response to atomoxetine and its clinical profile by altering its PK, blood samples were obtained from all patients to determine CYP2D6 genotype. This CYP2D6 genotype status obtained at study entry was kept blinded from the patients and the investigator until the conclusion of each study, and was ultimately used by the sponsor in comparing the results between groups.

The Phase III pediatric efficacy trials were dose-titration studies on a weight-adjusted basis according to clinical response with a maximum total daily dose of 1.8 mg/kg, with the exception of one dose–response study. The dose–response study compared three dose levels of atomoxetine (0.5, 1.2, and 1.8 mg/kg/day) and placebo. The adult efficacy trials compared atomoxetine and placebo, and atomoxetine was titrated according to clinical response up to 120 mg/day. The impact of these studies on dose selection is discussed in the following.

A key part of the dose optimization strategy for atomoxetine was a pediatric two-year open-label safety and efficacy Phase III study, which investigated the comparability of the safety and tolerability of atomoxetine among a large number of CYP2D6 EMs and PMs (data on file at Lilly Research Laboratories). The final mean dose and clinical response, and also safety and tolerability, were similar among both the groups. These results clearly suggested that when clinicians were blind to CYP2D6 status and titrated atomoxetine based on the clinical response, the final efficacious dose was independent of CYP2D6 status. These data also support the comparability of tolerability and safety for the groups.

The effects of CYP2D6 status on the efficacy, safety, and tolerability of atomoxetine in children and adolescents were examined in a retrospective meta-analysis (27, data on file at Lilly Research Laboratories). At the endpoint, PMs had markedly greater reductions in mean symptom severity scores compared with EMs (-14.1 for EMs; -20.9 for PMs, $p = 0.002$). Fewer PMs discontinued due to lack of efficacy than EMs (26% vs. 17.3%), again suggesting that this subgroup had greater improvement in ADHD symptoms than EMs. Analysis of vital signs demonstrated a greater increase in heart rate and diastolic blood pressure for PMs compared with the EMs. No difference was noted in effects on the corrected QT interval. Several adverse events were more frequent in PMs ($p < 0.05$), specifically decreased appetite, abrasion, and tremors. Although steady-state concentrations of atomoxetine in PMs are higher and more sustained than in EMs following administration of the same mg/kg/day dose, there are only modest differences observed in tolerability, which do not appear to have marked effects on overall clinical outcomes (27).

The data collected during atomoxetine's development, considered in its entirety, suggested that a pharmacogenetic test for CYP2D6 status was not necessary before treatment with atomoxetine. Instead, an initial starting dose (0.5 mg/kg/day in pediatric patients, 40 mg in adults) along with a dose-titration up to a target total daily dose (1.2 mg/kg/day and 100 mg, respectively) was recommended. A target dose more than 1.2 mg/kg/day was not shown to provide additional benefit, and therefore the 1.2 mg/kg/day dose was deemed as the appropriate initial target dose for most patients (32).

DOSE–RESPONSE AND PK/PD MODELING

The dose optimization strategy focusing on efficacy utilized a Phase III dose–response study with the following treatments: placebo, 0.5, 1.2, and 1.8 mg/kg/day. Statistical analyses of this study's data revealed a graded dose–response, where the dose of 0.5 mg/kg/day was associated with intermediate efficacy between placebo and the two higher doses. At the endpoint, atomoxetine doses of 1.2 and 1.8 mg/kg/day were consistently associated with superior outcomes in ADHD symptoms compared with placebo and were not different from each other. The 1.2-mg/kg/day dose seems to be as effective as 1.8 mg/kg/day and is thus the appropriate initial target dose for most patients (32).

Data from this study were used to evaluate the exposure–response relationship using PK/PD modeling for the purposes of further optimizing the dosing of atomoxetine (30). The PK/PD analysis utilized data from EMs only, since only a small number of PMs participated in this study due to their infrequency in the general population. Furthermore, the range of exposures observed in EMs was unique from the range in PMs, making the PK/PD analysis comparing EMs and PMs confounded. Therefore, this part of the dose optimization strategy for atomoxetine focused primarily on EM data. Based on statistical analysis discussed previously, PMs had greater reductions in mean symptom severity scores compared with EMs (-14.1 for EMs; -20.9 for PMs, $p = 0.002$). One hypothesis is that the greater efficacy in PMs may be due to the greater exposure to atomoxetine. On the other hand, the greater efficacy could be a result of the different PK profile in PMs, resulting from the longer half-life and more sustained exposure during the day, which may suggest a different PK/PD relationship in PMs. Further work on whether a different PK/PD relationship is observed based on CYP2D6 status is warranted and is ongoing for future publications.

In this study, the population PK model developed in a previous analysis of five studies was used to obtain empirical Bayesian clearance estimates for each patient. The final dataset used to conduct the population PK analysis contained data from 189 pediatric patients. The area under the concentration–time curve over the dosing interval ($AUC_{0-\tau}$) was calculated for each patient using the clearance estimates, and the relationship of $AUC_{0-\tau}$ with the ADHDRS-IV-Parent:Inv score was examined.

Figure 2 summarizes the distribution of $AUC_{0-\tau}$ values for the three dose groups. Although mean, median, and modal $AUC_{0-\tau}$ values were different for the three dose groups, there was a clinically significant overlap in exposures between the 0.5 and 1.2 mg/kg/day treatment groups, and between the 1.2 and 1.8 mg/kg/day treatment groups. Because of a limited number of capsule strengths and a moderate degree of PK variability, even with the use of weight-based dosing, this variation and overlap in exposures is not unexpected.

A non-linear model (inhibitory E_{max} model) was fit to the observed AUC and change from baseline ADHDRS-IV-Parent:Inv total scores data to explore the relationship between efficacy and AUC (Fig. 3). Patients randomized to placebo were used in this analysis by assigning an AUC of zero. The resulting fit of this model suggests that the expected maximum improvement from baseline would be -17.4 (compared to -6.2 for 8 weeks of placebo dosing). This suggests an overall maximum benefit of -11.2 over placebo. This analysis is useful for characterizing the shape of the exposure–response curve in order to estimate the dose that provides a near maximum improvement in ADHD symptoms. Based on the median AUC values for each dosing group, Figure 3 suggests that at a dose of 1.2 mg/kg/day (median AUC of 1.08 $\mu g \bullet hr/mL$), the curve begins to flatten and approach the maximum value. Therefore, this analysis provides additional evidence that a target dose of 1.2 mg/kg is desirable. This analysis shows there is a relationship between systemic exposure and efficacy, which is similar to that between dose and efficacy (32), and supports the dose selection of 1.2 mg/kg/day as an initial target dose.

DOSING RECOMMENDATIONS AND LABELING

Current labeling recommendations for atomoxetine in children and adolescent patients (up to 70 kg) initiate treatment at a total daily dose of approximately 0.5 mg/kg and is increased after a minimum of 3 days to a target total daily dose of approximately 1.2 mg/kg, administered either as a single daily dose in

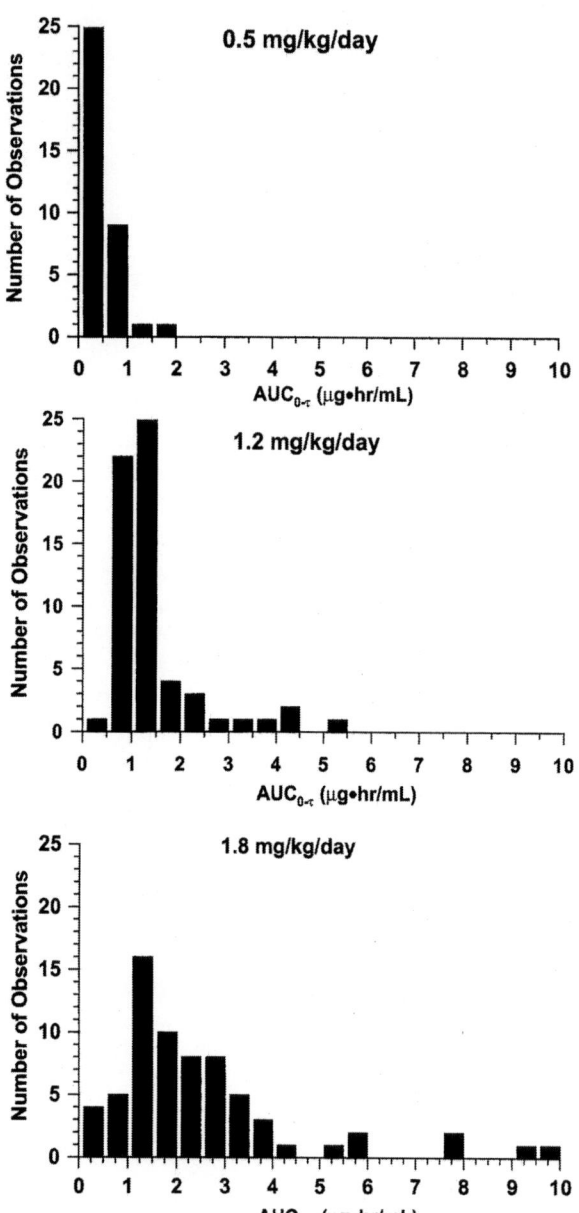

Figure 2 Frequency distribution of area under the atomoxetine plasma concentration versus time curve at the three dose levels in extensive metabolizer patients. *Abbreviation:* AUC, area under concentration–time curve.

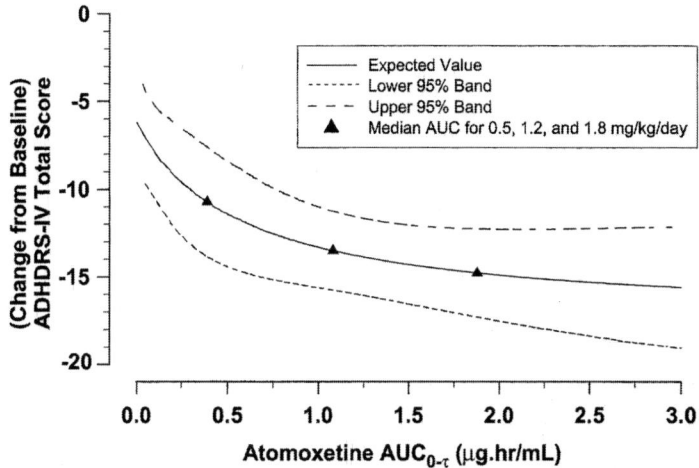

Figure 3 Model-predicted mean change from baseline to endpoint in ADHDRS-IV-Parent:Inv Total score and atomoxetine AUC for extensive metabolizer patients with confidence bounds. *Abbreviations*: ADHDRS-IV-Parent:Inv Total score, Attention-Deficit/Hyperactivity Disorder Rating Scale-IV-Parent Version: Investigator Administered and Scored; AUC, area under concentration–time curve.

the morning or as evenly divided doses in the morning and late afternoon/early evening. These dosage recommendations are without regard to an individual's CYP2D6 genotype.

Based on the cumulative amount of data in PMs, including evaluations of efficacy, safety, and tolerability, it was determined that this subpopulation could be safely and effectively treated using the same dosing regimen as the rest of the population. In the current labeling, there is extensive information describing various aspects of atomoxetine in PMs, which was possible since this subpopulation was purposefully included and evaluated during clinical development. Dose optimization based on safety and tolerability relied on data from all patients. However, final dose selection was based primarily on EM response, since greater efficacy is observed in PMs compared with EMs.

During the development of any drug that primarily relies on CYP2D6 for its clearance, it is unclear at the onset of development whether individuals will need to be prospectively identified before treatment and individualized dosing based on the genotype utilized. Applying pharmacogenetic information during drug development allows for the determination of whether individualized dosing is warranted and also the determination of the appropriate regimen for the subpopulation. In some cases, the knowledge related to genotype and clinical outcomes can increase the quality of a clinician's decision about individualizing drug treatment (45). However, as discussed in this chapter, differential dosing was not deemed necessary for Strattera based on the data as a whole.

REFERENCES

1. Wong DT, Threlkeld PG, Best KL, Bymaster FP. A new inhibitor of norepinephrine uptake devoid of affinity for receptors in rat brain. J Pharmacol Exp Ther 1982; 222:61–65.
2. Oberlender R, Nichols DE, Ramachandran PV, Srebnik M. Tomoxetine and the stereoselectivity of drug action. J Pharm Pharmacol 1987; 39:1055–1056.
3. Gehlert DR, Gackenheimer SL, Robertson DW. Localization of rat brain binding sites for [3H]tomoxetine, an enantiomerically pure ligand for norepinephrine reuptake sites. Neurosci Lett 1993; 157:203–206.
4. Gehlert DR, Schober DA, Gackenheimer SL. Comparison of (R)-[3H]tomoxetine and (R/S)-[3H]nisoxetine binding in rat brain. J Neurochem 1995; 64:2792–2800.
5. Wheeler WJ, Bymaster FP, Calligaro DO, et al. Strattera® (atomoxetine HCl), an inhibitor of the norepinephrine transporter. 1. The preparation of C-14 labeled atomoxetine, and two of its metabolites. 2. The preparation and biological evaluation of some additional putative metabolites of atomoxetine. In: Dean DC, Filer CN, McCarthy KE, eds. Synthesis and Applications of Isotopically Labelled Compounds. Vol. 8. New York, NY: John Wiley and Sons, 2004:357–360.
6. Spencer T, Biederman J, Wilens T, et al. Effectiveness and tolerability of tomoxetine in adults with attention deficit hyperactivity disorder. Am J Psychiatry 1998; 155:693–695.
7. Spencer T, Heiligenstein JH, Biederman J, et al. Results from 2 proof-of-concept, placebo-controlled studies of atomoxetine in children with attention-deficit/hyperactivity disorder. J Clin Psychiatry 2002; 63:1140–1147.
8. Michelson D, Allen AJ, Busner J, et al. Once-daily atomoxetine treatment for children and adolescent with attention deficit hyperactivity disorder: a randomized, placebo-controlled study. Am J Psychiatry 2002; 159:1896–1901.
9. Kratochvil CJ, Heiligenstein JH, Dittmann R, et al. Atomoxetine and methylphenidate treatment in children with ADHD: a prospective, randomized, open-label trial. Am Acad Child Adolesc Psychiatry 2002; 41:776–784.
10. Heil SH, Holmes HW, Bickel WK, et al. Comparison of the subjective, physiological, and psychomotor effects of atomoxetine and methylphenidate in light drug users. Drug Alcohol Depend 2002; 67:149–156.
11. Fuller RW, Hemrick-Luecke SK. Antagonism by tomoxetine of the depletion of norepinephrine and epinephrine in rat brain by alpha-methyl-m-tyrosine. Research Commun Chem Path Pharmacol 1983; 41:169–172.
12. Bymaster FP, Katner JS, Nelson DL, et al. Atomoxetine increases extracellular levels of norepinephrine and dopamine in prefrontal cortex of rat: a potential mechanism for efficacy in attention deficit/hyperactivity disorder. Neuropsychopharmacology 2002; 27:699–711.
13. Gasior M, Bergman J, Kallman MJ, Paronis CA. Evaluation of the reinforcing effects of monoamine reuptake inhibitors under a concurrent schedule of food and i.v. drug delivery in rhesus monkeys. Neuropsychopharmacology 2005; 30:758–64.
14. Wee S, Woolverton WL. Evaluation of the reinforcing effects of atomoxetine in monkeys: comparison to methylphenidate and desipramine. Drug Alcohol Depend 2004; 75:271–276.

15. Sauer JM, Ponsler GD, Mattiuz EL, et al. Disposition and metabolic fate of atomoxetine hydrochloride: the role of CYP2D6 in human disposition and metabolism. Drug Metab Dispos 2003; 31:98–107.

16. Ring BJ, Gillespie J, Eckstein JA, Wrighton SA. Identification of the human cytochromes P450 responsible for atomoxetine metabolism. Drug Metab Dispos 2002; 30:319–323.

17. Evans DAP, Maghoub A, Sloan TP, Idle JR, Smith RL. A family and population study of the genetic polymorphism of the debrisoquine oxidation in a white British population. J Med Genet 1980; 17:102–105.

18. Steiner E, Bertilsson L, Sawe J, Bertling I, Sjoqvist F. Polymorphic debrisoquine hydroxylation in 757 Swedish subjects. Clin Pharmacol Ther 1988; 44:431–435.

19. Madsen H, Nielsen KK, Brosen K. Imipramine metabolism in relation to the sparteine and mephenytoin oxidation polymorphisms—a population study. Br J Clin Pharmacol 1995; 39:433–439.

20. Abdel-Rahman SM, Leeder JS, Wilson JT, et al. Concordance between tramadol and dextromethorphan parent/metabolite ratios: the influence of CYP2D6 and non-CYP2D6 pathways on biotransformation. J Clin Pharmacol 2002; 42:24–29.

21. Guengerich FP. Human cytochrome P450 enzymes. In: Ortiz de Montellano PR, ed. Cytochrome P450: Structure, Mechanism, and Biochemistry. New York: Plenum Press, 1995:473–535.

22. Sachse C, Brockmoller J, Bauer S, Roots I. Cytochrome P450 2D6 variants in a Caucasian population: allele frequencies and phenotypic consequences. Am J Hum Gen 1997; 60:284–295.

23. Agundez JA, Ledesma MC, Ladero JM, Benitez J. Prevalence of CYP2D6 gene duplication and its repercussion on the oxidative phenotype in a white population. Clin Pharmacol Ther 1995; 57:265–269.

24. Masimirembwa C, Persson I, Bertilsson L, Hasler J, Ingelman-Sundberg M. A novel mutant variant of the CYP2D6 gene (CYP2D6*17) common in a black African population: association with diminished debrisoquine hydroxylase activity. Br J Clin Pharmacol 1996; 42:713–719.

25. Oscarson M, Hidestrand M, Johansson I, Ingelman-Sundberg M. A combination of mutations in the CYP2D6*17 (CYP2D6Z) allele causes alterations in enzyme function. Mol Pharmacol 1997; 52:1034–1040.

26. Sauer JM, Ring B, Witcher JW. Clinical pharmacokinetics of atomoxetine hydrochloride (Strattera®). Clin Pharmacokinetics 2005; 44(6):571–590.

27. Allen AJ, Wernicke J, Dunn D, et al. Safety and Efficacy of Atomoxetine in Pediatric CYP 2D6 Extensive vs. Poor Metabolizers. Biological Psychiatry 2002; 51(8S):37S. Abstract 109.

28. Witcher JW, Long AJ, Sauer JM, et al. Atomoxetine pharmacokinetics in children with attention deficit hyperactivity disorder. J Child Adolesc Psychopharmacol 2003; 13:53–64.

29. Witcher JW, Kurtz D, Heathman M, Sauer JM, Smith BP. Population pharmacokinetic analysis of atomoxetine in pediatric patients. Clin Pharmacol Ther 2004; 75:46.

30. Witcher JW, Kurtz DL, Sauer JM, Michelson D, Smith BP, Ruff D. Pharmacokinetic/pharmacodynamic relationship of atomoxetine exposure and efficacy in child and adolescent ADHD patients. Am Psych Assoc 2002; Philadelphia, PA, USA.

31. Spencer T, Biederman J, Heiligenstein J, et al. An open-label, dose-ranging study of atomoxetine in children with attention deficit hyperactivity disorder. J Child Adolesc Psychopharmacol 2001; 11:251–265.

32. Michelson D, Faries DE, Wernicke J, et al. (Atomoxetine ADHD Study Group). Atomoxetine in the treatment of children and adolescents with ADHD: a randomized, placebo-controlled dose–response study. Pediatrics 2001; 108:e83.

33. Allen AJ, Wernicke JF, Dunn D. Safety and efficacy of atomoxetine in pediatric CYP2D6 extensive and poor metabolizers. Biol Psychiatry 2001; 49(suppl 8):37S.

34. Reimann IW, Firkusny L, Antonin KH, Bieck PR. Oxaprotiline: enantioselective noradrenaline uptake inhibition indicated by intravenous amine pressor tests but not alpha 2-adrenoceptor binding to intact platelets in man. Eur J Clin Pharmacol 1993; 44:93–95.

35. Phillips MA, Bitsios P, Szabadi E, Bradshaw CM. Comparison of the antidepressants reboxetine, fluvoxamine and amitriptyline upon spontaneous pupillary fluctuations in healthy human volunteers. Psychopharmacology 2000; 149:72–76.

36. Chalon SA, Granier LA, Vandenhende FR, et al. Duloxetine increases serotonin and norepinephrine availability in healthy subjects: a double-blind, controlled study. Neuropsychopharmacology 2003; 28:1685–1693.

37. Linnoila M, Karoum F, Calil HM, Kopin IJ, Potter WZ. Alteration of norepinephrine metabolism with desipramine and zimelidine in depressed patients. Arch Gen Psych 1982; 39:1025–1028.

38. Farid NA, Bergstrom RF, Ziege EA, Parli CJ, Lemberger L. Single-dose and steady-state pharmacokinetics of tomoxetine in normal subjects. J Clin Pharmacol 1985; 25:296–301.

39. DuPaul GJ, Power TJ, Anastopoulos AD, Reid R. Reliability and validity. In: ADHD Rating Scale-IV: Checklists, Norms, and Clinical Interpretation. New York, NY: The Guilford Press, 1998:28–42.

40. American Psychiatric Association. Attention-deficit and disruptive behavior disorders. In: Diagnostic and Statistical Manual of Mental Disorders. 4th ed. Washington, DC: American Psychiatric Associaton, 1994:78–85.

41. Conners CK, Erhardt D, Sparrow E. Conners' Adult ADHD Rating Scales (CAARS). North Tonawanda: Multi-Health Systems Inc., 1999.

42. Glassman AH. Cardiovascular effects of tricyclic antidepressants. Annu Rev Med 1984; 35:503–511.

43. Wernicke JF, Faries D, Girod D, et al. Cardiovascular effects of atomoxetine in children, adolescent, and adults. Drug Safety 2003; 26:729–740.

44. Michelson D, Adler L, Spencer T, et al. Atomoxetine in adults with ADHD: two randomized, placebo-controlled studies. Biological Psychiatry 2003; 53:112–120.

45. Lesko LJ, Woodcock J. Translation of pharmacogenomics and pharmacogenetics: a regulatory perspective. Nature Rev Drug Discov 2004; 3:763–769.

12

Pediatric Dose Optimization Using Pharmacokinetics and Pharmacodynamics

Jun Shi

*Clinical Pharmacology and Drug Dynamics, Forest Laboratories, Inc.,
Jersey City, New Jersey, U.S.A.*

INTRODUCTION

The pediatric subject, representing the spectrum from prematurely born neonates to adolescents, is characterized by dynamic processes of physical, physiological, and psychosocial development. The influence of growth and maturation on a drug's pharmacokinetics (PK) and pharmacodynamics (PD) is as dynamic as children themselves. Prior to the end of the last century, most drugs had not been studied in children; therefore, there were no adequate age-defined dose recommendations in the labels. As a result, pediatricians had to use these drugs on a trial-and-error basis, which often led to either overdose or underdose, causing toxicity or ineffectiveness. In 1997, the U.S. Congress passed the Food and Drug Administration Modernization Act (FDAMA), which encouraged pediatric drug development by providing an incentive in the form of an additional six months' marketing exclusivity. We have now seen an unprecedented surge in research activity related to pediatric drug testing and labeling. The key issue of pediatric drug development is to determine how much data are required in pediatrics for establishing appropriate dosage regimen, given that the safety and efficacy of a drug is already established in adults.

One of the most important strategies of pediatric drug development is to characterize factors that influence PK and PD parameters, and thereby bridge the adult efficacy and safety to pediatrics so that the proper treatment can be determined for pediatric patients of various ages. Sufficient methodology is now available to minimize the number of PK/PD samples taken in pediatrics, and to estimate the population mean or typical parameters and their measures of variability, along with estimates of each subject's parameters on sparse and unbalanced data (1–3). This chapter will provide an overview of the PK/PD study design and data analysis in pediatrics. The focus of the chapter concentrates on two case studies: sotalol—a drug which is predominantly renally excreted, and leflunomide—a drug which is primarily metabolized, to illustrate the important features of these methodologies (4,5).

GENERAL CONSIDERATIONS OF PK/PD STUDY DESIGN AND DATA ANALYSIS IN PEDIATRICS

The Food and Drug Administration (FDA) constructs a decision tree, which maps out different study requirements (PK, PK/PD, safety, efficacy) according to assessments on similarity of disease progression, outcome of pharmacotherapy, PK–PD relationship between adults and pediatrics, and availability of a bio-marker for efficacy (Fig. 1) (6). The drug exposure is the fundamental linkage between adult and pediatric pharmacotherapy. This mandates the performance of PK studies in almost all scenarios of a pediatric drug development. For

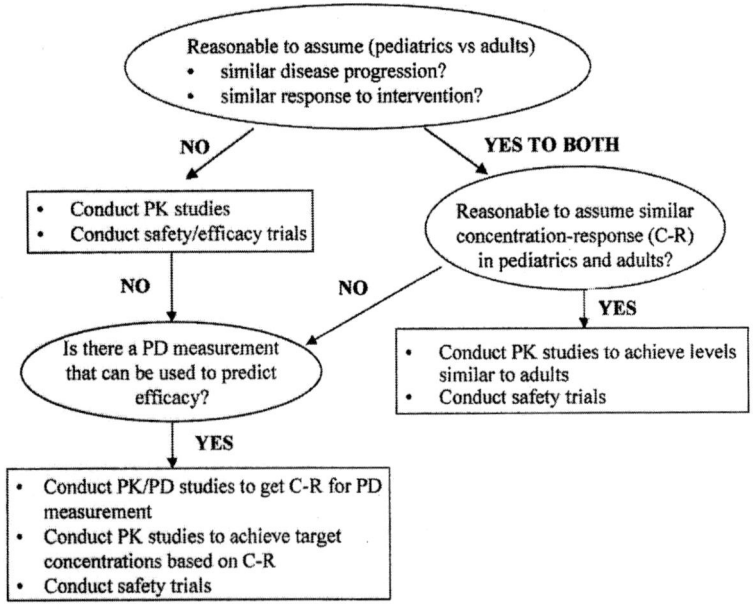

Figure 1 FDA-proposed pediatric study decision tree integration of pharmacokinetics–pharmacodynamics. *Source*: Courtesy of the Food and Drug Administration.

designing informative pediatric trials, available information in adults should be fully utilized. The following assumptions are usually made for a PK bridging:

- The disease etiology, progression, and outcome of the therapy are similar between adult and pediatric subpopulations.
- The exposure–response, including efficacy and safety, established in adults is similar to that in pediatric populations. If the clinical response to the exposure relationship is not clear or not applicable, a biomarker can be used as a surrogate.
- The safety and efficacy conferred from a recommended adult regimen can be conferred to pediatric populations, assuming that comparable drug exposure can be achieved.

A PK–PD study using a biomarker is often required to assess similarity of the exposure and response relationship between adults and pediatrics before a direct PK bridging can be deemed adequate. Model-based PK–PD analysis is a powerful tool to allow the exploration of dose and regimen scenarios and to probe the optimal one in pediatrics: (*i*) to match the adult drug exposure in pediatrics if their PK–PD relationship is similar, or (*ii*) to achieve the target concentration according to the exposure–response bridging if their PK–PD relationship is different. Well-controlled safety and efficacy studies have to be conducted if there are no biomarkers available for efficacy and safety or if the disease patho-physiology, progression, and outcome of pharmacotherapy are likely to be different between the two populations (e.g., bisphosphonates for osteoporosis in post-menopausal women and for osteogenesis inperfecta in pediatric patients), or there is little reason to assume continuity between adult and pediatric tested indication (e.g., depression).

There are numerous challenges in the design, conduct, and data analysis of PK–PD studies in pediatric patients that are distinctively different from issues encountered in similar studies for adult patients. One of the most important strategies of pediatric trials is to effectively utilize prior adult PK information for dose selection and sampling design. The dose is usually calculated based on adult parameters plus empirical scaling models, assuming that clearance and volume of distribution are proportional to either body surface area (BSA) or body weight (BW). This empirical dosing adjustment is known to have many drawbacks. A sequential design could offer an opportunity of dosing refinement in which a small PK study is conducted prior to a large-scale safety and efficacy study. The dose selection is critical when one fixed dose is employed to compare study drug against placebo or active comparator. If a dose-ranging study with multiple dose levels is to be conducted to obtain safety and efficacy data or to define PK–PD relationship, a parallel design can be applied where PK is an add-on investigation to the trial. A major challenge in pediatric studies arises from the ethical and logistic constraints on the number of blood samples and the effect of measurements that can be obtained, especially, in neonates and young infants. Limited sampling approaches coupled with population-based non-linear mixed-effects modeling methodology have been explicitly recommended in the draft guidance documents on pediatric studies by the U.S. FDA (7) and have been widely applied to pediatric studies to handle sparse and unbalanced PK–PD data. The goal of the sparse sampling is to provide convenient schedules with minimal blood draws and reduced load on bioanalytical assays, while maintaining accuracy in determining important PK information without bias. The general technique is to use the prior PK data in adults plus a scaling model along with D-optimality sampling methods (8,9). Varying sampling times with time windows could protect against the ill effects of misspecification in scaling models (10). If the PK of the drug is complex, with multiple informative time points or segments, a composite sampling strategy can be applied. This approach randomly assigns a subject to one of a few sampling groups with times or time windows pre-selected. The samples should be collected on more than one occasion to allow estimation of inter-occasional variability. The development of the limited sampling model can be guided and validated by Monte-Carlo simulations (11).

In addition to lack of dense datasets, other challenges in pediatric data analysis are: (*i*) scaling for body size adjustment, (*ii*) collinearity of covariates (Fig. 2), and (*iii*) time-varying covariates. Empirical body size adjustment

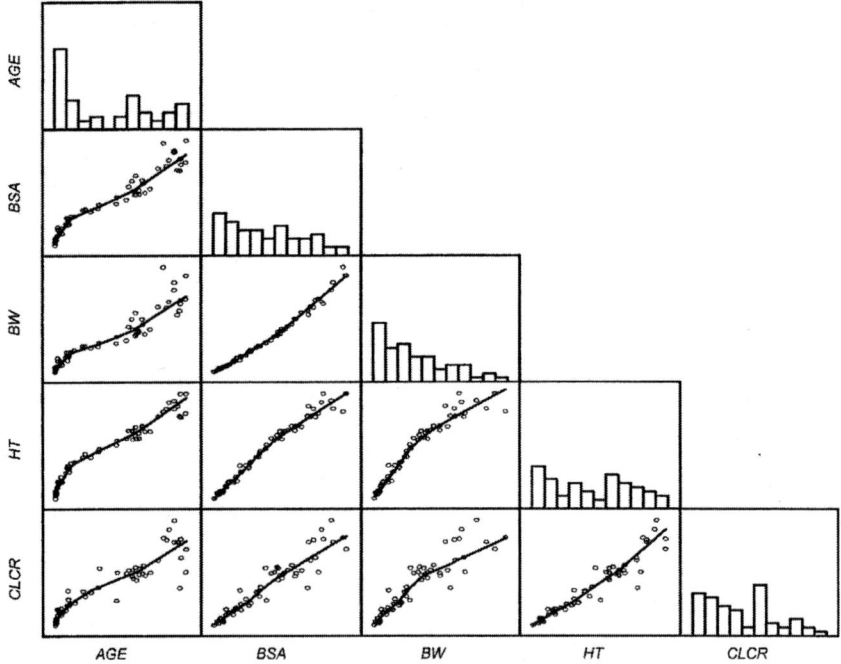

Figure 2 Collinearity of the covariate variables in the sotalol pediatric population PK dataset (age ranged from <1 month to 12 years). Creatinine clearance (CL_{CR}) was calculated based on age, height, and serum creatinine according to Schwartz (44). *Abbreviations*: BSA, body surface area; BW, body weight; HT, height.

using either BSA or BW is often applied in the trials for dosing administration, but the results may show that the empirical approach is not adequate for certain age groups. Allometric size adjustments (with exponent of 0.75 for clearance and 1 for volume of distribution using BW) provide a more mechanistic, physiologically based approach that, if used a priori, allows delineating the effect of other covariates, for example, organ function or concomitant medication, from the size variables and avoids collinearity between the size variables (11). Perhaps a more appropriate size adjustment approach is to fit all the parameters of the full model and let the data decide the optimal scaling. However, this approach cannot be applied to a covariate model with two covariates showing a high degree of collinearity (12). Potential body size covariates should be measured at each PK/PD visit and captured in the dataset. There are pitfalls for simultaneously fitting pediatric data with adult data: different formulations and bio-availabilities, different meals and food effects on absorption and bioavailability of drugs, different compliances of dosing, and different data quantity in terms of number of subjects and number of samples per subject between the two populations. Modeling pediatric data and adult data together should be carefully conducted by tackling these potential issues and other hidden extrinsic

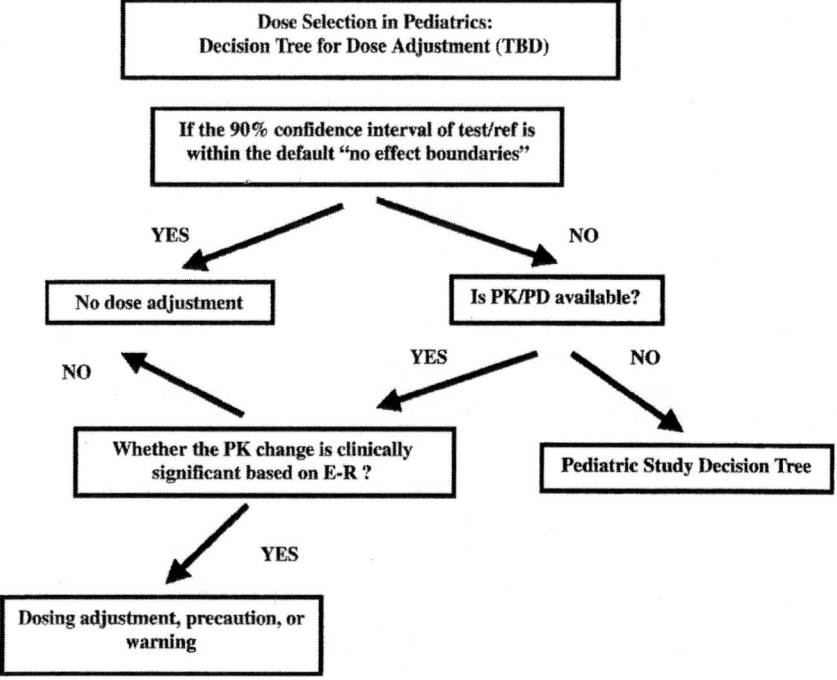

Figure 3 FDA-proposed criteria for dose adjustments in pediatric populations. *Abbreviations*: PK, pharmacokinetics; PD, pharmacodynamics; E–R, exposure–response.

factors. Bayesian methods can be used to analyze the combination of sparse pediatric data and informative prior distributions estimated from adult data plus appropriate scaling models (13).

Once a statistically significant difference in PK is identified between pediatrics and adults, the necessity of dose adjustment for pediatric subpopulations should be judged based on whether or not the PK difference will likely lead to a clinically significant PD difference. The FDA's proposed decision tree could guide this process (Fig. 3). Population PK/PD models, if used for bridging the recommended dose, should be carefully validated or evaluated.

POPULATION PK–PD OF SOTALOL IN PEDIATRIC PATIENTS WITH SUPRAVENTRICULAR OR VENTRICULAR TACHYARRHYTHMIA

d,l-sotalol hydrochloride is an antiarrhythmic agent with Class III and non-selective β-blocking properties. In adults, sotalol is labeled for life-threatening ventricular fibrillation and tachycardia and for maintenance of sinus rhythm in patients with symptomatic atrial fibrillation or atrial flutter (14). In pediatric patients, sotalol was considered to be efficacious for similar indications because of the similar electrophysiologic basis of the arrhythmias (15–18). However, demonstrating benefit based on clinical outcomes is challenging for antiarrhythmics, especially in pediatrics. The PK and PD of sotalol have been extensively studied in adults (19). Sotalol is nearly completely absorbed after oral administration. It has negligible plasma protein binding and is not metabolized. It is mainly eliminated unchanged by the kidneys. The PK of sotalol is dose-proportional. The respective biomarkers for the Class III and β-blocking actions are the QTc and RR interval, recorded in the surface ECG, and their respective relations to the drug concentration are well established in adults (20,21). As sotalol is predominantly eliminated unchanged by the kidneys in adults, an important impact of maturation of renal function on the PK of sotalol in the pediatric population can be anticipated. In addition, the relationships between drug concentrations and QTc or RR interval prolongation in the pediatric patients are unknown. The FDA agreed with the sponsor, as part of the pediatric written request, to use biomarker data to derive dosing guidelines in pediatrics, such that the effects are consistent with adults. This was a strategy to leverage wealthy safety and efficacy data obtained in adults to pediatrics.

A PK study and a PK–PD study were conducted to investigate the impact of maturation of renal function and body size-related changes and also other demographic characteristics on the PK and PD of sotalol in pediatric patients of various age groups with ventricular tachyarrythmia (VT) and supraventicular tachyarrythmia (SVT).

An extemporaneously compounded formulation made by dissolving sotalol HCl tablets in syrup (5 mg/mL) was used. In the PK–PD study, each patient received a total of nine oral doses with an upward titration without a washout period. Three dose levels, 30, 90, and 210 mg/m^2/day, were studied. The daily doses were divided into three doses. Doses were given every 8 hours in pediatrics instead of every 12 hours in adults, because of the notion that children usually have a half-life shorter than adults, which may lead to breakthrough arrhythmias if the trough level is too low. The mid-dose (i.e., 90 mg/m^2/day) was selected because it was the BSA-normalized initial adult daily dose (160 mg/1.73 m^2). In the PK study, each patient received a single dose of 30 mg/m^2 of BSA. In the PK study, blood samples were collected at 0.5, 1, 2, 3, 5, 8, 12, 16, 22, and 36 hours following the dose. In the PK–PD study, blood samples were taken at 0.5, 2, 4, and 8 hours following the third, sixth, and ninth doses. Electrocardiogram (ECG) measurements were taken at the same time as the PK sampling during these visits with two additional timepoints, 1.5 and 3 hours following the doses. Baseline electrocardiograms (ECGs) were determined on the same six occasions on the day prior to the first dose of sotalol.

A total of 59 patients, from birth to 12 years old, were enrolled in the studies. Of these, 34 were in the PK study and 25 were in the PK–PD study. Fifty-four were diagnosed to have SVT only, three VT only, and two SVT and VT. All had normal renal function ($\geq 80\%$ of normal creatinine clearance, CL$_{CR}$, for age).

Table 1 summarizes the characteristics of the patients with analyzable PK and PD data by age category. All patients younger than three months had a normal birth weight and gestational age. The PK database consisted of 611 plasma sotalol concentration measurements. Of those, 328 were collected from the PK study, and 283 were collected from the PK–PD study. There were 499 observed RR intervals from 22 patients (22.7 per patient), and 477 observed QTc values from 23 patients (20.7 per patient) available for analysis.

The results of population PK modeling showed that sotalol kinetics underwent significant development and body-size-related changes in the pediatric population tested, which ranged from newborns to 12-year-old school-age children. The body surface area (BSA) was the most important single covariate for both CL/F (total oral clearance) and V/F (apparent volume of distribution), followed by body weight (BW) and age. The relationship of BSA to CL/F and V/F can be described better by a linear model with a negative intercept (Fig. 4) than by an exponential model. After taking BSA into consideration, the remaining inter-subject variabilities in CL/F and V/F were fairly small (about 20%, dropped from over 200% and 60%, respectively). The inter-subject variability in k_a and in t_{lag} were relatively large, and could not be accounted for by demographic factors. The data also showed no impact of gender on the CL/F. The race effect could not be reliably assessed due to an unbalanced distribution across age groups. CL$_{CR}$ was also an important single covariate for CL/F, after BSA and similar to BW. Because there were no patients with renal dysfunction in the study, the individual impact of CL$_{CR}$ on CL/F could not be evaluated. In light of the collinearity between BSA or BW and normal CL$_{CR}$, CL$_{CR}$ was not included in the final model.

Table 1 Demographics of Patients with Analyzable Data by Age Category

		Age group			
	Neonates ≤1 month	Infants >1 to ≤24 months	Children >2 to <7 years	Children ≥7 to 12 years	Total
PK from both studies					
N	9	17	9	23	58
Sex, M/F	5/4	10/7	5/4	10/13	30/28
Race, C/B/H/O	8/1/0/0	12/5/0/0	8/0/1/0	19/1/2/1	47/7/3/1
BSA, m²	0.23 ± 0.03	0.41 ± 0.10	0.70 ± 0.10	1.10 ± 0.22	0.70 ± 0.38
BW, kg	3.6 ± 0.8	8.4 ± 2.9	17.2 ± 3.3	32.4 ± 9.7	18.5 ± 13.6
Height, cm	52.0 ± 2.8	71.6 ± 10.6	104.2 ± 10.5	135.3 ± 16.1	98.9 ± 35.5
CCr, mg/dL	0.5 ± 0.2	0.3 ± 0.1	0.4 ± 0.1	0.6 ± 0.1	0.47 ± 0.17
CL_{CR}, mL/min/1.73 m²	51.8 ± 19.9	103.2 ± 26.3	134.8 ± 29.8	134.0 ± 23.8	112.3 ± 38.3
PK–PD Study[a]					
N	7[b]	9[b]	3	6[c]	25
Sex, M/F	3/4	6/3	2/1	2/4	13/12
Race, C/B/H/O	6/1/0/0	7/2/0/0	2/0/1/0	5/0/0/1	20/3/1/1
BSA, m²	0.224 ± 0.029	0.409 ± 0.102	0.700 ± 0.080	1.17 ± 0.216	0.576 ± 0.389
CL_{CR}, mL/min/1.73 m²	51.3 ± 22.8	101 ± 14.1	121 ± 35.3	129 ± 20.5	96.3 ± 36.6

[a]All patients in the PK–PD study had analyzable PK data.
[b]One patient in the group had no analyzable QTc and RR interval data.
[c]One patient in the group had no analyzable RR intervals.

Abbreviations: C, Caucasian; B, Black; H, Hispanic; O, other; BSA, body surface area; BW, body weight; PK, pharmacokinetics; PD, pharmacodynamics; CL_{CR}, creatinine clearance; CCr, serum creatinine concentration.
Source: Adapted from Ref. 4. Courtesy of Springer Publications.

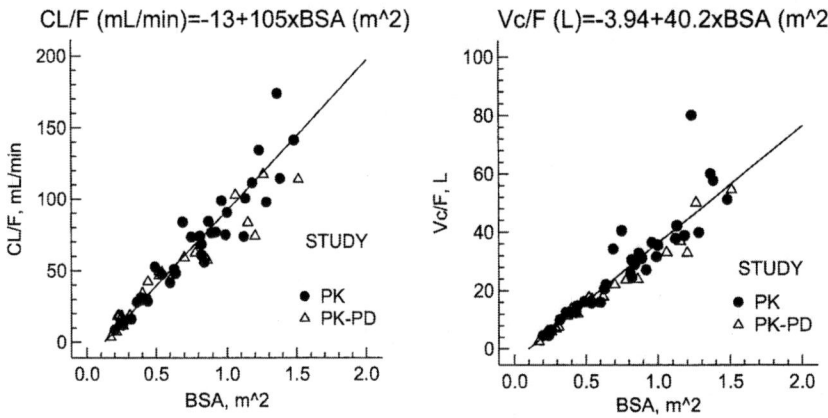

Figure 4 Plots of individual CL/F and V/F based on the final pharmacokinetic model versus BSA for 58 patients from the PK (*filled circle*) and PK–PD (pharmacodynamic) (*open triangle*) studies. The dispersion of individual parameter values about the regression model is only modestly less than seen for individual parameters based on the PK model without BSA as a covariate. *Abbreviations*: BSA, body surface area; CL/F, total oral clearance; V/F, apparent volume of distribution. *Source*: Adapted from Ref. 4. Courtesy of Springer Publications.

Sotalol is mainly renally excreted (19). Much attention has been paid to the PK and dosage regimens of such drugs in neonates and young infants because of an underdeveloped renal function. Ideally, an appropriate dosage adjustment should produce a constant AUC throughout the different age groups. However, the plots of the predicted C_{max} and AUC values against BSA indicated that neonates or young infants with a BSA < 0.33 m^2 tended to have a greater drug exposure (C_{max} and AUC) compared with the rest of the pediatric population (Fig. 5). Immaturity of the kidney in the smallest children is a possible reason for the difference. This result indicated that the empirical BSA adjustment applied in this study, which assumes a direct proportional relationship between CL/F and BSA, may not be adequate for the smallest children with a BSA < 0.33 m^2 from the point of view of the drug's exposure.

Pharmacodynamic analysis indicated that pediatric patients were more sensitive to the β-blocking effect than to the Class III effect at the same dose (Fig. 6), which was similar to adult population (20). Children with BSA < 0.33 m^2 represent a sub-population not only with larger drug exposures (Fig. 7), but also larger pharmacological effects than the larger children (Fig. 8).

The population PK–PD modeling results clearly indicated that the QTc and RR intervals were linearly related to sotalol plasma concentration. The slope for the QTc interval was 0.02 ± 0.002 (standard error) msec·mL/ng (Fig. 9), which was similar to that (0.02 msec·mL/ng) in adults (21). The inter-subject variability in the slope, expressed as percent CV, was also similar (58% vs. 54%, in pediatrics and adults). The slope for the RR interval was

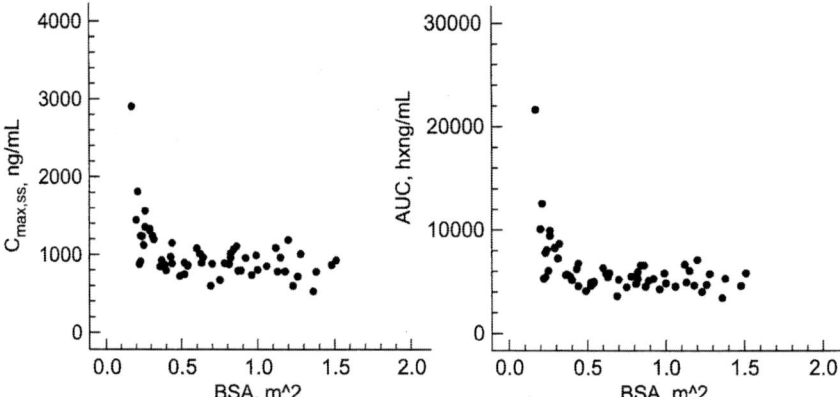

Figure 5 Plots of $C_{max,ss}$ and AUC against BSA. [The $C_{max,ss}$ values were obtained by simulations using individual post hoc Bayesian PK parameter estimates. AUC values were obtained from AUC = Dose × F/CL, where CL/F was obtained by the post hoc Bayesian method. Dose = 30 mg × 0.882 × BSA (m²) for both calculations.] *Abbreviations*: BSA, body surface area; AUC, area under concentration time curve; CL/ F, total oral clearance. *Source*: Adapted from Ref. 4. Courtesy of Springer Publications.

0.03 ± 0.008 msec·mL/ng for a typical three-year-old child. The RR interval was age-dependent, that is, age was a significant covariate for both baseline RR interval (strong) and the slope of the β-blocking effect (weak). Figure 10 shows the relationship between the RR interval and drug concentrations for four children from different age groups. A 2D plot of the pooled data as in

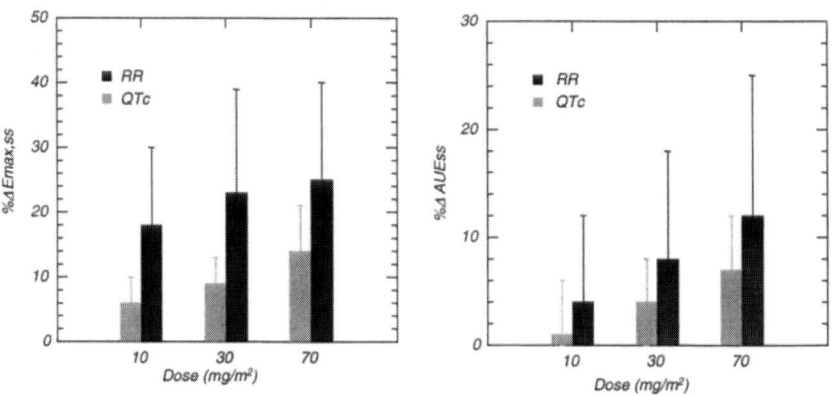

Figure 6 Relative sensitivity of the Class III and β-blocking effects to sotalol in pediatric patients. *Abbreviations*: %ΔE_{max}, percentage of increase of observed maximum QTc or RR interval; %ΔAUE$_{ss}$, percentage of increase of area under the QTc or RR interval time curve at steady-state, represents average percent prolongation of QTc or RR interval during a dose interval.

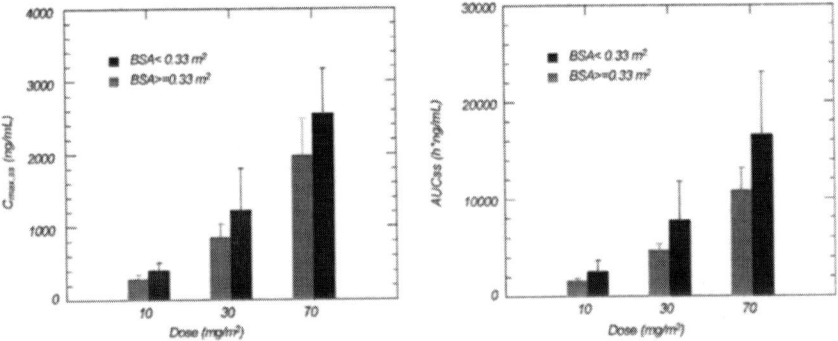

Figure 7 Higher exposures to sotalol (C_{max} and AUC) are observed in children with BSA < 0.33 m² compared with larger children. *Abbreviations*: BSA, body surface area; AUC, area of concentration under the curve.

Figure 9 for QTc would not demonstrate the impact of age on the relationship between RR interval and drug concentration. In order to compare the β-blocking activity of sotalol in the pediatric patients with that in the adults, the same PD model (i.e., E_{max}) was applied to pediatric data (heart rate at resting) without age as a covariate; the fit was equivalent or slightly better than that by the linear model without age (12). The EC_{50} was estimated to be 790 ng/mL in pediatric patients, which was similar to 804 ng/mL reported in literature with adults undergoing exercise (20,22).

On the basis of the PK–PD data, sotalol syrup was approved by the FDA for patients aged two years and above (30 mg/m² t.i.d. as starting dose with subsequent titration to a maximum of 60 mg/m²). The FDA recommended specific dosing regimens for neonates and infants. Instead of using 0.33 m² BSA as a cut-off, an age cut-off of two years was applied as a more conservative

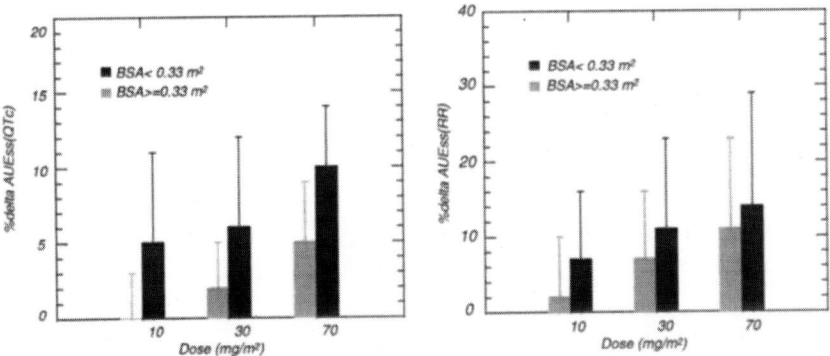

Figure 8 Greater Class III and blocking effect observed in neonates and young infants with BSA < 0.33 m². *Abbreviations*: BSA, body surface area; %delta AUE$_{ss}$, percentage of increase of area under the QTc or RR interval time curve at steady-state.

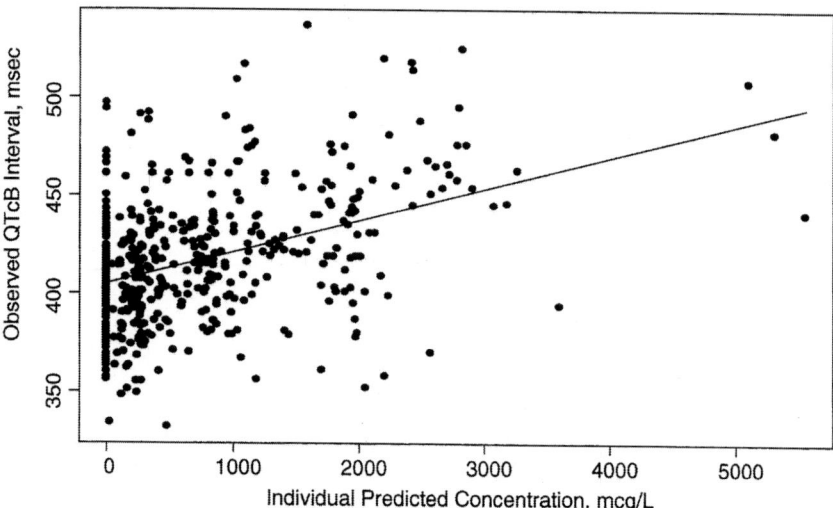

Figure 9 Observed QTc interval versus the individual (empirical Bayes) predicted sotalol concentration for all patients in the PK–PD study. QTc(msec) = 405 + 0.02 Cp (ng/mL). *Abbreviations*: PK, pharmacokinetics; PD, pharmacodynamics. *Source*: Adapted from Ref. 4. Courtesy of Springer Publications.

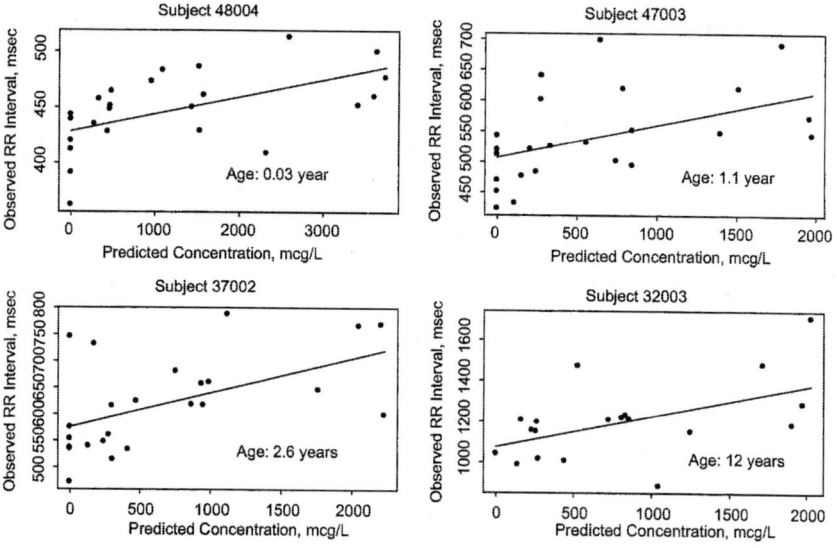

Figure 10 Four representative individual plots of observed RR interval versus individual (empirical Bayes) predicted sotalol concentrations. *Source*: Adapted from Ref. 4. Courtesy of Springer Publication.

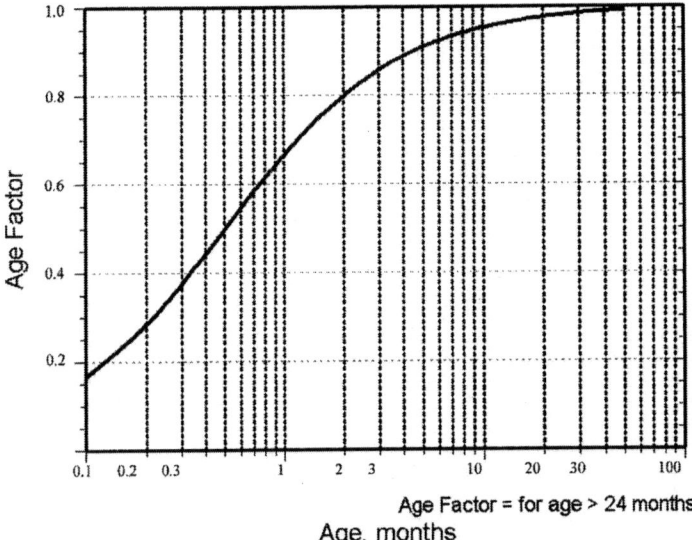

Age Factor = for age > 24 months

Age, months

Figure 11 Dose adjustment factor for sotalol in pediatrics aged 2 years or younger. For children aged about 2 years and greater with normal renal function, doses normalized for body surface area are appropriate for both initial and incremental dosing. For children aged about 2 years or younger the dosing regimen should be reduced by a factor that depends heavily upon age. For a child aged 1 month, the starting dose should be multiplied by 0.68; the initial starting dose would be $(30 \times 0.68) = 20 \text{ mg/m}^2$, administered three times daily. *Source*: Adapted from approved label for Betapace™ in the *Physician's Desk Reference*.

approach from the safety perspective. The PD effects of sotalol in pediatrics were similar to those in adults for a given exposure. Hence the exposure in the adults was a reasonable target in pediatrics. The systemic clearance of sotalol increases until the patient reaches two years of age independent of body-size, owing to the maturation process of the kidneys. After about two years, sotalol's clearance predominantly depends on body size. Based on the model findings, a dose, which was not directly studied in trials, was recommended in patients less than two years of age that included an age factor (Fig. 11) (14,23).

Since the population PK model established was to recommend dosage regimen for pediatric use of sotalol, the model was evaluated by a predictive check using Monte-Carlo simulations. The results revealed that the population PK model adequately described the central tendency of the observed plasma sotalol concentration data (Fig. 12).

In conclusion, using PK–PD for bridging adult safety and efficacy data to pediatric patients, the dosing recommendations for sotalol in pediatrics aged one month to 12 years are made and incorporated in the labeling.

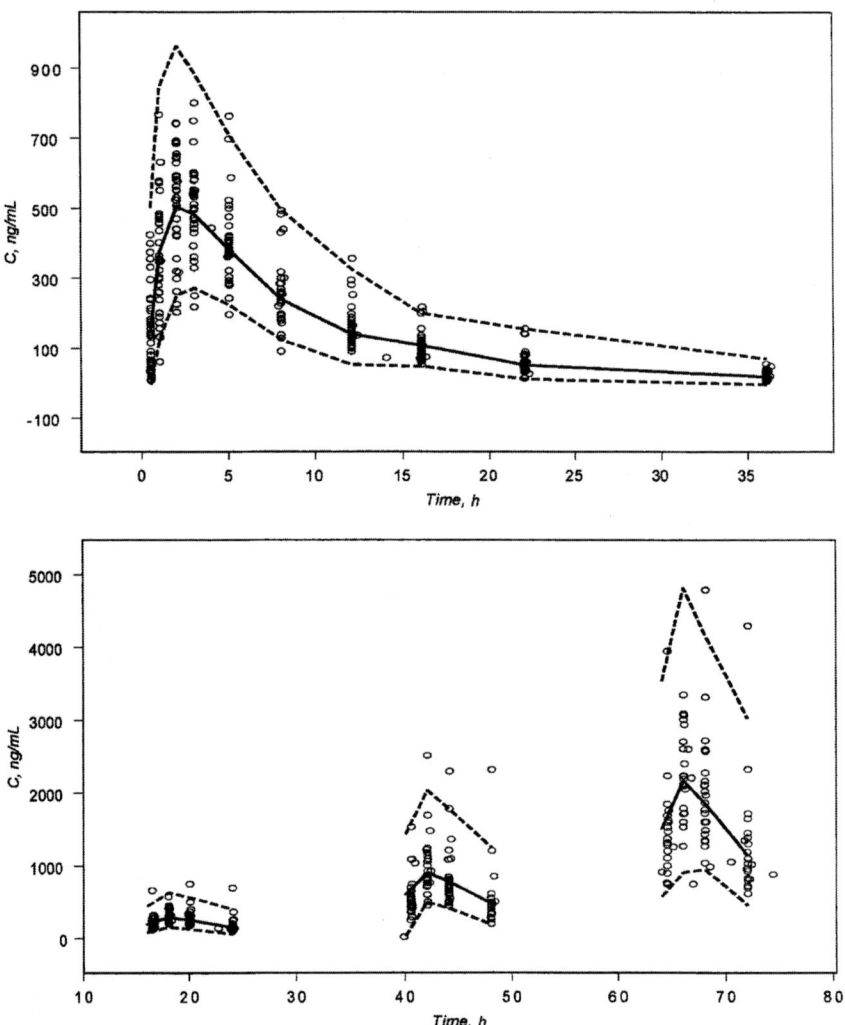

Figure 12 Results of the evaluation of sotalol population pharmacokinetic model using predictive check. *Source*: Adapted from Ref. 4. Courtesy of Springer Publications.

POPULATION PK OF THE ACTIVE METABOLITE OF LEFLUNOMIDE IN PEDIATRIC SUBJECTS WITH POLYARTICULAR-COURSE JUVENILE RHEUMATOID ARTHRITIS

Leflunomide is a disease-modifying antirheumatic drug, which effectively reduces the signs and symptoms of active rheumatoid arthritis (RA) in adults, while inhibiting joint damage and improving physical function (24). In clinical trials of adults, leflunomide (20 mg/day) demonstrated efficacy equivalent to that of methotrexate (7.5–15 mg/wk) and sulfasalazine (2 g/day) for improving individual signs and symptoms of active RA (25–28) and slowing disease progression (29–31). The PK of leflunomide has been characterized in healthy adults and adults with active RA (32–34). Following oral administration, leflunomide, a highly non-polar pro-drug, is rapidly and completely absorbed and is converted largely to its active metabolite A77 1726 (M1) during the first pass. M1 is responsible for essentially all antirheumatic activity in vivo. Peak concentrations of M1 occur between 6 and 12 hours after dosing. M1 displays linear PK at the doses from 5 to 25 mg/day. M1 has a low volume of distribution ($V_{ss} = 0.13$ L/kg) and it binds extensively to albumin (>99.3%) in healthy subjects; protein binding is linear at therapeutic concentrations. M1 has a long half-life ($\sim$2 weeks) but can be much longer in some patients. The elimination is complex, involving both biliary and renal excretion, with biliary recycling contribution to the drug's long half-life.

Juvenile rheumatoid arthritis (JRA) is an inflammatory disease defined as a chronic, idiopathic arthritis with onset before the sixteenth birthday. Although the etiology of JRA is unknown, many of the etiological factors associated with adult RA are also associated with JRA. Similarities in T cell, B cell, and macrophage abnormalities have been demonstrated (35). Evidence of complement activation and abnormal production and regulation of cytokines are common features of both diseases (35). The relationship between dosage and clinical effect suggests that leflunomide should be given at a daily rate of 20 mg to obtain near maximum probability of clinical success in adult RA patients (60%) (36). At this dose, the median value of the average steady-state concentration in adults was about 34 mg/L.

Due to a lack of validated biomarkers for the efficacy or safety of leflunomide in adults, two clinical trials, one PK and another safety and efficacy, were undertaken sequentially to evaluate the PK, efficacy, and safety of leflunomide in the treatment of JRA.

Study I, open-label, non-controlled, multicenter study, included a six-month treatment period with up to a 24-month extension phase in pediatric subjects (6–17 years) with active, polyarticular-course JRA, who had previously failed or were intolerant of methotrexate therapy. Leflunomide treatment was initiated with a loading dose equivalent to 100 mg/day in a standard adult with a BSA of 1.73 m^2 (57.8 mg/m^2/per day), administered on days 1 through 3. Thereafter, maintenance doses of leflunomide were given daily, based on an equivalent of 10 mg/day/1.73 m^2 (the low adult maintenance dose). Because of the restricted number of milligrams that can be reliably administered using the 10-mg tablets, BSA categories were used to determine the dose. In subjects without clinical response on or after eight weeks based on Definition of Improvement responder analysis for JRA subjects published by Giannini et al. (37), escalation to the equivalent of leflunomide 20 mg/day/1.73 m^2 BSA was allowed at the discretion of the investigator. On day 3, weeks 4, 12, and 26, serial blood samples were collected prior to the dose and at 2, 4, 8, and 24 hours following dosing. In addition, single blood samples were collected on several pre-defined event-related occasions, including dose change, early discontinuation, or severe leflunomide-related adverse event. The objective of this small-scale study was to learn the PK of leflunomide in the target pediatric patient population so that a revised dose for the later efficacy and safety can be made if needed.

Study II was a randomized, double-blind, parallel-group, 16-week safety and efficacy trial comparing leflunomide with methotrexate in pediatric subjects (age 3–17 years) with active, polyarticular-course JRA, who were naïve to both methotrexate and leflunomide. A simplified treatment regimen was developed based on the PK results of Study I. Loading doses with 100-mg tablets and maintenance doses with 10-mg tablets were assigned based on actual BW as described in Table 2. Subjects unable to swallow the tablet(s) as a whole were permitted to crush the tablet(s) and mix it in apple sauce or jam. In Study II, one or two blood samples were obtained during weeks 2, 4, 8, 12, and 16. Fixed sample collection times were not specified.

The evaluable PK population consisted of 73 subjects: 27 subjects in Study I and 46 subjects in Study II. Among them, 57 subjects were female and 16 subjects were male, which was consistent with the epidemiology of RA (35,38). Age ranged from 3 to 17 years, weight ranged from 13 to 75 kg, and BSA ranged from 0.56 to 1.83 m^2. A total of 674 concentrations of M1 were included in the database, including 493 from Study I and 181 from Study II. The number of concentrations of M1 collected per subject averaged 9.2 (range, 1–23). Fewer samples of M1 were collected in Study II (3.9 samples per subject) than in Study I (18.3 samples per subject).

A previously established structural PK model for M1 concentration–time data from adults was fitted to the M1 data from the pediatric population as the base model. Population analyses indicated that age and gender of pediatric subjects did not influence M1 concentrations significantly, but body size (BW or BSA) correlated strongly with V/F and weakly with CL/F in children (Fig. 13), as defined in the following:

$$V/F(L) = 5.8 \cdot (BW/40\,kg)^{0.769} \tag{1}$$

$$CL/F(L/h) = 0.020 \cdot (BW/40\,kg)^{0.430} \tag{2}$$

Table 2   Weight-Based Leflunomide Dosing Regimen in Study II

Actual body weight (kg)	Loading dose (100 mg/day)	Maintenance dose (mg/day)
<20	× 1	5
20–40	× 2	10
>40	× 3	20

Note: 5 mg/day was given as 10 mg every other day.
Source: Adapted from Ref. 5. Courtesy of Springer Publications.

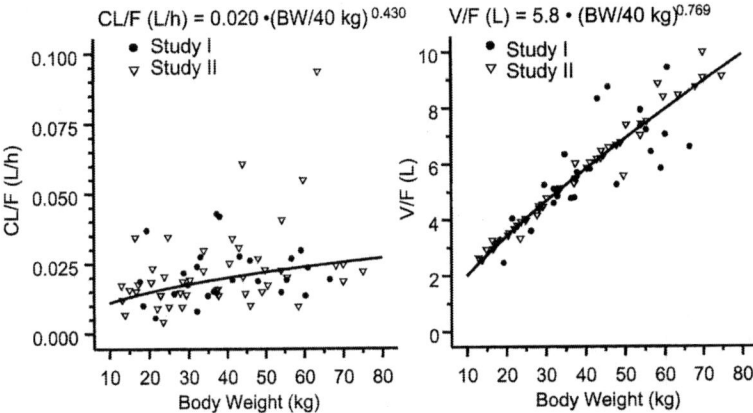

Figure 13 Relationships between clearance and body weight (*left panel*) and volume of distribution and body weight (*right panel*). *Abbreviations*: CL/F, total oral clearance; V/F, apparent volume of distribution; BW, body weight. *Source*: Adapted from Ref. 5. Courtesy of Springer Publications.

The inter-subject variation in CL/F and V/F, expressed as the coefficient of variation for CL/F and V/F, were 50% and 19%, respectively.

To examine the uniformity in exposure produced by the leflunomide maintenance regimens investigated in Study II, M1 C_{ss} data in 2000 JRA patients with a uniform distribution of BW from 10 to 80 kg were simulated using the established population PK model. The results indicated that only the maintenance dose of leflunomide of 20 mg/day in pediatric subjects weighing >40 kg achieved systemic exposures to M1 comparable with those previously observed in adults who received leflunomide of 20 mg/day (32,36). The leflunomide doses prescribed for subjects <20 kg (10 mg every other day) or between 20 and 40 kg (10 mg/day) resulted in lower predicted values for C_{ss} (Fig. 14, *left panel*). Simulation of C_{ss} values using a single leflunomide dose adjustment for a body weight <30 kg provided more comparable exposure to M1 than the dosing regimen tested in Study II (Fig. 14, *middle panel*). However, a dose of leflunomide of 10 mg/day in pediatric subjects who weighed <30 kg would slightly underexpose them to M1 on average, compared with that in adult patients or the pediatric group, which weighed from 30 to 80 kg. A third simulation was performed using the weight-based doses suggested by the optimal regimens from the graphic exploration (Fig. 14, *right panel*). With this dosing regimen, median C_{ss} for M1 was around 34 μg/mL in each of the weight groups, matching the median C_{ss} previously observed in adult patients with RA who received leflunomide of 20 mg daily in Phase II and Phase III studies (32,36).

An exposure-versus-response relationship was further examined: among the 47 pediatric subjects treated with leflunomide for 16 weeks in Study II, 32 were categorized as responders and 15 were categorized as non-responders

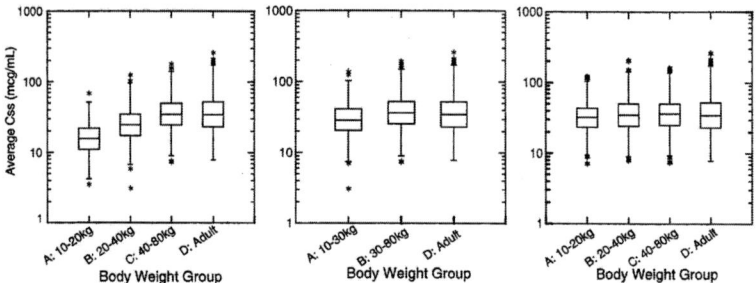

Figure 14 Simulations of steady-state concentrations of M1 in 2000 pediatric "patients" compared with observed values in adults. Predicted concentrations were derived for leflunomide dose regimens from Study II (i.e., the Phase III study) (*left panel*), leflunomide dosing based on body weight above or below 30 kg (*middle panel*), or the refined leflunomide dose recommendations derived from the population pharmacokinetic models (*right panel*). An outside value is defined as a value that is smaller than the lower quartile minus 1.5 times the inter-quartile range, or larger than the upper quartile plus 1.5 times the inter-quartile range (*inner fences*). These values are plotted with an *asterisk*. *Abbreviation*: C_{ss}, concentration at steady-state. *Source*: Adapted from Ref. 5. Courtesy of Springer Publications.

when assessed by JRA Definition of Improvement >30% (37). Comparison of M1 concentrations with response or non-response revealed a trend for lower exposures in the group of subjects who failed to respond to leflunomide (Fig. 15, *left panel*). The majority of subjects (80%) in the non-responder group had concentrations of M1 that were less than the median exposure in the responder group. Lighter subjects also tended to be less likely to respond to leflunomide (Fig. 15, *right panel*), but the trend was less pronounced than that for the M1 concentrations. These analyses suggest that the leflunomide doses in Study II may be sub-optimal among subjects who weighed less than 40 kg, providing supporting evidence that the concentration versus response relationship between pediatrics and adult patients is similar. Logistic regression analysis also showed a slight trend of higher C_{ss} and higher probability of the response as defined by Giannini et al. (37) (Fig. 16). However, the relationship was not statistically significant by *t*-statistics due to the small sample size of the study.

The relationship between the C_{ss} of M1 and clinical effect previously determined in adult RA patients showed that the maximum probability of clinical success (60%) would be obtained by choosing a dose rate that maintains a C_{ss} above the target concentration of 13 mg/L for the majority of the patients. To achieve the maximum probability of clinical success in 95% of the patients treated with leflunomide, the dose rate would have to be adjusted to achieve a median plasma concentration of 30 mg/L (95% CI: 13; 67), requiring a daily dose of 16 mg leflunomide. The dose rate recommended is 20 mg daily, and this dose rate should achieve the maximum probability of clinical success in

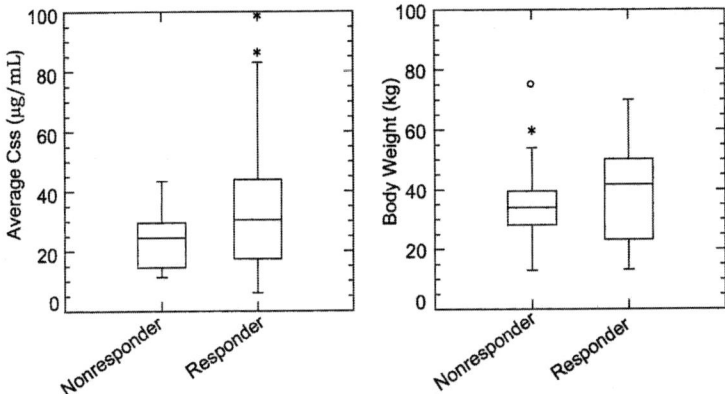

Figure 15 Steady-state concentration (C_{ss}) of the M1 metabolite and body weight in pediatric responders and non-responders to leflunomide. Data were taken from a Phase III study in subjects with juvenile rheumatoid arthritis (42,43). Response was defined >30% improvement as defined by Giannini et al. (37). An outside value is defined as a value that is smaller than the lower quartile minus 1.5 times the inter-quartile range, or larger than the upper quartile plus 1.5 times the inter-quartile range (*inner fences*). These values are plotted with an *asterisk*. A far out value is defined as a value that is smaller than the lower quartile minus three times the inter-quartile range, or larger than the upper quartile plus three times the inter-quartile range (*outer fences*). These values are plotted with an *open circle*. *Source*: Adapted from Ref. 5. Courtesy of Springer Publications.

99% of the patients. The plateau effect in the relationship between the C_{ss} and clinical effect shows that higher dosages of leflunomide would not increase the probability of clinical success to any significant degree (36).

Multiple pathways are involved in leflunomide metabolism and M1 elimination, and the PK of M1 in pediatrics cannot be reliably predicted from the PK in

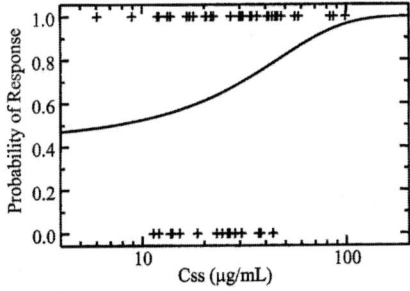

Figure 16 Results of logistic regression model prediction, plotted as probability of the response defined as responders (1) or non-responders (0) as defined by Giannini et al. (37) versus average steady-state M1 concentration (C_{ss}).

adults simply by normalizing a body size covariate (BW or BSA) in an empirical way. Human liver microsomes studies suggested P450 CYP 1A2 as the principal P450 isozyme responsible for leflunomide metabolism. Studies with human recombinant CYP isozymes also indicated a role for CYP 2C19 and CYP 3A4 in leflunomide metabolism (39). M1 is eliminated by further metabolism and subsequent renal excretion and also by direct biliary excretion. After oral administration of leflunomide, approximately 43% of the dose is excreted in the urine, primarily as leflunomide glucuronides and an oxalinic acid derivative of M1, and 48% is excreted in the feces, primarily as M1 (24). M1 has an extremely long $t_{1/2}$, largely due to enterohepatic recycling. A sequential design was implemented in the program to first derive the PK information in JRA patients in a small scale and then to examine the efficacy and safety in a large scale with regimens recommended from the earlier study.

The strong correlation that was observed between body size and V/F, reducing the inter-subject variation in V/F from 35.9% to 18.6%, indicates that a loading dose regimen for pediatric patients should be adjusted, if indeed a loading dose is administered. Due to the very long half-life of M1 ($\sim$2 weeks), a loading dose of 100 mg for 3 days was used in clinical studies of adult patients to facilitate the rapid attainment of steady-state concentrations of M1. However, since leflunomide is a chronic treatment for a chronic disease for which full response to therapy may take several months, the true benefit of the loading dose has been debated and has been shown to be associated with an increased risk of treatment discontinuation in adults (40,41). Furthermore, a disproportionate number of gastrointestinal adverse events, headaches, and cases of alopecia were reported within the first four weeks of leflunomide therapy in Study II, the Phase III study of JRA (42,43). Beginning leflunomide therapy for JRA without a loading dose may delay the initial onset of response in some patients, but it permits a better opportunity for pediatric patients with JRA to tolerate early leflunomide therapy. In addition, the gradual accumulation provides an opportunity for a routine clinical monitoring of the safety during the accumulation. In pediatric patients with polyarticular-course JRA, CL/F was only correlated weakly to BW with an exponent significantly smaller than standard allometric coefficient, that is, 0.75, indicating that maintenance dose adjustments for BW should be more modest than the 50% dose reductions often applied empirically in practice. Even with the most influential covariate identified (i.e., BW) and included in the model, the inter-subject variation in CL/F was reduced only slightly (from 53.6% to 50.4%, expressed as percent CV), indicating that dosage reduction by half should only be required when the BW distribution is wide, that is, in JRA patients, and only for those with a low body weight. Either measure of body size (BW or BSA) provided similar prediction power on CL/F, but BW can be measured more easily and more accurately, and it was selected to be the sole covariate in the final population PK model.

Using the commercially available formulation strengths of leflunomide, the adjusted dosage regimen derivation was a trial and error process. First, the number of body weight groups was determined based on: (*i*) the therapeutic index of the drug, and (*ii*) the possible regimens, given the available formulation strengths. Second, the partitioning of the BW groups was determined by considering: (*i*) the correlation between the CL/F and BW and the variability in CL/F, (*ii*) the BW distribution of JRA patients, and (*iii*) clinical convenience (20, 30, 40 kg). Finally, simulation was used to examine the performance of each possible dosage regimen. Through this process, the optimal weight-based protocol for dose adjustment was identified (Table 3). Although 15 mg/day would mean 10 and 20 mg on alternating days due to the lack of a 5-mg tablet, the inclusion of this regimen resulted in comparable exposure to M1 (median and range) across BW categories. This may trade some convenience for a gain in a better overall balance between efficacy and safety compared with the other dose adjustment protocols that were tested.

The final optimal population model was evaluated by a cross-study comparison and a predictive check. The cross-study evaluation (Table 4) shows the substantial agreement in the estimated PK parameters for the final model fitted to the data of the two studies individually and the combined data set. The predictive check (Fig. 17) revealed that the population PK model based on BW adequately described both the central tendency and variability of the observed plasma M1 concentration data. Most of the observed data points fell within the range defined by the 95% prediction interval simulated by the model (*shaded area*).

In summary, this present study assessed PK data collected during an uncontrolled Phase I trial (Study I) and a controlled Phase III trial (Study II) of leflunomide for the treatment of pediatric subjects with JRA to create a model for the population PK of the active metabolite, M1, and then use this model in conjunction with efficacy and safety data obtained to determine appropriate dosing regimens in pediatric patients with JRA. Analysis of M1 concentrations and treatment response in Study II revealed a trend for lower exposures to M1 in the group of children who failed to respond to leflunomide. The doses summarized in Table 3, recommended based on the population PK model, provide

Table 3 Doses that Would Achieve a Uniform Range of M1 Exposure for Pediatric Patients with JRA

Actual body weight (kg)	Initial maintenance dose (mg/day)
10–20	10
20–40	15
>40	20

Note: 15 mg/day was given as 10 mg and 20 mg rotation every other day. *Source*: Adapted from Ref. 5. Courtesy of Springer Publications.

Table 4 Cross-Study Comparison of the Final Population Pharmacokinetic Model

Study	CL/F (L/hr)	V/F (L)	k_a (hr^{-1})	Exponent[b] for V/F	Exponent[b] for CL/F	IIV$_{CL}$ (%)	IIV$_V$ (%)	IIV$_{ka}$ (%)	Residual error (%)
Study I	0.0191	5.67	1.07	0.811	0.377	46.7	18.4	170.7	17.7
Study II	0.0206	6.37	1.00[a]	0.719	0.452	52.7	19.3	0[a]	19.5
Study I + Study II	0.0200	5.80	1.13	0.769	0.430	50.4	18.6	171.5	18.2
SE	(0.00127)	(0.23)	(0.455)	(0.0989)	(0.192)	(22.0)	(10.0)	(101.5)	(6.3)

[a]Due to lack of data obtained from the rising phase, k_a and its variance were fixed to 1 and 0, respectively.

[b]The format of the covariate model was: $P_j = P_{typical} (BW/40)^{exponent}$, where P is the parameter (CL/F or V/F).

Abbreviations: CL/F, total oral clearance; V/F, apparent volume of distribution; k_a, first-order input-rate constant; IIV, inter-individual variation in PK parameters, expressed as %CV; SE, standard error of the estimate.

Source: Adapted from Ref. 5. Courtesy of Springer Publications.

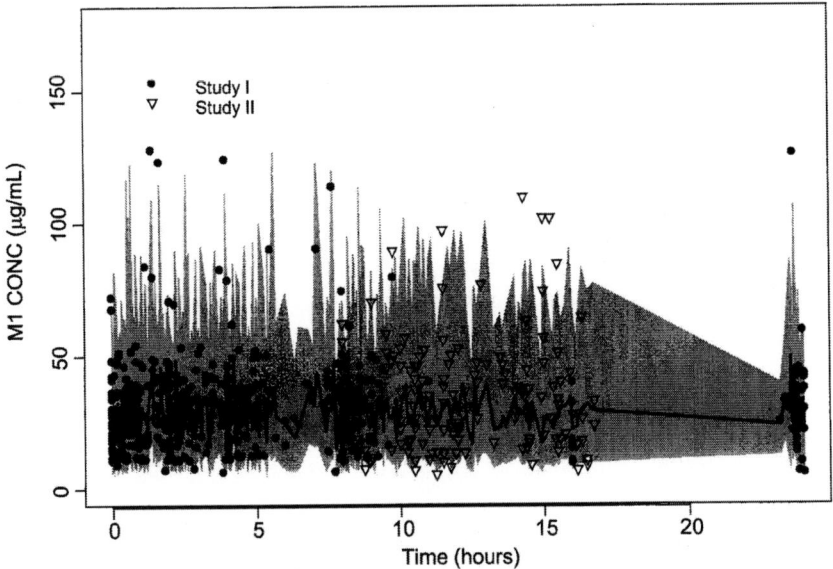

Figure 17 Plot of the predictive check evaluation on the final model. The *solid curve* represents the median concentrations of the 500 simulated datasets and the *upper* and the *lower boundar*ies of the *shaded area* represent the 97.5th and 2.5th quantiles of the simulated data, respectively. Time after dose is used for the plot and the plot only displays the data within 24-hour post-dosing in order to show individual data points. *Source*: Adapted from Ref. 5. Courtesy of Springer Publications.

exposure to M1 comparable with that achieved in adults with a dose of leflunomide at 20 mg/day.

CONCLUSION

Children cannot simply be regarded as "miniature" adults; they differ from adults and even from other children with regard to drug absorption, distribution, metabolism, and elimination. Furthermore, age-related differences in receptor-binding characteristics are also evident. PK/PD studies play a key role in pediatric clinical programs and are a central contributor to define pediatric dose adjustments specified in the product labeling.

Populations in pediatric PK–PD studies frequently cover a much wider range in body size than similar studies in adults. Therefore, appropriately applying a size adjustment approach is critical in dose selection of the trials, optimal sampling design, and PK–PD modeling for other covariates, and, ultimately, in dosage regimen recommendations. Limited sampling designs are a frequently used feature in population PK–PD analysis in pediatric populations. Sufficient methodology is now available to allow for the design of D-optimality or random sampling-based schemes and validation of these schemes. Furthermore, reliable and unbiased results can be obtained using various Bayesian and non-linear mixed effects modeling approaches, even though the data is sparse and unbalanced.

The recent regulatory initiatives and policies have stimulated pediatric clinical studies resulting in improved understanding of the PK/PD of drugs prescribed in pediatrics. The pursuit of relationships between exposure and response specifically in pediatric populations represents the frontier in limited sampling design, population PK/PD modeling, and dose optimization. The integration of model-based techniques as a tool in these investigations is both rational and necessary.

ACKNOWLEDGMENT

The author would like to thank Dr. Thomas M. Ludden for his review and helpful suggestions.

REFERENCES

1. CDER/FDA. Population Pharmacokinetics: US Department of Health and Human Services, Food and Drug Administration, Center for Drug Evaluation and Research, 1999.
2. Beal SL, Sheiner LB. The NONMEM system. Am Statistician 1980; 34:118–119.
3. Sheiner LB, Beal SL, Boeckmann AJ. NONMEM Users Guide, NONMEM Project Group. San Francisco: University of California, 1994.
4. Shi J, Ludden TM, Melikian AP, Gastonguay MR, Hinderling PH. Population pharmacokinetics and pharmacodynamics of sotalol in pediatric patients with supraventricular or ventricular tachyarrhythmia. J Pharmacokinet Pharmacodyn 2001; 28(6):555–575.
5. Shi J, Kovacs SJ, Wang Y, Ludden TM, Bhargava VO. Population pharmacokinetics of the active metabolite of leflunomide in pediatric subjects with polyarticular course juvenile rheumatoid arthritis. J Pharmacokinet Pharmacodyn 2005; 32(3–4):419–439.
6. CDER/FDA. Exposure—Response Relationships—Study Design, Data Analysis, and Regulatory Applications. Rockville: US Department of Health and Human Services, Food and Drug Administration, Center for Drug Evaluation and Research, 2003.
7. CDER/FDA. General Considerations for Pediatric Pharmacokinetic Studies for Drugs and Biological Products—Draft Guidance. Rockville: US Department of Health and Human Services, Food and Drug Administration, Center for Drug Evaluation and Research, 1998.
8. Panetta JC, Wilkinson M, Pui CH, Relling MV. Limited and optimal sampling strategies for etoposide and etoposide catechol in children with leukemia. J Pharmacokinet Pharmacodyn 2002; 29(2):171–188.
9. Panetta JC, Iacono LC, Adamson PC, Stewart CF. The importance of pharmacokinetic limited sampling models for childhood cancer drug development. Clin Cancer Res 2003; 9(14):5068–5077.
10. Hashimoto Y, Sheiner LB. Designs for population pharmacodynamics: value of pharmacokinetic data and population analysis. J Pharmacokinet Biopharm 1991; 19(3):333–353.

11. Bernd Meibohm, Stephanie Läer, John C. Panetta, Jeffrey S. Barrett. Population pharmacokinetic studies in pediatrics: issues in design and analysis. The AAPS J. May 4, 2005. In press.

12. Bonate PL. The effect of collinearity on parameter estimates in nonlinear mixed effect models. Pharm Res 1999; 16(5):709–717.

13. Gastonguay MR, Gibiansky L, Gillespie WR, Khoo K, the PPRU Network. Population Pharmacokinteics in Pediatric Patients Using Bayesian Approaches with Informative Prior Distributions Based on Adults. AAPS Meeting (1999).

14. The current labeling for Betapace® (sotalol HCl). In: Physicians' Desk Reference, 54th ed. Montvale, NJ: Medical Economics, 2000:739–745.

15. Maragnes P, Tipple M, Fournier A. Effectivenness of oral sotalol treatment of pediatric arrhythmia. Am J Cardiol 1992; 69:751–754.

16. Pfammatter JP, Paul T, Lehmann C, Kallfelz HC. Efficacy and proarrhythmia of oral sotalol in pediatric patients. Am Coll Cardiol 1995; 26:1002–1007.

17. Tanel RE, Walsh EP, Lulu JA, Saul JP. Sotalol for refractory arrhythmias in pediatric and young adult patients: initial efficacy and long-term outcome. Am Heart J 1995; 130:791–797.

18. Beaufort-Krol GCM, Brink-Boelkens MTE. Effectiveness of sotalol for atrial flutter in children after surgery for congenital heart disease. Am J Cardiol 1997; 79: 92–94.

19. Hanyok JJ. Clinical pharmacokinetics of sotalol. Am J Cardiol 1993; 72:19A–26A.

20. Woosley RL, Barbey JT, Wang T, Funck-Brentano C. Concentration–response relations for the multiple antiarrhythmic actions of sotalol. Am J Cardiol 1990; 65(2):22A–27A; discussion 35A–36A.

21. Barbey JT, Sale ME, Woosley RL, Shi J, Melikian AP, Hinderling PH. Pharmacokinetic, pharmacodynamic, and safety evaluation of an accelerated dose titration regimen of sotalol in healthy middle-aged subjects. Clin Pharmacol Ther 1999; 66:91–99.

22. Bhattaram VA. Role of biomarkers in drug development. AAPS Workshop on Clinical Biomarkers in Drug Development: Efficacy Assessment, Pharmacokinetics/ Pharmacodynamics and Regulatory Insights. November 5–6, 2004. Holiday Inn Inner Harbour, Baltimore, MD.

23. Bhattaram VA, Booth BP, Ramchandani RP, et al. Impact of pharmacometrics on drug approval and labeling decisions—a survey of 42 new drug applications. AAPS J. 2005; 7(3):E503–512.

24. Prescribing Information for Arava Tablets (Leflunomide). March 2004.

25. Strand V, Cohen S, Schiff M, et al. Treatment of active rheumatoid arthritis with leflunomide compared with placebo and methotrexate. Arch Intern Med 1999; 159:2542–2550.

26. Tugwell P, Wells G, Strand V, et al. Clinical improvement as reflected in measures of function and health-related quality of life following treatment with leflunomide compared with methotrexate in patients with rheumatoid arthritis: sensitivity and relative efficiency to detect a treatment effect in a twelve-month, placebo-controlled trial. Arthritis Rheum 2000; 43:506–514 (2000).

27. Kalden JR, Scott DL, Smolen JS, et al. Improved functional ability in patients with rheumatoid arthritis: long-term treatment with leflunomide versus sulfasalazine. J Rheumatol 2001; 28:1983–1991.

28. Smolen JS, Kalden JR, Scott DL, et al. The European Leflunomide Study Group. Efficacy and safety of leflunomide compared with sulfasalazine in active rheumatoid arthritis: a double-blind, randomized, multicenter trial. Lancet 1999; 353:259–266.

29. Larsen A, Kvien TK, Schattenkirchner M, et al. Slowing of disease progression in rheumatoid arthritis patients during long-term treatment with leflunomide or sulfasalazine. Scand J Rheumatol 2001; 30:135–142.

30. Scott DL, Smolen JS, Kalden JR, et al. Treatment of active rheumatoid arthritis with leflunomide: two year follow up of a double blind, placebo controlled trial versus sulfasalazine. Ann Rheum Dis 2001; 60:913–923.

31. Sharp JT, Strand V, Leung H, Hurley F, Loew-Fridrich I. Treatment with leflunomide slows radiographic progression of rheumatoid arthritis: results from three randomized controlled trials of leflunomide in patients with active rheumatoid arthritis. Leflunomide Rheumatoid Arthritis Investigators Group. Arthritis Rheum 2000; 43:495–505.

32. Rozman B. Clinical pharmacokinetics of leflunomide. Clin Pharmacokinet 2002; 41:421–430.

33. Weinblatt ME, Kremer JM, Coblyn JS, et al. Pharmacokinetics, safety, and efficacy of combination treatment with methotrexate and leflunomide in patients with active rheumatoid arthritis. Arthritis Rheum 1999; 42:1322–1328.

34. Li J, Yao HW, Jin Y, et al. Pharmacokinetics of leflunomide in Chinese healthy volunteers. Acta Pharmacol Sin. 2002; 23:551–555 (2002).

35. Nepom B. The immunogenetics of juvenile rheumatoid arthritis. Rheum Dis of No Amer 1991; 17: 825–842.

36. Weber W, Harnisch L. Use of a population approach to the development of leflunomide: a new disease-modifying drug in the treatment of rheumatoid arthritis. Hoechst Marion Roussel COST B1 medicine, Geneva 1997. 239–244.

37. Giannini EH, Ruperto N, Ravelli A, Lovell DJ, Felson DT, Martini A. Preliminary definition of improvement in juvenile arthritis. Arth Rheum 1997; 40:1202–1209.

38. Cassidy JT. Juvenile rheumatoid arthritis. In: Kelley WN, Harris ED, Ruddy S, Sledge CB, eds. Textbook of Rheumatology. 5th Ed. WB Saunders, 1996:1207–1254.

39. Kalgutkar AS, Nguyen HT, Vaz AD, et al. In vitro metabolism studies on the isoxazole ring scission in the anti-inflammatory agent lefluonomide to its active alpha-cyanoenol metabolite A771726: mechanistic similarities with the cytochrome P450-catalyzed dehydration of aldoximes. Drug Metab Dispos 2003; 31:1240–1250.

40. Geborek G, Crnkic M, Peterson IM, Saxne T. Etanercept, infliximab, and leflunomide in established rheumatoid arthritis: clinical experience using a structured follow up program in southern Sweden. Ann Rheum Dis 2002; 61:793–798.

41. Siva C, Eisen SA, Shepherd R, et al. Leflunomide use during the first 33 months after Food and Drug Administration Approval: experience with a national cohort of 3,325 patients. Arthritis & Rheumatism (Arthritis Care & Research) 2003; 49:745–751.

42. Silverman E, Mouy R, Spiegel L, et al. Leflunomide in Juvenile Rheumatoid Arthritis (JRA) Investigator Group. Leflunomide or methotrexate for juvenile rheumatoid arthritis. N Engl J Med 2005; 352(16):1655–1666.

43. Silverman E, Spiegel L, Hawkins D, et al. Long-term open-label preliminary study of the safety and efficacy of leflunomide in patients with polyarticular-course juvenile rheumatoid arthritis. Arthritis Rheum 2005; 52(2):554–562.

44. Schwartz GJ, Brian LP, Spitfire A. The use of plasma creatinine concentration for estimating glomerular filtration rate in infants, children, and adolescents. Pediatr Clin North Am 1987; 34:571–590.

Index